Prentice Hall's Basic Ethics in Action series in normative and applied ethics is a major new undertaking edited by Michael Boylan, Professor of Philosophy at Marymount University. The series includes both wide-range anthologies as well as brief texts that focus on a particular theme or topic within one of four areas of applied ethics. These areas include: Business Ethics, Environmental Ethics, Medical Ethics, and Social and Political Philosophy.

Anchor Volume
Michael Boylan, *Basic Ethics*, 2000

Business Ethics
Michael Boylan, ed., *Business Ethics*, 2001
Patrick Murphy, Gene R. Laczniak, Norman E. Bowie, & Thomas A. Klein, *Ethical Marketing*, 2005
Edward Spence, *Advertising Ethics*, 2005
James Donahue, *Ethics for Professionals*, forthcoming
Dale Jacquette, *Journalistic Ethics*, forthcoming
Joseph Des Jardin, *Business, Ethics, and Sustainability*, forthcoming

Environmental Ethics
Michael Boylan, ed., *Environmental Ethics*, 2001
Lisa H. Newton, *Ethics and Sustainability: Sustainable Development and the Moral Life*, 2003
J. Baird Callicott & Michael Nelson, *American Indian Environmental Ethics: An Ojibwa Case Study*, 2004
Mary Anne Warren, *Obligation to Animals*, forthcoming

Medical Ethics
Michael Boylan, ed., *Medical Ethics*, 2000
Michael Boylan & Kevin Brown, *Genetic Engineering: Science and Ethics on the New Frontier*, 2002
Rosemarie Tong, *New Perspectives in Healthcare Ethics*, 2007
David R. Cummiskey, *International Perspectives on Medical Ethics*, forthcoming

Social and Political Philosophy
Seumas Miller, Peter Roberts, & Edward Spence, *Corruption and Anti-Corruption: An Applied Philosophical Approach*, 2005
R. Paul Churchill, *Human Rights and Global Diversity*, 2006
Kia Nielsen, *Social Justice*, forthcoming

Please contact Michael Boylan (michael.boylan@Marymount.edu) or Prentice Hall's Philosophy & Religion Editor to propose authoring a title for this series!

New Perspectives in Health Care Ethics

An Interdisciplinary and Crosscultural Approach

ROSEMARIE TONG, PH.D.
University of North Carolina at Charlotte

Upper Saddle River, New Jerssey 07458

Library of Congress Cataloging-in-Publication Data

Tong, Rosemarie.
    New perspectives in health care ethics: an interdisciplinary and crosscultural approach/
Rosemarie Tong.
        p. ; cm. — (Basic ethics in action)
    Includes bibliographical references.
    ISBN-13: 978-0-13-061347-9 (pbk.)
    ISBN-10: 0-13-061347-9 (pbk.)
    1. Medical ethics. 2. Medical ethics—Cross-cultural studies.
[DNLM: 1. Ethics, Medical. 2. Bioethical Issues. 3. Delivery of Health Care—ethics. W 50 T665n
2007] I. Title. II. Series.
R724. T564 2007
174.2—dc22   2005035711

Editor-in-chief: Sarah Touborg
Acquisitions Editor: Mical Moser
Editorial Assistant: Carla Worner
Senior Managing Editor: Joanne Riker
Production Liaison: Fran Russello
Manufacturing Buyer: Christina Amato
Art Director: Jayne Conte
Composition/Full-Service Project Management: Babitha Balan/GGS Book
Services
Printer/Binder: LSC Communications, Inc.

Pearson Education LTD. London
Pearson Education Singapore, Pte. Ltd
Pearson Education, Canada, Ltd
Pearson Education–Japan
Pearson Education Australia PTY, Limited

Pearson Education North Asia Ltd
Pearson Educación de Mexico, S.A. de C.V.
Pearson Education Malaysia, Pte. Ltd
Pearson Education, Upper Saddle River,
New Jersey

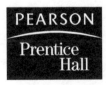

ISBN : 0-13-061347-9

9 2020

Contents

Preface

When I set out to write this book four years ago, I thought it would be a relatively easy task for me to accomplish. My reason for thinking so was simply that health care ethics is my area of expertise. For over 20 years I have taught, researched, and written about ethical issues that arise in the realm of health care. My supposed strength proved to be my undoing, however. I had a hard time deciding which intriguing and important health care subjects to include in the book without writing the proverbial tome. I knew I could not include all the subjects that interest me, but I did not know which ones to exclude. Fortunately, Prentice-Hall assigned four excellent anonymous readers to my initial manuscript and with their help I managed to organize my reflections on health care ethics into a reasonably sized volume.

As reconceived, the book is divided into five parts. Part One probes different conceptual frameworks for health care ethics ranging from those that stress the tried-and-true principles of autonomy, beneficence, nonmaleficence, and justice to those that emphasize the virtues of trust, fidelity, and caring. Among the concepts probed in Part One are (1) confidentially and privacy; (2) truthfulness, veracity, and full disclosure; and (3) *bona fide* informed consent. In addition, a variety of health care professionals are asked to come center stage to discuss their competencies and qualities of character.

Part Two of the book analyzes the concepts of health and disease, asking whether our society is guilty of "medicalizing" moral weaknesses, personal foibles, and lifestyle choices. To what degree is a condition like erectile dysfunction a true disease and to what extent is it instead the result of a lack of desire for sexual intimacy with one or more persons? This section of the book also examines the benefits and burdens of biomedical and behavioral research. Before we die, many of us may have participated in a clinical research study and played a role in the development of a miracle drug or surgical intervention meant to enhance or prolong our lives. Will we have done so fully informed and without unknowingly risking our health? How will we react if we discover that we have been assigned to receive a placebo (colloquially called a "sugar pill") instead of the experimental drug? Will we be content to accept our assignment or will we instead exit the study?

Part Three of the book is probably the longest section of the book and deliberately so. Not only are the beginning-of-life issues discussed there of general interest to the public, they are also of special personal interest to me as a woman, mother, and feminist. Using pivotal ethical and legal cases, I examine the moral dilemmas generated by health care's most controversial reproduction-controlling technology: abortion. Is destroying a blastocyst for the purposes of embryonic stem-cell research really the moral equivalent of taking a morning-after pill or using RU-486 to terminate an early pregnancy? Having a second-trimester abortion subsequent to discovering one's fetus has a severe genetic disease? Agreeing to a third-trimester partial-birth abortion? Why is our society so anxious and polarized about beginning-of-life issues? Why do controversies about issues involving the moral status of human embryos threaten to tear us apart? Having raised questions such as these about abortion, I proceed to discuss some major reproduction-assisting technologies (*in vitro* fertilization, donor insemination, embryo transfer). When, with whom, and how should someone participate in the human procreative process? As a gamete donor, as a surrogate or gestational mother who bears but does not rear the children she gestates, or as a rearing parent who deliberately selects key genetic traits for his or her child?

Part Four of the book examines end-of-life issues, beginning with the process of aging. The number of elderly people in our society is growing by leaps and bounds as people live longer and often healthier lives. Yet our society's health care and social policies are ill-equipped to provide adequate care for millions of octogenarians with chronic diseases. Relatively few people have the kind of health care insurance that can pay the bills for decades of hospital, skilled-nursing home, and/or assisted-living care. In addition, only a small percentage of Americans have the money to purchase out-of-pocket home health care for themselves for a decade or more. Although relatively well-to-do people may view their years after retirement as a golden opportunity to try new things and to explore the world, many poor people approach their old age with great apprehension. Somehow our society needs to address the funding of long-term care for everyone who needs it. Providing subsidies for prescription drugs is a good start, but it is not enough. People in their 80s, 90s, and 100s need help with tasks of daily life. A miracle drug cannot feed, wash, put to bed, turn over, or diaper a failing body.

Over and beyond confronting the diminishment that almost always accompanies the aging process, our society needs to deal with the dying process more honestly and more compassionately. No matter how healthy a person is, he or she will have to die one day or another. None of us are immune to unexpected life-shortening disease, serious accidents, and the cumulative effects of how we have taken care of our bodies and psyches throughout our lives. Moreover, some of us are born with genetic diseases that medicine has not found a way to treat, let alone cure. Therefore, we all need to prepare ourselves and our families for our demise and death, making it clear how much or how little we want medicine to use its arsenal—its technologies, surgeries, and drugs—to keep us alive. Some of us will want to give way to the forces of death as soon as we find ourselves unable to relate to others and/or to enjoy even the simplest of life's pleasures. But others of us will want to stay biologically alive no matter what, even if we are no longer conscious. Important questions still trouble us about the moment of death and whether it makes sense for health care professionals to aggressively treat people whose days are numbered and who are on the verge of death. Perhaps we need to focus less on keeping people breathing an additional day or two at the very end of their lives, and more on helping them begin to die when it is clear their lives will end in a year or less. For this reason, the availability of hospice care and palliative care is especially important. We need the help of others as we work through the physical, psychological, spiritual, and practical issues that confront us as we say our final goodbyes to those whom we love.

Part Five of the book broaches the politically as well as personally volatile issues surrounding just micro- and macro-allocations. As most of us know, there is a severe lack of organ donors. Ironically, this shortage vexes us at the very same time medicine is achieving great success in the technological aspects of organ transplantation. Were organ donors in plentiful supply, many more people who need organs would be able to live 5, 10, or even 20 years longer than they might otherwise live. To be sure, there are cost problems associated with organ transplantation. It is not clear, for example, that there are ways for us as a society and/or as individuals to pay for everyone's organ transplant as well as everyone's drugs, therapies, surgeries, and more. Thus, sooner or later, we need to reform our health care system and make rational as well as compassionate decisions about which health care goods and services are luxuries and which ones are instead necessities to which everyone is somehow "entitled" whether or not they can personally pay for them. The United States needs to join the rest of the developed nations of the world and provide health care for all its citizens. Concomitantly, the United States needs to ask itself why quality health care seems to cost so much more here than in comparable developed nations. Why are we spending nearly 16% of our GNP on health care? Do we really need to be spending so much? Is there an argument to make that we should be spending even more, or far less?

As readers might suspect, *New Perspectives in Health Care Ethics* is meant to raise more questions than it answers. It is a work that demands readers' engagement. Not surprisingly, it is also the kind of book that I could not have finished single-handedly. Reggie Raymer of the University of North Carolina at Charlotte, a dedicated teacher and persistent researcher, helped me gather material for this book as did my loyal, utterly competent off-campus assistant, Lisa Singleton. Lisa also worked hard to help me copyedit the book. Without her help and that of Babitha Balan, my book would still be a manuscript on my desk. Also in the background of this book is Dr. Michael Boylan, the series editor. His humane, interdisciplinary, and multicultural worldview of ethics inspired me throughout the process of writing this book. Finally, I want to acknowledge everyone at Prentice-Hall who helped bring this book to press. In particular, I extend my thanks to Carla Worner, Russ Miller, and Mical Moser.

Acknowledgments

Pages and/or sections from books or articles I have published earlier have been reproduced here with the permission of the publishers, namely, Perseus Press, MIT Press, and The World and I. I thank these three publishers for their spirit of cooperation and kind support.

chapter one

Introduction

This book is different from a **medical ethics** book that focuses exclusively on bedside or clinical ethics issues such as the physician–patient relationship, the diagnosis and treatment of disease, and the relief of pain and suffering. It is also different from a **bioethics** book that adds to the favored topics of medical ethics other topics where biology affects human affairs—for example, environmental and public health issues, such as clean water and air, safe food (who among us has not been scared by the threat of mad cow disease or mercury-laden fish?), and disposal of toxic wastes.[1] Rather, this book is a **health care** ethics book that aims to encompass not only most medical ethics and bioethics issues but also a wide variety of other health-related issues characterizing the times in which we live. It is likely to be of primary interest to health care professionals and students seeking careers in health care, but it is meant to serve the general public as well. After all, the United States is probably one of the most health-focused (though by no means the healthiest) nations in the world. In fact, scarcely a day goes by when we or someone in our lives does not broach a health-related issue.

I. POINTS OF EMPHASIS

During the course of writing this book, I was struck by several recent developments in the U.S. health care system. First, physicians are no longer the sole or necessarily the most important health care professionals with respect to patients' treatment or care, nor is their power as great as it used to be. Presently, physicians are members of health care teams, and their treatment of patients represents only a fraction of the total care a patient receives. For example, consider a patient who needs a mastectomy because she has been diagnosed with breast cancer. Before she agrees to have the surgery, the patient will probably ask her physician numerous questions about the surgery, including how successful it is likely to be and how disfiguring. In addition, the patient will probably consult the Internet or a self-help book for detailed information about the physical and psychological benefits and risks of this type of surgery. If the patient decides to have the surgery, one or more physicians will perform the actual procedure, but they will be assisted by several nurses and a variety of technicians. Prior to and/or after her operation, the patient may be counseled or consoled by a member of a breast cancer survivors group, a psychologist, or even a chaplain. Moreover, she may be assisted by a social worker or case manager who will help her find ways to pay not only for all the costs associated directly with her operation but also for any further treatment or medication she may need.

Although some patients and physicians may long for the intense, nearly familial sort of physician–patient relationship that supposedly existed in the early half of the twentieth century, the fact of the matter is that this type of relationship—if it ever truly existed as the rule—currently exists only as the exception. As I stressed above, health care decisions are no longer private transactions between patients and physicians but quasi-public transactions involving patients, a team of health care professionals, and a bevy of administrators and insurers. In the past, the term "health career professional" almost always evoked the image of a physician or perhaps a nurse. But now this same term may bring to mind people with careers in a wide variety of health-related areas including behavioral medicine, clinical and laboratory science, dentistry, dietetics and nutrition, health information and communication, health promotion and kinesiology, health services administration and research, genetic diagnosis and counseling, mental health, nursing, pastoral care, pharmacy, public health, physical and occupational therapy, speech therapy, and social work. Clearly, health care has become a major industry in the United States, and it is one of the few segments of the market in which the demand for workers continuously outstrips the supply. In fact, so great is the demand for health care workers in the United States that it has recently started to employ health care professionals from other nations, including developing nations. So noticeable is this trend that when my father was a patient in a skilled nursing home a few months ago, he and I could not help noticing that the patient population was served mainly by immigrant nurse aides from African nations.

Depending on how commodious one's understanding of a profession is—and mine is very commodious—most of the health careers listed above can be viewed as bona fide **health care professions** for several reasons. First, most of them require individuals to master certain skills, competencies, proficiencies, and techniques; maintain standards of excellence; be regularly evaluated; and train or, in some instances, even school new members. In addition, most of them have some means of systematic and regular communication, ranging from proceedings and newsletters to meetings and conferences, to electronic listservs and chat rooms. Finally, a large number of the health careers listed above have either a code of ethics or a sense of mission that requires them to set aside personal concerns in order to meet the needs of those whom they profess to serve.[2]

A second striking development in U.S. health care is the fact that health care professionals no longer have the option of limiting their responsibilities exclusively to medical ethics, understood as bedside or clinical ethics—that is, an ethics focused on serving the best interests of individual patients by providing them state-of-the-art medical treatment competently and compassionately. Increasingly, health care professionals are required to think in terms of the aggregate good of all the patients they serve and to add to clinical ethics so-called organizational ethics issues. Among these latter issues are practice guidelines, profiling, and salary structures to influence health care professionals' behavior. Also present on the typical list of organizational ethics issues are items such as fair and truthful marketing of health care goods and services, hiring and promotion criteria, bidding and contracting policies, conflicts of interest, accounting practices, and financial auditing and reporting.[3]

In addition to being asked to recognize their organizational as well as clinical duties, health care professionals are also urged to consider their social and political responsibilities. Gunshot and knife wounds, addictive behaviors, child, spouse, and elder abuse, sexually transmitted diseases, poor nutrition, and lack of exercise have become subjects of great concern for many health care professionals. Moreover, social and political issues such as access to health care, quality and cost of health care, Medicare and Medicaid funding levels, and the challenge of providing culturally-sensitive health care to diverse populations have become regular subjects of conversations among health care professionals. As these latter issues expand in size and scope, the relationship between micro- and macro-issues in health care is highlighted. Individual decisions at the bedside are embedded in complex organizations and social networks, and unless health care professionals understand these systems, they cannot hope to serve the best interests of their patients, themselves, and society in general.

Yet another change in contemporary U.S. health care is health care professionals' increasing conviction that health and its maintenance, rather than disease and its treatment, are the main focus of health care, and that the term "health" should not be confined to physical and mental health but instead be expanded to include spiritual and social health. Preventive and alternative medicines increasingly challenge curative and scientific biomedicine. Moreover, there is growing interest in emphasizing the important role public health plays in health care. Although the bread and butter issues of public health—clean water, good hygiene, unpolluted air, adequate nutrition, proper exercise, ample rest, and minimal stress and tension—are not nearly as exciting as the latest life-extending technologies and life-altering genetic breakthroughs, these common sense basics, more than their dramatic counterparts, are probably the main determinants of individuals' and societies' overall health status.

A final noteworthy development in contemporary U.S. health care is the increasing shift of health care from inpatient care in hospitals to outpatient care in clinics and even back to homes. During the second half of the twentieth century, the hospital became the center of patient care. There, researchers and physicians worked the miracles medicine previously could not work. Lives were saved and prolonged. But as inpatient hospital care becomes prohibitively costly, and as a variety of technologies become exportable to the home, there is less reason to make the hospital the main site of health care service and physicians the main deliverers of health care. Many of the procedures physicians had to perform in the hospital in the past can now be done by nurses and technicians at outpatient centers and even in patients' own homes. Moreover, as medical treatments become more user-friendly, patients are able to engage more in self-care. Home remedies are coming back into fashion.

II. CONCLUDING THOUGHTS

Clearly, this is an extraordinary period of time in the history of health care. Old paradigms are giving way to new paradigms; the boundaries between medicine and business are being rethought; and the very concept of health is being reconceived. Those who are presently in or entering one of the health care professions will meet many challenges. But they will also have an extraordinary opportunity to substantially improve people's physical, mental, spiritual, and social health. I, for one, am grateful to be a **health care ethicist** at this particular time. The conversations in which I participate provide me with a sense of meaning and purpose, of being more than an armchair philosopher pontificating arcane and exceedingly abstract thoughts to bewildered and/or bored listeners.

To be sure, it is not always easy to participate in meaningful health care conversations. We live in a pluralistic society in which people do not share all values. In the United States, there is a real divide between people labeled "conservative" and people labeled "liberal." Taken to the extreme, neither the conservative position nor the liberal position represents my position. If the term "conservative" describes a set of values that require everyone to be a fundamentalist Christian and/or supporter of an unfettered market system, then I am not a conservative. Similarly, if the term "liberal" describes a set of values that require everyone to be a secular humanist and/or an advocate of a totally socialist state in which the government provides people with all of their needs, then I am not a liberal. Rather, I like to think of myself as a reflective moderate who thinks that where important matters are involved— matters such as health care—conservatives and liberals can and should work together, recognizing each other as well-intentioned, intelligent, and decent human beings who probably are more similar than they have come to think.

Readers who want the one right answer to the pressing health care issues that trouble our society will not find this book satisfying. But readers who want to think about these issues from a variety of perspectives will. The best we can do in a democratic, pluralistic society is to listen to each other attentively, to express our views respectfully, and to change our minds occasionally. Given the enormous problems our health care system faces, none of us has the luxury of digging in our heels or getting our own way all of the time. The time for compromising and consensus building is here; and I see my role as helping people solve our health care system's problems in ways that almost everyone can recognize as reasonable, or as the best human beings can do under trying circumstances. Even if we are not health care professionals or students aspiring to become health care professionals, as members of an extremely health-focused society that seeks health care continuously, we all need to be informed about what medicine can and cannot do to heal our bodies, psyches, and spirits.

Endnotes

1. Van Rensselaer Potter, *Bioethics: Bridge to the Future* (Englewood Cliffs, NJ: Prentice-Hall, Inc., 1959), p. 1.
2. Nancy D. Berkman, Matthew K. Wynia, and Larry R. Churchill, "Gaps, conflicts, and consensus in the *Ethics* statements of professional associations, medical groups, and health plans," *Journal of Medical Ethics*, 30, no. 4 (August 2004): 395.
3. Mark P. Aulisio, Robert M. Arnold, and Stuart J. Youngner, Society for Health and Human Values–Society for Bioethics Consultation, and Task Force on Standards for Bioethics Consultation, *Core Competencies for Health Care Ethics Consultation* (Lake View, IL: American Society for Bioethics and Humanities, 1998), pp. 20–21.

chapter two

Ethical Theories and Principles in Health Care

I. INTRODUCTION

Health care ethics is a type of normative, applied ethics. It is based on the assumption that, despite all of our differences, we can determine what is right and wrong within the constraints of a human condition prone to error. Even in a pluralistic society—perhaps especially in a pluralistic society—the goal of health care ethics is to provide health care professionals, students who seek health care careers, and members of the general public with moral guidelines that any rational person would recognize as worthy ones to follow. At the low end of the moral spectrum, such guidelines simply tell us what we must not do to other individuals. Do not kill, cheat, lie, steal, or otherwise harm anyone. However, at the high end of the moral spectrum, such guidelines also suggest ways we can positively benefit other persons by increasing their well-being. Both inside and outside the professional world, our challenge is to follow these guidelines so that we can flourish together as human beings.

II. ETHICAL RELATIVISM, ETHICAL PLURALISM, AND ETHICAL WORLDVIEWS

In the United States a wide variety of ethical theories, including utility-based ethics, duty-based ethics, virtue-based ethics, law-based ethics, rights-based ethics, and feminist ethics have played significant roles in shaping contemporary health care ethics. An unfortunate, but common effect of realizing that ethical theories are plural rather than singular in number is the feeling that, when all is said and done, ethics is a very relative or highly subjective practice in all realms of human activity. After all, if ethics experts disagree among themselves about the norms that should guide people through the process of moral decision-making, what hope is there for people whose busy workdays give them limited time for moral reflection? Thus, it is not surprising that many people, including many health care professionals, are driven to the position that there are no universal moral standards, that ethics is without foundations, and that moral differences cannot be resolved.

Before I dismiss ethical relativism as wrong-headed, I think it is important to describe this view at some length. There are two types of ethical relativism: (1) **ethical subjectivism**, according to which supposed moral truths are only personal views or individual opinions about what is right and wrong; and (2) **cultural relativism**, according to which supposed moral truths are merely the norms societies create and maintain to regulate themselves. For the most part, ethical subjectivists and cultural relativists are driven to their respective positions by their desire not to be ethical "know-it-alls" or cultural imperialists who mistake their particular moral views for the absolutely right moral views for everyone, everywhere. Although this desire is laudable, it can go to extremes. Some relativists refuse to make any moral judgments at all, a refusal that strikes me as a deleterious conversation stopper. At the very least, I want to be able to say that it is wrong to torture children for personal gratification. And I think I can make this assertion in a morally humble manner. To accomplish this feat, all I need to remember is the times I have made a wrong or partially wrong moral judgment and have benefited from the corrections of others.

Fortunately, most people in the United States are not really ethical relativists and opportunities for moral reflection, debate, and revision are many. Ours is a multicultural, pluralistic society in which relatively small groups of people have the opportunity to test their particular norms against those that are prevalent in the nation or even the world. Because we have inherited a wide variety of moral perspectives, most of which have several grains of truth, we are often put in the position of debating their relative merits. That this is indeed the case has been persuasively argued by philosopher Alasdair MacIntyre. He invites us to consider, for example, the three arguments made most often in the abortion debate, arguments we will consider at length in Chapter 6. He points out that, even though each one of these arguments has different implications for abortion policy, we are probably unwilling to *totally* reject any one of them. The three arguments are as follows:

> (1) Everybody has certain rights over his or her own person, including his or her own body. It follows from the nature of these rights that at the stage when the embryo is essentially part of the mother's body, the mother has a right to make her own uncoerced decision on whether she will have an abortion or not. Therefore abortion is morally permissible and ought to be allowed by law.

> (2) I cannot will that my mother should have had an abortion when she was pregnant with me, except perhaps if it had been certain that the embryo was dead or gravely damaged. But if I cannot will this in my own case, how can I consistently deny to others the right to life that I claim for myself? I would break the so-called Golden Rule unless I denied that a mother has in general a

right to an abortion. I am not of course thereby committed to the view that abortion ought to be legally prohibited.

(3) Murder is wrong. Murder is the taking of innocent life. An embryo is an identifiable individual, differing from a newborn infant only in being at an earlier stage on the long road to adult capacities and, if any life is innocent, that of an embryo is. If infanticide is murder, as it is, abortion is murder. So abortion is not only morally wrong but ought to be legally prohibited.[1]

According to MacIntyre, arguments one through three share several features in common. First, each argument is based on a set of premises, which—though fundamentally different from those in the other arguments—are nonetheless compelling to rational persons. We cannot deny the force of an argument based on rights, nor one based on the principle of universalizability, nor one based on the value of human life, because all of these values are of importance to us. Second, each argument is made as impersonally and objectively as possible. Considerations related to gender, race, ethnicity, religion, and social class are screened out so as to block the objection that ethical arguments are nothing but "a clash of antagonistic wills, each will determined by some set of arbitrary choices of its own."[2] Third, each argument has a distinctive, historical origin. MacIntyre notes "a concept of rights which has Lockean antecedents is matched against a view of universalizability which is recognizably Kantian and an appeal to the moral law which is Thomist."[3] Moral principles and concerns do not descend on human beings from on high, in MacIntyre's estimation; rather human beings pull them out of one or another spatiotemporal nexus.

MacIntyre's third point is particularly important. It brings to mind philosopher Michael Boylan's comments on the importance of developing a personal worldview. According to Boylan, each of us is bound by a so-called **Personal Worldview Imperative**. This imperative states: "All people must develop a single, comprehensive and internally coherent worldview that is good and that we strive to act out in our daily lives."[4] Boylan insists we reflect long and hard on which ethical theories shape our lives, and whether the lives we lead would be recognized as good ones by any rational person.

Developing a personal worldview that is comprehensive, internally consistent, and recognizable by any rational person as a good way to live is no easy task, however. Nevertheless, we must each accomplish this task if we want to live worthwhile lives. The philosopher Socrates probably said it best centuries ago when he stated, "The unexamined life is not worth living." However, Boylan adds to Socrates's words the important elaboration that:

> It is not enough to exist like a piece of driftwood floating on the sea of life. This is true because free, rational deliberation is an essential part of our ability to be autonomous individuals. And unless we are autonomous agents, we have no real participation in ethics. Where there is no real participation in ethics, we give up a fundamental aspect of what it means to be a human being.[5]

If Boylan is correct, and I think he is, we must all consider a wide variety of ethical theories, and then decide which one(s) not only best reflects our personal worldview but also meets the standard of rational acceptability.

In general, a personal worldview will meet the rational acceptability standard if it accords with the norms typically expressed in most codes of professional ethics, or if it can be voiced without meeting immediate and total rejection for being "off the wall." I realize the rational acceptability standard will not satisfy persons who seek as their moral guidelines an absolute set of values, defined in detail and subject to one and only one interpretation. I also recognize that persons who want to live life strictly on their own terms will reject this same standard. But I am not bothered by these reactions, simply because I believe that in a multicultural, pluralistic society, the best we human beings can do is to carefully construct a personal worldview for ourselves that makes moral sense to thoughtful people. Will we make mistakes and will there be room for improvement? Of course! But here the words of the ancient Greek philosopher Aristotle should be of comfort to us. Centuries ago, he wrote:

> . . . Our discussion will be adequate if it has as much clearness as the subject-matter admits of, for precision is not to be sought for alike in all discussions, any more than in all the products of the crafts. Now fine and just actions, which political science investigates, admit of much variety and fluctuation of opinion, so that they may be thought to exist only by convention, and not by nature. And goods also give rise to a similar fluctuation because they bring harm to many people; for before now men [sic] have been undone by reason of their wealth, and others by reason of their courage. We must be content, then, in speaking of such subjects and with such premises to indicate the truth roughly and in outline, and in speaking about things which are only for the most part true and with premises of the same kind to reach conclusions that are no better. In the same spirit, therefore, should each type of statement be *received*; for it is the mark of an educated man [sic] to look for precision in each class of things just so far as the nature of the subject admits.[6]

Ethics is not a science; it is an art that requires every ounce of moral imagination, emotion, and thought we can muster.

III. MAJOR ETHICAL THEORIES IN THE WESTERN WORLD: FORGING A PERSONAL WORLDVIEW

A. Utility-based Ethics (Utilitarianism)

Utilitarianism is one of the most widely-embraced ethical theories in the United States and elsewhere. Utilitarians believe that the desire for happiness or pleasure is universal, and that people intuitively view the attainment of happiness or pleasure as their ultimate goal in life. Thus, according to utilitarians, it is only reasonable to think that actions are right to the degree they promote overall happiness or pleasure and wrong to the degree they promote overall unhappiness or pain. It is important to stress that when utilitarians refer to overall happiness they have something very special in mind. Unlike ethical egoists who are preoccupied with their individual happiness, utilitarians are concerned about the aggregate happiness of *all* sentient beings—that is, any and all beings capable of experiencing pleasure or pain, including nonhuman animals.

In their quest to do whichever action is most likely to promote overall happiness or pleasure, utilitarians consider both the happiness-producing and unhappiness-producing consequences of several alternative actions before deciding on one. For example, assume that a genetic counselor has a 30-year-old client who has tested positive for Huntington's Disease (HD), a degenerative and fatal neurological condition, the symptoms of which remain unmanifested until age 40 or so. The client, who happens to be an airline pilot, refuses to tell his employer that he has the HD gene. Should the genetic counselor breach confidentiality and reveal the pilot's HD status to the pilot's employer, or should she instead maintain the pilot's privacy for as long as possible (until, for example, the pilot actually starts to manifest such symptoms of HD as hand tremors)?

According to utilitarians, in deciding what to do, the genetic counselor should weigh the relative harms and benefits of *not* breaching confidentiality against the relative harms and benefits of breaching confidentiality. On the one hand, if she stays silent, many plane passengers may lose their lives. On the other hand, if she turns the pilot in, he will probably lose his livelihood. Also relevant to the genetic counselor's moral calculations is the importance of medical confidentiality, without which patients are not likely to fully disclose intimate information about their psyches and bodies to health care professionals. If genetic counselors routinely divulged their patients' secrets, few patients would choose to be tested for a presymptomatic genetic condition.

To help the genetic counselor make her moral decision, utilitarians will probably provide her with one or another checklist. One of the most controversial of these checklists is nineteenth-century philosopher Jeremy Bentham's **hedonic calculus**. Bentham (1748–1832), a founder of utilitarianism, designed what he termed a hedonic calculus to enable people to measure the overall happiness- or pleasure-producing consequences of actions in terms of their duration, intensity, certainty, propinquity, fecundity, purity, and extent.[7] Like most people in the eighteenth and nineteenth centuries, today's genetic counselor would probably find Bentham's decision-making tool too complex to use. Happiness or pleasure is, as we know, incredibly difficult to rank on a numerical scale.

Unable to measure in strictly quantitative terms the amount of happiness/pleasure she will net for the pilot and others if she reveals/keeps private the pilot's secret, the genetic counselor may seek further guidance in the thoughts of Bentham's successor, John Stuart Mill (1806–1873).[8] Mill urged people to distinguish between the quality, as opposed to the quantity, of goods available to them, and not to accept the idea that all pleasures or happinesses are of equal quality. He claimed less of something excellent—for example, a single piece of Lady Godiva chocolate—is generally better than more of something mediocre—for example, a bag of stale Halloween candy. In addition to making this point, Mill emphasized that we are not alone in our struggle to do the right thing. The genetic counselor, for example, can turn to other genetic counselors or to her professional organization for advice. She can ask her peers what respected and reasonable genetic counselors have done about similar cases in the past. In particular, she can ask them how well or poorly they think their judgments have served the **principle of utility**, according to which persons should act so as to produce the greatest balance of good over evil, all sentient beings—nonhuman as well as human—considered equally.

Yet, no matter what the genetic counselor decides to do, she cannot escape the main criticism that has been raised against utilitarianism; namely, that in some instances it will be necessary to sacrifice one person's or a few persons' interests in order to serve the interests of many people. However, even if it is right to sacrifice an HD-diagnosed pilot's personal good to prevent harm befalling a plane full of people, is it right, for another example, to end the life of one patient because five other patients will die unless her organs are immediately distributed among them? Assume that Sally, who is destined to die in less than a month, is unemployed and without family or friends, whereas five other patients, each of whom needs an organ transplant, are powerful persons with large families and many friends. Also assume that only Sally can provide the needed organs, since alternative organ sources are unavailable. The circumstances being such, so-called **act utilitarians** (who directly apply the principle of utility to each and every case as it arises) would probably be inclined to terminate Sally's life immediately. They would claim that individual rights, even Sally's right not to be killed, are not absolute and must give way to the group's interest in life.

In contrast to act utilitarians, so-called **rule utilitarians** would probably view killing Sally as a morally wrong action. Rule utilitarians, as the name implies, apply the principle of utility to general rules of action rather than to particular actions. For this reason, they would be inclined to argue that even if the particular act of killing Sally produces overall happiness or pleasure in the immediate circumstances, a general rule permitting, let alone requiring, such an act would not produce more overall happiness or pleasure in the long run. On the contrary, it would probably lead to radical social instability, to a fear that what happened to Sally could happen to a family member, a friend, or oneself.

In its emphasis on rules, rule utilitarianism seems to represent an improvement over act utilitarianism. Yet, it is doubtful whether rule utilitarians are prepared to follow their rules no matter what. I very much doubt, for example, that a rule utilitarian would insist it is clearly wrong (disutilitarian) to deprive an octogenarian of a marginally life-extending but extremely costly organ transplant, in order to fund primary health care for 100,000 children who would otherwise be at risk for serious disease or even death. The overall benefit of enabling the octogenarian to live a few more weeks probably does not outweigh the overall benefit of enabling 100,000 children to reach adulthood in healthy shape. Along the same lines of reasoning, I also suspect that a rule utilitarian would not fault understaffed health care professionals for using the method of triage in order to save as many victims of a school bus accident as possible. On the contrary, the rule utilitarian would support their decision to give first priority to those children who can be saved but only if they are immediately treated, second priority to those whose treatment may be delayed without great risk, and third priority to those who seem doomed to die no matter what.

To be sure, the desperate conditions described above are not everyday occurrences in U.S. emergency rooms. As medicine is typically practiced in the United States, most health care professionals have the luxury of practicing **nonutilitarian** medicine; that is, of providing what they perceive as the best care for *each* one of their patients. In the United States, the best interests of the individual patient are still paramount and will probably remain so, unless health care professionals adopt another *ethos* that requires them to put the interests of their collective patient population above those of any one individual in it. Sadly, this group-focused *ethos* taken to the extreme is the one that currently prevails in much of the developing world, where health care resources are extremely limited. In some African nations, for example, it would take a community's entire health care budget to provide one HIV/AIDS patient with the treatment she needs. Under such circumstances, her life, however worthy, will probably be sacrificed so that the group is not left without health care resources to meet all the rest of its needs.

B. Duty-based Ethics (Deontology)

The question of balancing individual rights against group well-being prompts a discussion of deontology (from *deon*, the Greek word for duty), an ethical system that relies heavily on the work of Immanuel Kant (1724–1804) and that stresses the importance of doing one's duty and following rules. As noted in the triage example above, utilitarian theory sometimes allows the sacrifice of one or more individuals so that the group can in some important way benefit. The end, it seems, would justify the means in some circumstances. According to Kant and most deontologists, however, respect for individual persons is key. One must never treat a person merely as a means to some other person's happiness. A case in point here would be conjoined twins, one of whom cannot live without using the other's body. In a case where the dependent twin is not only less healthy than the other twin but also worsening his or her twin's condition, utilitarians might reason that the way to achieve overall happiness or pleasure is to separate the conjoined twins so that the healthier one has a shot at a normal life. The fact that the less healthy twin will almost surely die as a result of the surgery is simply the price that must be paid to achieve overall happiness or pleasure, according to utilitarians. Deontologists would take exception to utilitarians' justification for killing one of the twins so that the other can have a normal life, however. The twins should remain conjoined, in deontologists' estimation. Better they both die than one be used to save the other.

Interestingly, utilitarians recently won the day in just such a case. British physicians separated month-old conjoined twins, named Jodie and Mary, after their parents failed to legally block the operation. In an article entitled "Killing Mary to Save Jodie: Conjoined Twins and Individual Rights," lawyer David Wasserman describes the twins' condition as follows:

> Joined at the abdomen, with partially fused spines and a shared bladder, the twins were kept alive by a single working heart and pair of lungs, both on Jodie's side, and presumably both controlled by Jodie's brain. The heart and lung on Mary's side did not function but the aorta on Jodie's side fed directly into the aorta on Mary's side, supplying Mary with oxygenated blood. Physicians estimated that if they remained conjoined, both would be likely to die in six months to a year from the strain of the single working heart. Separated, Mary was likely to die immediately, which she did, while Jodie was estimated to have a ninety-five percent chance of leading a normal life.[9]

For religious reasons, the parents saw their daughters' fates as bound together by God and insisted that it would be wrong to sacrifice one of their twins for the other's sake. The physicians disagreed. They thought it better that Mary's life be sacrificed for Jodie. Indeed, says Wasserman, some of the physicians seemed to view Mary as a mere "parasite" feeding off Jodie, implying that Jodie was of more value than Mary. When a British court of appeals agreed with the physicians, utilitarians cheered the decision on the grounds that it is better that one person lives than two persons (or is it one person and one "parasite"?) die. In contrast, deontologists booed the decision, concurring with Wasserman, "We should be terribly wary of ordering the death of a child, even a sickly, oddly-formed, and barely sentient child, because we see her as a parasite on a child with greater health, vigor, and cognitive potential."[10]

A second contrast between utilitarianism and deontology is that the former is a **consequentialist** ethical theory (which holds that the intended or actual consequences of an ethical choice determine its rightness), whereas the latter is a **nonconsequentialist** ethical theory (which holds that not consequences but adherence to principles determines the rightness of an ethical choice). In other words, unlike utilitarians, who insist that what makes an action wrong or right is its happiness-producing or pleasure-producing consequences, deontologists maintain that an action's moral worth depends on the reasons behind it, specifically whether it is performed for duty's sake or for some reason other than duty. Kant is particularly adamant on this point, as are those deontologists who claim with him that only actions performed from duty are truly moral.

In order to understand what Kantians mean by performing an action from duty, the following example may prove helpful. Consider a group of nursing home aides who have been told it is the policy of their institution not to subject patients to uncomfortable and sometimes dehumanizing tube feedings prematurely, but instead to spoon-feed patients for as long as possible. According to deontologists, if an aide spoon-feeds a frail patient who takes a very long time to eat because that is what a good aide is supposed to do under the circumstances, the aide acts in a morally worthy or "right" manner. In contrast, if another aide acts in precisely the same way not because it is her duty to do so but simply because she feels sorry for vulnerable patients or wants to score points with her supervisor, she acts in a morally insignificantor "neutral" manner. As deontologists see it, although the second aide's actions have good consequences, her imperfect, self-serving motives for spoon-feeding the patient diminish the moral worth of her action. Of course, if yet another aide refuses to spoon-feed the patient on the grounds that it takes too long and the patient is going to die anyway, deontologists will judge the aide's actions not merely morally insignificant or neutral, but instead morally unworthy or "wrong."

Despite the fact that fine-grained distinctions between morally worthy, morally neutral, and morally unworthy actions may initially strike us as ethical hairsplitting, further reflection on the complexity of human motivations may cause us to reconsider this initial reaction. Most people have very mixed motives for doing their jobs—some of them morally worthy, but others very self-serving. All too often, we let the wrong sort of feelings, emotions, biases, and prejudices determine how well or poorly we do our jobs and relate to each other. Realizing this, Kant sought to ground morality upon a foundation steadier than emotion. He chose reason, an instrument capable, in his estimation, of generating the ultimate guideline for moral decision-making. He termed this guideline the **Categorical Imperative** and articulated it in three different ways:

(1) Act only on that maxim through which you can at the same time will that it should become a universal law;

(2) Act in such a way that you always treat humanity, whether in your own person or in the person of another, never simply as a means but always at the same time as an end; and

(3) Never . . . perform an action except on a maxim such as can be a universal law, and consequently such that the will can regard itself as at the same time making universal law by its maxim.[11]

Although applying the Categorical Imperative to concrete situations can be challenging, it is easy enough to understand how it is supposed to work. Consider, for example, a physician who wonders whether it is morally permissible for him to lie to a patient with liver cancer about her grim prognosis for fear she will not be able to handle the bad news about her imminent death. Among the questions the physician should ask himself before he lies to the patient and tells her she is going to be "just fine" are the following: (1) Is lying consistently universalizable, in the sense that any rational person is willing to endorse the rule, "Lie, whenever telling the truth may upset a patient grievously?" (2) Is lying compatible with treating the patient lied to as one who needs truthful information to chart the course of her destiny?; and (3) Is lying under such circumstances motivated by a sense of duty to the patient or by one's dislike of emotionally-charged situations? Chances are, say deontologists, that if the physician asks himself these questions and answers them honestly, he will recognize that he has a duty to tell the truth to his patient.

To be sure, like utilitarianism, deontology has its flaws. There do, after all, seem to be times when it is right to violate supposedly absolute and exception-less rules, such as "Do not lie," "Do not kill," and "Do not commit suicide." For example, is it really the case that all rational persons cannot will as a universal law of nature, the law "Do not commit suicide except when your disease is terminal and there is no way for your physician to assuage your pain and suffering short of putting you into a terminal coma, which— for all practical purposes—is not much different from being dead?" Moreover, strictly interpreted, Kant's version of deontology appears to have another weakness. It offers no clear guidance for handling conflicts between two supposedly absolute moral rules. For example, assume that a social worker agrees to hide a battered woman from her husband. If the husband, brandishing a loaded gun, comes to the social worker and demands to know the location of his wife, should the social worker tell him where his wife is, or should she instead lie to him about her whereabouts? No matter which choice the social worker makes, it would seem that she will do something wrong. She will break either the rule, "Never tell a lie," or the rule, "Never bring harm to another person." To be sure, deontologists might argue that one or the other of these rules is not really absolute; or that God would never permit two really absolute moral rules to conflict; or that the social worker has a third option—she can refuse to say anything to the husband and hope that he does not shoot her. However, none of these responses provide a clear procedure by which to prioritize genuinely conflicting, supposedly absolute moral rules.

Moreover, as we noted in the example of the nursing home aide, deontologists claim that our feelings neither add to nor subtract from the moral worth of our actions. But is this really the case? Is it really morally better to spoon-feed a patient *only* because it is one's professional duty to do so and not also because one feels empathy for a fragile man who, though he could wolf down a 16-inch pizza in his prime, can now eat little more than a small bowl of oatmeal? It would seem that patients do not want caregivers to view them simply as "duties" for whom they are responsible as professionals. Rather it would seem that patients want to be viewed as unique persons for whom caregivers have some genuine human feelings. Perhaps, then, Kant was wrong: doing one's duty simply because it is one's duty may not be enough. On the contrary, moral worth may ultimately depend on what is in one's heart, as one does one's duty.

Dissatisfied with some, though certainly not all, aspects of Kant's ethical theory, philosopher W. D. Ross (1877–1940) developed a version of deontology that seems both less absolutistic and more friendly to human emotions than Kant's version of deontology.[12] To avoid irresolvable conflicts between two supposedly absolute moral duties, such as, "Never tell a lie" and "Never bring harm to another person," as in the case of the husband who demands access to the wife he has battered on numerous occasions, Ross distinguished between **actual moral duty** and *prima facie* (at first sight) **moral duty**. In Ross's estimation, ethical conflicts arise when two *prima facie* duties (not two actual duties) conflict. For example, physicians have a *prima facie* duty not to lie to their patients about their medical condition. But they also have a *prima facie* duty not to harm their patients. Thus, if a physician fears that his patient may commit suicide if he tells her she has liver cancer, the physician will need to determine his actual duty under the circumstances. His decision will depend on his moral intuitions about the importance of lying/not lying to this particular patient. Much will turn on the physician's knowledge about his patient's values and virtues. But no matter what the physician decides, he will, according to Ross, have to defend his choice to his peers by appealing to their moral intuitions—to what they would have judged to be their actual duty in the same situation. Would they agree, in other words, that "benevolent deception" is warranted in this case?

For Ross, moral intuitions play a role not only in determining which of our *prima facie* duties are actual, but also in revealing our *prima facie* duties to us in the first place. Ross claims that we just know by means of our moral intuitions that fidelity, reparation, gratitude, justice, beneficence, self-improvement, and nonmaleficence are our *prima facie* duties. Although critics of Ross concede that his list of *prima facie* duties is a plausible one, they nonetheless doubt that all rational persons would necessarily accept it as authoritative for them. In other words, critics of Ross suspect he is either an ethical subjectivist or, worse, an arrogant elitist who mistakes his peer group's preferred values for universal values. As they see it, such a mistake is of enormous consequence in the health care realm, where appeals to "our" moral intuitions could easily invite abuses of power in the name of some arrogant group's self-proclaimed ethical superiority. For example, given their status and prestige, some health care professionals may be tempted to view their moral judgments about what is in a patient's best interests as better than the patient's.

C. Virtue-based Ethics

Virtue ethics differs from both utility-based and duty-based ethics in its focus on the goodness or badness of people's characters rather than on the rightness or wrongness of people's actions. Perhaps the most well-known virtue ethicist is the Greek philosopher Aristotle (384–322 B.C.E.) who claimed that the ultimate goal of human action is personal happiness, *eudaemonia*, understood as a state of total well-being.[13] Given that we all desire this state of affairs, said Aristotle, we all want to know how to attain it. Although eating, drinking, having sex, and the like will help us achieve happiness, in Aristotle's estimation, we cannot achieve full and true happiness unless we use and enjoy the capacity that distinguishes us from both plants and animals. This capacity is the human ability to reason.[14]

In Aristotle's thought system, reason is variously defined and linked to two sorts of wisdom: theoretical wisdom, reason directed toward contemplation, and practical wisdom, reason directed toward action. Of these two sorts of wisdom, the latter one is the most important in our daily struggle to be decent human beings. Practical wisdom enables us to determine which goals in human life are worthy of pursuit. It helps us to see, for example, that a life spent playing video games is not as worthwhile as a life spent caring for patients. In addition, practical wisdom enables us to organize our activities and relate them to the activities of other human beings. Many times, we experience life as if we were running around in circles, unable to find the center of our own circle—the point of calm where we can find our elusive "true self" and get our acts together. It is practical wisdom that helps us find our center and to answer questions such as "for whom? how much? when? why? and how?"[15]

Yet another way that practical wisdom helps us is by keeping the lid on our passions or raw emotions so that we can become morally good, in the sense of virtuous people. As Aristotle saw it, each moral virtue is a mean or midpoint between its defect and excess, and it is practical wisdom that helps us strike this delicate balance point. So, for example, practical wisdom helps us be courageous instead of rash or cowardly. Similarly, it helps us be truthful about ourselves instead of boastful or self-deprecating.

In order to fully appreciate how Aristotle envisions practical wisdom working in everyday life, imagine a nurse who thinks another health care professional is not acting in patients' best interests. She wonders whether she should blow the whistle on her colleague or keep her thoughts to herself. According to Aristotle, if the nurse routinely rushes to judgment, she should think twice about blowing the whistle, for fear of acting rashly rather than courageously. In contrast, if she knows she usually hesitates to take a stand, she should think twice about not blowing the whistle, for fear of acting in a cowardly rather than courageous manner. Of course, the nurse cannot go on thinking forever. At some point, she will have to make a decision. In choosing either to blow the whistle or not to blow the whistle, the degree to which the nurse is practically wise will, in Aristotle's estimation, determine whether her action choice is rash, cowardly, or courageous.

At this point, the objection may be made that an ethics of virtue, which relies so heavily on practical wisdom, is an unrealistic action guide anywhere, but especially in a heterogeneous society where individuals do not always agree on the worth of various ends.[16] Arguably, the more heterogeneous a society is, the more necessary an ethics of rules is. Although this objection to virtue ethics is a serious one, virtue ethicists stress that ethics is more than a matter of rules; it is also a matter of ideals. Whereas rules indicate which activities and behaviors are forbidden, permitted, or required, ideals encourage us to put our best foot forward even when we do not have to do so. Ideals are, arguably, a stronger means of behavior control than punishment-backed laws. By imposing moral ideals upon ourselves freely, we provide ourselves with the opportunity to become moral giants; that is, our best selves.

Given the fact that ideals have guided the practice of healing through the ages, virtue ethics should appeal to health care professionals. Echoing the Hippocratic Oath, contemporary codes of professional ethics stress that the strength of medicine's moral foundation depends on health care professionals cultivating a certain set of virtues. Among these essential virtues are respect for human dignity, compassion, and respect for human life.[17] Embodying these virtues in oneself clearly requires more in the way of thought, effort, practice, and dedication than merely adhering to hospital policies, government standards, and legal rules. Where virtue is at stake, compliance is not enough. Only continual striving to be a good human as well as a skilled professional is acceptable.

D. Natural Law–based Ethics

Like virtue-based ethics, natural law–based ethics emphasizes the role that reason plays in moral life. According to Ronald Munson, the basic idea behind natural law–based ethics is probably best expressed by the Roman philosopher Cicero: "Law is the highest reason, implanted in Nature, which commands what ought to be done and forbids the opposite. This reason, when firmly fixed and fully developed in the human mind, is Law."[18] If rational persons reflect upon their essential purposes in life—about what they are meant to do before they die—they will conclude that Nature (or God) has hard-wired them to live, to procreate, to love, to know, and so forth. Therefore, people defy nature whenever they ignore or refuse to fulfill their human destiny by deliberately choosing death over life, childlessness over procreating, ignorance over knowledge, hating over loving, and so on. This line of reasoning usually leads to views such that it is wrong to practice voluntary active euthanasia, to use contraceptives, or to have an abortion.

Critics of natural law–based ethics point out that, nowadays, very few people believe that some sort of natural law determines their nature and functions. For example, most contemporary people reject the view that the main purpose of the sexual organs is procreation, and that they, therefore, do wrong when they use birth control. As they see it, if the sexual organs have any purpose, it is the purpose of providing people with physical pleasure and/or the means to intimately bond with each other. Thus, if anything is a violation of the sexual organs' supposed purpose, it is most likely rape and not contraception, sterilization, or abortion.

But even if one rejects the underlying assumptions of natural law–based ethics, the fact of the matter is that certain principles of natural law have shaped the practice of health care as we know it today. Among the legacies of natural law is the **principle of totality**, according to which it is not morally permissible for human beings to submit to surgeries and the like, unless they do so for the good of their entire bodies. For example, although it is morally permissible for a woman to have a cancerous uterus removed so she can go on living, it is not permissible for her to have a liposuction simply because she wants her thighs to look like a fashion model's. Because such risky sculpting of the body is undertaken not for health's sake but merely for vanity's sake, it is wrong, according to exponents of natural law–based ethics.

Another major principle of natural law, and one that is commonly invoked in the world of health care, is the **principle of double effect**. According to this principle, if an action has two effects—namely, an intended good one and an unintended bad one that is nonetheless foreseen as possibly occurring—the action may be performed for the sake of the good effect provided that (1) the intended good effect is at least equal in value to the unintended bad effect and (2) the bad effect is not the means of producing the good effect. For example, it is morally acceptable for a physician to administer adequate pain relief to suffering patients, even if doing so might hasten or precipitate their death. So long as the physician's intention is to relieve pain and not to hasten death, the physician does no wrong.

The major appeal of natural law theory is precisely its emphasis on maintaining that which is "natural" and somehow resisting that which is "artificial." Leon Kass, M.D. claims that a proper understanding of our nature as human beings is necessary for the wise practice of medicine. He states:

> Appreciating the meaning of our embodiment, institutionalized already in our taboos on cannibalism and incest, would lead us to oppose the buying and selling of human organs or the practice of surrogate motherhood. Understanding the virtues of mortality would show us the folly of seeking to prolong life indefinitely and the wisdom of self-sacrifice against the narcissistic prejudices connected with a strictly survivalist principle of life. Recognizing our body's immanent and purposive activities toward wholeness and well-working would instruct and restrain our willful self-manipulation by illuminating which possible alterations of bodies and media might be helpful or harmful to human well-being.[19]

Whatever the merits of Kass's plea, its message is likely to fall on more than a few unreceptive ears. Organ selling, surrogate motherhood, elective cosmetic surgery, and research on extending the life span to 100-years plus are not typically viewed in the United States with the same horror that meets cannibalism and incest. Moreover, the very distinction Kass wishes to maintain, namely, the distinction between the natural and the artificial, is one that makes increasingly less sense in the contemporary health care arena, where technology routinely performs miracles. Still without some sense of health care's proper limits, health care professionals might find themselves regularly helping people like Orlan, a French performance artist and professor of fine arts at the École des Beaux Arts in Dijon, who views her face as a painting entitled "The Ultimate Masterpiece: The Reincarnation of St. Orlan." Since 1990, a team of plastic surgeons have been using a computer-generated blueprint designed by Orlan to replace her facial features with the forehead of Mona Lisa, the eyes of Gérôme's Psyche, the chin of Botticelli's Venus, the mouth of Boucher's Europa, and the nose of a sixteenth-century painting of Diana.[20] Suffice it to say that most health care professionals do not applaud Orlan's team of plastic surgeons, sensing that even if no natural law forbids their assisting people like Orlan, some law or code of professional ethics should.

E. Rights-based Theories (Contractarianism)

Yet another ethical theory that plays a role in the health care realm is contractarianism and the rights-based theories to which it is linked. In the United States it is assumed that all persons have individual rights, some of them nearly absolute. According to George J. Annas, J. D., rights ". . . help people prevent people from being treated as interchangeable, inanimate objects and insist that they be treated as unique persons."[21] Some theorists insist that the only kind of rights we have are so-called **negative rights**—that is, rights of noninterference which specify what ought not be done to a person. John Hospers, a libertarian philosopher, espouses this view of rights. He states:

> Each man [sic] has the right to life: any attempt by others to take it away from him, or even to injure him, violates this right, through the use of coercion against him. Each man [sic] has a right to liberty: to conduct his life in accordance with the alternatives open to him without coercive action by others. And every man [sic] has the right to property: to work to sustain his life (and the lives of whichever others he chooses to sustain, such as his family) and to retain the fruits of his labor.[22]

Thus, Hospers reasons that a competent adult person has, for example, the negative right to refuse any drug, test, procedure, or treatment she does not want. Some theorists embrace the right to refuse medical intervention so fiercely that they insist no one should be forced to submit to unwanted treatment even to save someone else. Specifically, Annas provides the example of a pregnant woman, about to deliver her child, who refuses to submit to an unwanted Caesarean section that physicians believe is necessary to save the child's life. He comments:

> Forcing surgery degrades pregnant women and dehumanizes them, treating them like inert containers . . . The law provides no more support for these decisions than it would for one that would force a mother to 'donate' a kidney or bone marrow to her child.[23]

For Annas, bodily integrity is nearly an absolute right. One's body is not just a piece of property; it is, for Annas, something akin to sacred space.

As important as negative rights are, they provide little comfort to someone, for example, who very much wants medical treatment—say, a life-saving liver transplant—and does not have the insurance or out-of-pocket funds to pay for it. Unless persons have so-called **positive rights**—that is, rights to receive certain goods and/or services from identifiable persons or organizations—they may have to go without shelter, food, clothing, health care, and/or education. To be sure, those who support negative rights only are not necessarily opposed to helping destitute people. But, as they see it, helping such people is a matter of charity and not of duty. In contrast, those who support positive as well as negative rights believe that, in a just society, everyone has a duty to help sustain everyone else's life. Because we are each other's equals, they say, we owe each other whatever a human being needs to lead a recognizably human life.

In his *Theory of Justice* (1971) John Rawls finds space for positive as well as negative rights. Hypothesizing that all rational persons want to live in just, rather than unjust, societies, Rawls proposes that we ask ourselves what kind of society a perfectly rational group of individuals would construct if they were brought together to set up a society from scratch. Specifically, he asks us to imagine ourselves in an "original position," prior to the inception of society, wherein we would know nothing about ourselves except that we are rational creatures who wish to be as free and happy as possible. Comments Rawls:

> Among the essential features of this situation is that no one knows his place in society, his class position or social status, nor does anyone know his fortune in the distribution of natural assets and abilities, his intelligence, strength, and the like . . . [T]he parties do not know their conception of the good or their special psychological propensities. The principles of justice are chosen behind a veil of ignorance.[24]

Rawls suggests that, under such uncertain circumstances, it is in our best interest to guide our deliberations with the "maximin" rule of choice. According to this rule, if we are not sure whether we are going to get the long or short end of the stick, so to speak, we should proceed on the assumption that we are likely to be the losers rather than the winners of the draw.[25] Haunted by the vision of ourselves as existing at the bottom of society's pecking order, says Rawls, we will be motivated to construct a just society—that is, the kind of society in which each person has "an equal right to the most extensive liberty compatible with a similar liberty for others"[26] and which arranges social and economic equalities so that they are "reasonably expected to be to everyone's advantage."[27]

Although it may not be psychologically possible for some people to set aside their vested interests long enough to put their psyches into an original position, the idea of a veil of ignorance may still be useful in the realm of health care. Consider a woman who has been asked to participate in a health care reform project. The health care insurance system she and her team conceive de novo will be enacted into law. In order to ensure that the system they conceive is just, the woman and her team mentally step behind the veil of ignorance. There, the woman imagines herself as not knowing whether she is a hard-working poor woman who cannot afford health care insurance, a single mother with Medicaid, an elderly widow with Medicare, or the high-salaried, fully-insured hospital Vice President she actually is. Under such circumstances of imposed uncertainty, or so the Rawlsian argument goes, the woman would be inspired to conceive a system of health care insurance that covers everyone equally, just in case she turns out to be not a privileged person but a disadvantaged person.

F. Feminist Approaches to Ethics

Quite different from the ethical theories we have discussed so far are feminist approaches to ethics. Although these ethical perspectives are many and diverse, most of them tend to emphasize either issues related to care or issues related to power. **Care-focused** feminist approaches to ethics have as their primary task the validation and/or reinterpretation of such culturally-associated feminine values as compassion, empathy, nurturance, and kindness. In contrast, **power-focused** feminist approaches to ethics have as their first concern the elimination or modification of any system, structure, or set of norms that contributes to the oppression of vulnerable people, beginning with women, particularly women at the bottom of their respective societies.

Among the most well-known, care-focused feminist thinkers is psychologist Carol Gilligan. In her path-breaking book *In a Different Voice*,[28] Gilligan developed an account of moral development that challenged the one her mentor, Lawrence Kohlberg, had developed. According to Kohlberg, whether we are referring to men or women, moral development is a six-stage, progressive process. It begins, he said, with Stage One, "the punishment and obedience orientation." In order to avoid the stick of punishment or receive the carrot of reward, individuals do as they are told. Stage Two is "the instrumental relativist orientation." Based on a limited principle of reciprocity—"You scratch my back and I'll scratch yours"—individuals do what satisfies their own needs and occasionally the needs of others. Stage Three is "the interpersonal concordance or 'good boy–nice girl' orientation." Individuals conform to social expectations simply because they want other people to like them. Stage Four is "the law and order orientation." Individuals do their duty in order to be recognized as honorable as well as likable people. Stage Five is "the social contract legalistic orientation." In return for freedom to do as they please most of the time, individuals promise not to harm others. Finally, Stage Six is "the universal ethical principle orientation." Individuals who achieve this highest stage of moral development are no longer governed primarily by self-interest, the opinions of others, or even the particular laws of their nation. Rather, they are motivated by self-legislated and self-imposed universal principles such as those of justice, reciprocity, and respect for the dignity of human beings as equally valuable persons.[29]

Puzzled by the fact that women rarely climbed past the good boy–nice girl stage, whereas men routinely ascended at least to the social contract stage, Gilligan hypothesized that the deficiency lay not in women but in Kohlberg's scale. She alleged his scale provided a way to measure not *human* moral development but only *male* moral development; if women were measured on a scale that accommodated women's typical style of moral reasoning as well as men's, women would prove just as morally developed as men.

In order to bring into clear focus the nature and merits of women's typical style of moral reasoning, Gilligan conducted several empirical studies. On the basis of these studies, she concluded that for a variety of cultural reasons, women typically speak a language of care that stresses communal relationships and responsibilities, whereas men typically speak a language of justice that emphasizes individual autonomy and rights. Later, Gilligan added the observation that, increasingly, U.S. society is able to accept atypical "masculine" women who prefer the language of justice over the language of care but not atypical "feminine" men who prefer the language of care over the language of justice. If Gilligan's observation is more than a matter of personal conjecture, its implications in the realm of health care are many and serious.[30] Whether a health care professional is a man or a woman, they should not only be encouraged to act in a caring way but also be respected for so acting.

Although power-focused feminists agree with Gilligan that the ethics of care deserves to be recognized as legitimate, they do not want to privilege, even slightly, the ethics of care over the ethics of justice. As power-focused feminists see it, precisely because we live in an increasingly uncaring world, the value of justice cannot be overemphasized. It is, they say, absolutely necessary for our defense against not only sexism (the inequity that is of traditional concern to feminists) but also classism, ethnocentrism, heterosexism, ableism, ageism, and all the other "isms" that plague our poorly integrated, multicultural society. Power-focused feminist ethicists agree with philosopher Alison Jaggar that they should (1) articulate moral critiques of actions and practices that perpetuate women's subordination; (2) prescribe morally justifiable ways of resisting such actions and practices; and (3) envision morally desirable alternatives that will promote women's emancipation.[31] However, they do not think they should limit the scope of their concern and action to women only. Rather, the ultimate goal of power-focused feminist ethicists is to identity and eliminate the *kind* of oppression that women, conceived as a class or group, have traditionally experienced. Although power-focused feminist may begin with a question like "How does this health care policy affect women?," they will generally conclude with a question like "How does this health care policy affect other equally vulnerable or even more vulnerable groups than women?" Often, it takes an oppressed group or formerly oppressed group to recognize the oppression of another group and to seek justice for it.

IV. ETHICAL PRINCIPLES IN HEALTH CARE

Clearly, the ethical theories described above provide more than enough raw material for each of us to develop a personal worldview. Mixing and matching ethical theories may seem like a daunting task (explaining why some people give in to the seductive call of ethical relativism too quickly), but the fact of the matter is that it can be accomplished quite well. For example, reflecting on the ethical theories we discussed above, bioethicists Tom Beauchamp and James Childress have forged an ethical theory termed **principlism** that fits the world of health care particularly well.

According to Beauchamp and Childress, four historically-grounded, nonuniversal, co-equal principles govern health care ethics. These principles are nonmaleficence, beneficence, autonomy, and justice.[32] Beauchamp and

Childress claim that at least in the United States, most people subscribe to these principles as part of their common morality. They point out that the principle of nonmaleficence finds voice in the often-quoted ancient Hippocratic Oath, "At least, do no harm," and that the principle of beneficence is operative whenever the best interests of a patient are at stake. In addition, they note that autonomy and justice, individual rights and the common good, are bread-and-butter staples in the kitchen cabinet of American values.

Because the principles of nonmaleficence, beneficence, autonomy, and justice probably do strike most of us as the basic building blocks of morality, it is tempting to think that health care professionals, students seeking careers in health care, and members of the general public do not, afterall, need to forge their own personal worldview or ethics for health care. They can simply rely on Beauchamp and Childress's. But this temptation must be resisted. Just because Beauchamp and Childress have forged a personal worldview for themselves does not mean that we do not have to forge one for ourselves, even if it turns out to be substantially congruent with Beauchamp and Childress's. Although we may think we understand the concepts of nonmaleficence, beneficence, autonomy, and justice, the fact of the matter is that each one of these concepts is both difficult to define and to apply, particularly in the realm of health care, where patients' lives often depend on health care professionals' ethics.

A. The Principle of Nonmaleficence and the Standard of Due Care

Nonmaleficence is a principle which Americans endorse. Most of us are committed to the view that we should be free to do as we please provided that we do not harm anyone else as we go about our business. Unfortunately, harm is one of those terms that is difficult to delimit. Does harm include psychological and spiritual harm as well as physical harm? Does it include harm to oneself as well as to others? Does it include minor as well as major harm? Thus, it is not surprising that health care professionals do not view the Hippocratic Oath as a "no-brainer." Rather, they regard it as a motto requiring them to adhere to the standard of due care—that is, the kind of care health care professionals give patients when they treat them attentively and vigilantly so as to avoid mistakes.

Like most standards in health care, the **standard of due care** has changed over time. The current standard of due care is quite high because of the enormous amount of medical information that is readily available to health care professionals and because of how specialized the practice of medicine has become. Fifty years ago, most health care professionals were generalists, and patients expressed surprise when their physician managed to diagnose and treat their condition with a marginally good outcome. Today an ever-increasing number of health care professionals are specialists or even sub-specialists. There are some cardiac surgeons, for example, who perform only angioplasties, and they are not easily forgiven when they make a mistake. "Being perfect" is replacing "doing one's best" as the standard of due care in contemporary medicine, a fact that may explain, at least in part, why so many patients readily sue health care professionals for malpractice. Regrettably, fear of a malpractice suit leads some health care professionals to practice **defensive medicine**. They order more tests than are probably necessary for fear of exposing a patient to an unnecessary risk. Or they hesitate to give a newly-marketed pharmaceutical to a patient for fear that their patient may experience a rare side-effect. Or they treat only patients with minor problems, eschewing patients with major problems for fear they will get a bad "report card" if a patient dies on their watch. Even worse, when health care professionals do make a mistake, they and/or the institutions to which they are linked hesitate to admit the failure to the patients harmed. In fact, in November 1999, the National Academy of Sciences estimated that medical errors, including performing surgery on the wrong side of a patient's body, providing a fatal overdose of drugs, and performing unnecessary surgery were responsible for 98,000 deaths of hospital patients per annum.[33] Yet only 16% of HMOs and 40% of hospitals were forthright enough to report one or more "adverse actions" to the government.[34]

B. The Principle of Beneficence and the Risk of Paternalism

Clearly related to the principle of nonmaleficence is beneficence. Patients want more than not to be harmed; they want to be benefited—that is, taken good care of and, if possible, healed. Fortunately for patients, most people who become health care professionals do so precisely because they want to help people. Their work is motivated by the thought of saving lives, relieving human suffering, and increasing people's well-being. But because health care professionals have private as well as professional lives, they cannot be expected to devote themselves entirely to serving their patients' good. They have their families', friends', and institutions' good to serve as well. Thus, all that duty may demand of health care professionals is to do a reasonable amount of good for patients.

Determining what constitutes a reasonable amount of good for patients is no easy matter, and is probably best approached by way of example. For instance, it may be reasonable to expect health care professionals to do some charity work, particularly in an affluent nation that pays its health care professionals quite well, but unreasonable to ask them to treat only uninsured people or only people on Medicaid or Medicare. Health care professionals should not be expected to work for free or for very modest salaries because citizens are unwilling to be taxed to support universal, government-provided basic health care insurance. Similarly, although it may be reasonable to expect health care professionals to get patients in and out of their offices roughly on schedule, communicate test results as quickly as possible, and schedule routine appointments, it is probably unreasonable to ask them to be at patients' beck and call, spending half the day listening to trivial health complaints. Likewise, although it may be reasonable to require health care professionals to accept grumpy, senile, and incontinent patients, it may be unreasonable to expect them to welcome noncompliant, abusive, or violent patients. Finally, although it is usually reasonable to expect health care professionals to risk their health and even lives to treat patients with infectious diseases, there exist sets of circumstances that may exempt them from this heavy obligation.

Significantly, the limits of reasonable beneficence have been questioned in particularly intense ways in recent decades. For example, in the 1970s and 1980s, health care professionals vigorously debated whether they had a clear duty to treat patients with HIV-AIDS. Traditionally, health care professionals espoused the view that they had a moral duty to treat patients even at risk to themselves because of patients' vulnerability and the ideal of medicine as dedicated to goals that transcend self-interest and sometimes even call for self-sacrifice. But they formulated this view before the development of antibiotics and vaccines, when everyone, including health care professionals were at high risk for early death from killer diseases. Thus, dying in the line of duty struck nineteenth-century physicians, for instance, as a real possibility.

By contrast, after the development of antibiotics and vaccines, twentieth-century physicians stopped worrying about dying from killer diseases. A miracle drug would be able to save them if one of their patients infected them with deadly germs. Thus, when the fatal disease AIDS appeared on the American scene, and medical researchers were unable to control the infectious HIV virus which causes it, health care professionals suddenly had to confront the fact that they could actually die as a result of treating patients with HIV-AIDS. Because HIV-AIDS is transmitted through the exchange of bodily fluids including blood, something as small as a needle-stick accident or blood splashing could begin a health care professional's journey into the jaws of death. Shocked by this realization, many health care professionals initially protested that the duty of beneficence did not really include caring for patients with deadly, infectious, difficult to treat, and untreatable diseases such as HIV-AIDS; but, as it became clear that the risk of transmission of HIV-AIDS through occupational exposure was quite small, the great majority of health care professionals came to share the consensus opinion of the American Medical Association (AMA), namely, ". . . a physician may not ethically refuse to treat a patient whose condition is within the physician's current realm of competence solely because the patient is seropositive."[35]

As just indicated, most health care professionals take their duty of beneficence very seriously. For example, in Charlotte, North Carolina, many members of the Mecklenburg County Medical Society participate in a program called Physicians Reach Out that provides no-cost or very-low-cost health care to uninsured people. In addition, physicians and other health care professionals shuttle patients to and from their offices, schedule office hours late into the night, give noncompliant patients repeated opportunities to reform, and willingly work to the point of exhaustion. However, like many health care professionals, Charlotte health care professionals do not always carefully distinguish between acting beneficently on the one hand and acting paternalistically on the other. To act beneficently is to do for the patient the good the *patient* desires; to act paternalistically is to do for the patient the good the *health care professional* thinks the patient should desire.

Paternalism is best defined as "the intentional limitation of the autonomy of one person who limits autonomy appeals exclusively to grounds of benefit to the other person."[36] Because health care professionals want to help patients, they find it extremely frustrating when patients refuse medication and treatments that could substantially improve the quality of their lives or even save their lives. It troubles them not only when patients refuse medically necessary blood transfusions because of their religious convictions, for example, but also when patients with diabetes or cardiac disease refuse to change their diets because they like sweets and fats too much to do so. Truth be told, most health care professionals are not truly satisfied unless they get their patients to follow their advice. Thus, beneficence sometimes goes wrong, as it did in the case of Donald "Dax" Cowart, a burn patient, whose experience is summarized below:

> In 1973, "Dax" Cowart, age twenty-five, was severely burned in a propane gas explosion. Rushed to the Burn Treatment Unit of Parkland Hospital in Dallas, he was found to have severe burns over sixty-five percent of his body; his face and hands suffered third degree burns and his eyes were severely damaged. Full burn therapy was instituted. After an initial period during which his survival was in doubt, he stabilized and underwent amputation of several fingers and removal of his right eye. During much of his 232 day hospitalization at Parkland, his few weeks at Texas Institute of Rehabilitation and Research at Houston, and his subsequent six months' stay at University of Texas Medical Branch at Galveston, he repeatedly insisted that treatment be discontinued and that he be allowed to die. Despite this demand, wound care was continued, skin grafts performed and nutritional and fluid support provided. He was discharged totally blind, with minimal use of his hands, badly scarred, and dependent on others to assist in personal function.[37]

The health care professionals justified overriding Dax's wishes for no treatment on the grounds that he was not able, at least in the early period of his treatment, to fully understand what was in his best interests. They felt vindicated because despite his diminished physical condition, Dax eventually went on to become a lawyer and got married subsequent to leaving the hospital. Yet the fact remains that even though Dax says he is happy to be alive at present, he still maintains that the decision to die was one he could have made and should have been permitted to make when he was in the hospital. Health care professionals should not have substituted what they thought was good for Dax—namely, life—for what Dax thought was good for himself—namely, death. Just because actions have good consequences does not mean that they are right.

C. The Principle of Autonomy

Dax's case and cases far less egregious than his invite careful consideration of the principle of autonomy. The word autonomy is derived from the Greek words *auto* (self) and *nomos* (law). It finds dramatic expression in nineteenth-century philosopher John Stuart Mill's oft-quoted lines, according to which the only reason for which state power can be rightfully exercised over an individual against his or her will is to prevent harm to other individuals:

> His own good, either physical or moral, is not a sufficient warrant. He cannot be compelled to do or forebear because it will be better for him to do so, because it will make him happier, because, in the opinion, to do so would be wise or even right. These are good reasons for remonstrating with him, but not for compelling him or visiting him with any evil in case he does otherwise. To justify that, the conduct from which it is desired to deter him must be calculated to produce evil to someone else.[38]

Not only do autonomous persons have their own set of values and goals, they are also able to deliberate and reason about alternative courses of action, and to communicate their decisions to others. As we shall discuss at length in Chapter 3, the principle of autonomy is intimately connected to patients' right to refuse treatment and to be informed of the "medical consequences" of [their] actions.[39] Because U.S. patients are becoming both more aware of their rights and less trusting of health care professionals' beneficence, the importance of the principle of autonomy is growing exponentially in the realm of health care.

D. The Principle of Justice

Equally important as the principles of nonmaleficence, beneficence, and autonomy is the principle of justice. We Americans are convinced that it is unjust to treat one person better or worse than another similar person in similar circumstances unless there is a good reason for the differential in treatment. In the realm of health care, concerns about patients being treated fairly are likely to be particularly high if the supply of a medically necessary

treatment or drug outstrips the demand for it. Thus, health care professionals seek objective criteria for the just allocation of scarce medical resources.

Although checklists for the just allocation of scarce medical resources are many and diverse, they generally include criteria such as the
following six:

(1) To each, an equal share

(2) To each, according to need

(3) To each, according to effort

(4) To each, according to contribution

(5) To each, according to merit

(6) To each, according to ability to pay.[40]

In the abstract, each of the above criteria has something to recommend it; in
concrete situations, however, only some of them are appropriate to invoke.
For example, imagine there is only one dose of a life-sustaining drug in the
hospital pharmacy and that each of five patients have requested it be given
to them. To which one (or more) of these patients should health care professionals give the precious pharmaceutical?

If health care professionals give each of the five patients an equal share
of the drug, then none of the patients will receive the intended benefit of the
life-sustaining drug. All of them will die. Similarly, if health care professionals give the drug to whomever requested it first, they may "waste" it on a patient who has become so medically compromised that he or she can no longer
truly benefit from the drug. Allocating the drug on the basis of which patient
both needs it most and can benefit from it the most seems to be the fairest
way to proceed. Yet health care professionals might have second thoughts
about this criterion for justly allocating the drug, when they discover that the
selected patient is a chronic alcoholic who is fully responsible for his miserable health status, or a serial killer, or an indigent patient unable to pay even
a fraction of the drug's very high cost.

Such thoughts are understandable, but they are also incompatible with
a serious quest for justice. To allocate scarce medical resources to patients on
the basis of their social worth, moral goodness, or economic condition rather
than on the basis of their medical condition is more often than not wrong.
When kidney dialysis machines first became available to patients in 1964,
tens of thousands of patients needed these machines, but less than three
hundred were able to gain access to them. Most of the lucky patients were
selected from hundreds of applicants by hospital selection committees consisting of health care professionals and relatively privileged townspeople.
Sometimes labeled "God Committees," these selection committees chose patients on the basis of social worth criteria such as occupation, family, and
even religion and morality. Not surprisingly, financially-successful, church-
going citizens with intact, loving families had a better chance of being

selected for dialysis than "ne'er-do-well" single men or "down-and-out" divorced women. Rather than focusing on the equal worth of human beings as human beings, some selection committees mistook their "middle-class values" for "eternal verities"[41] thereby violating the principle of justice egregiously. Justice needs to be blind for it to do its work.

V. BALANCING THE PRINCIPLES OF NONMALEFICENCE, BENEFICENCE, AUTONOMY, AND JUSTICE

As we saw in the case of Dax and the other cases discussed above, the principles of nonmaleficence, beneficence, autonomy, and justice sometimes conflict. When this happens, is there some sort of "super principle" or set of guidelines to which we can appeal for guidance? As it turns out, Beauchamp and Childress offer us five guidelines to determine which principle is most important to heed in hard cases. They are as follows:

> (1) Better reasons can be offered to act on the overriding norm than on the infringed norm (for example, typically if persons have a right, their interests deserve a special place when balancing those interests against the interests of persons who have no comparable right).
>
> (2) The moral objective justifying the infringement has a realistic prospect of achievement.
>
> (3) No morally preferable alternative actions can be substituted.
>
> (4) The form of infringement selected is the least possible, commensurate with achieving the primary goal of the action.
>
> (5) The agent seeks to minimize the negative effects of the infringement.[42]

In order to determine whether Beauchamp and Childress's guidelines are really useful, we may wish to apply them to an actual case. The case I have in mind is the case of Armando Dimas, as reported by Lisa Belkin in a *New York Times Magazine* article entitled, "The high cost of living."[43]

According to Belkin, the night Armando was shot, the emergency room of Houston's Hermann Hospital was crowded to capacity. This fact caused some of the hospital staff to speculate that Armando, an indigent, undocumented Mexican immigrant, secured a hospital bed only because hospital authorities viewed him as a potential organ donor. After a preliminary examination of Armando, Dr. David MacDougall, the neurosurgeon on call, concluded, "This guy should be dead."[44] But Armando was not dead. He had been resuscitated, returned to consciousness, and put on a ventilator for life support. Gathered around his bed were his immediate family: a fourteen-member group of undocumented Mexican immigrants who had recently applied for residency in the United States. Although most of the hospital staff believed that Armando would ask to be removed from the ventilator if he knew his actual condition, his mother refused to let anyone tell her son that he was a quadriplegic. Dr. MacDougall finally broke the silence. He asked social worker Cindy Walker to convene a meeting between Armando's health care team and his family. Looking straight at Armando's mother, Dr. MacDougall told her it was time to face reality: her son was not miracle material. Armando's mother responded angrily to Dr. MacDougall, exploding in Spanish that it was wrong to "lie" to her son: "He can walk, he will walk. He can breathe; he will not need that machine."[45] The meeting ended abruptly and without resolution.

Informed about the confrontation that had just occurred, hospital authorities decided it was best to tell Armando about his condition, his mother's protests notwithstanding. They selected nurse Norma McNair to tell him the truth. To everyone's surprise, Armando did not opt for a do-not-resuscitate order. On the contrary, using two blinks of his eyes for "yes" and one for "no," he communicated a desire for full treatment. He wanted it all—cardiopulmonary resuscitation, antibiotics, ventilators, feeding tubes. Armando's health care team was caught off guard. In their experience, patients in Armando's condition almost always refused aggressive treatment. They did not know how to respond to a quadriplegic patient who demanded a "full-court press" of treatments.

The longer he stayed in the hospital, the more of a problem Armando became for the hospital's cost comptroller, former nurse Hazel Mitchell. Because Armando lacked health care insurance and his family was too poor to pay even a fraction of his bill out of pocket, the hospital had to absorb the total cost of Armando's care. Armando was also a major challenge for occupational therapist Mary Coffey. She knew that Armando would remain little more than a "head in a bed" unless she could order him a very expensive, custom-made wheelchair to support his back and head, thereby enabling him to use a mouth stick to blow commands to a computer. With this device, Armando could learn marketable skills. Although cost comptroller Mitchell initially refused to order the special wheelchair for Armando on the grounds that the hospital had already spent too much money on Armando, she later relented and ordered the chair (which turned out not to fit him). But at the same time, she decided to transfer Armando from Hermann Hospital to Hermina Bartkowski's Total Life Care Center ("Bart's," for short). There, the bills would be $300 a day instead of $890, largely because the staff consisted of Polish immigrant physicians and nurses willing to work for very low salaries.

Armando liked Bart's, where the standard of care was high due to the efforts of Director Bartkowski. Compared to the dangerous neighborhood in which his family home was located, Bart's was a safe and comfortable haven; however, after four and one-half years and approximately $750,000 worth of treatment, Hermann Hospital got tired of paying Armando's bills and gave his family one month to learn how to care for him at home. Although Armando's family objected to this turn of events, claiming they could not master the skills necessary to care for Armando adequately, he was nonetheless sent home in his ill-fitting special wheelchair without the ability to use the mouth stick. Gradually, Armando's mother, a woman with serious health problems of her own, became her son's 24-hour-a-day health care attendant. As for Armando, to this day he sits in his chair or lays in his bed, alternately, watching television and listening to the radio.[46]

VI. CONCLUSION

In reflecting on Armando's case, which pits the principle of justice against the principle of beneficence and, to a lesser extent, the principle of autonomy, the question to ask is whether Hermann Hospital did the right thing when it sent Armando home from Bart's. An application of Beauchamp and Childress's guidelines suggests that Hermann Hospital did no wrong; indeed that it acted "justly." Public hospitals like Hermann Hospital cannot underwrite the total care of all quadriplegic patients indefinitely. If they tried to do so, their doors might have to close for lack of funds. The fact that Armando and his family liked Bart's is not a good enough reason to keep Armando at Bart's, not if, as was the case, a disproportional amount of Hermann Hospital's total budget for indigent care was being spent on Armando. Sending Armando home saved Hermann Hospital hundreds of thousands of dollars to use for many other poor patients desperate for care.

Although home care for Armando was not ideal, since home consisted of a five-room trailer with an on-again, off-again electrical system, a dysfunctional heating system, and three times as many occupants as its rooms, it was the only reasonable option for Armando's long-term care. There were no less expensive nursing home facilities than Bart's to which to send him, and no charitable group had volunteered to pick up the tab for an undocumented Mexican immigrant who had a reputation for being on the "wild side" before being shot. Hermann Hospital trained Armando's family the best it could to deliver home care to Armando and, arguably, could not be held responsible for the fact that his sickly mother wound up as his primary caregiver. Pressed as it was to think of its entire patient population and not just Armando, Hermann Hospital determined that Armando had received more than his fair share of its resources and would have to rely on the generosity of others for the foreseeable future.

Even if Hermann Hospital technically passed the test of Beauchamp and Childress's guidelines when it chose to privilege the principle of justice over the principles of beneficence and autonomy in Armando's case, we may still wonder if total justice was served in his case. Had Armando been insured, he might have qualified for long-term care at Bart's; or if his family had been people of means, they could have used their own finances to pay the bill at Bart's. Minimally, had Armando had enough money, he could have paid for a special chair that actually fit him, so that he could have learned marketable skills. As it stands, Armando's future is bleak. It is not clear how long he can tolerate the boredom of his endless days nor what will happen to him in the event that his mother dies before he does.

Cases like Armando's remind us that in any realm, particularly, the realm of health care where so much can be at stake, the "right" answer is not necessarily perfectly right. In order to serve one principle, some other principles may need to be sacrificed; the sacrifice of these values, even when they are justified, will be a cause of great sadness for morally reflective people.

Discussion Questions

1. Using the ethical theories discussed in this chapter, formulate your own personal worldview. Is it different from all these theories or very similar to one or more of them?

2. Do you consider yourself a "practically wise" person? Why or why not?

3. Do you think the principles of nonmaleficence, beneficence, autonomy, and justice are the best ones to use in the realm of health care? Why or why not? Can you think of other principles to add to them? If so, what are they and why do you think they are so important?

4. Referring to the following quote by Leon Kass, "Recognizing our body's immanent and purposive activities toward wholeness and well-working would instruct and restrain our willful self-manipulation by illuminating which possible alterations of the bodies and media might be helpful or harmful to human well-being," what are the pros and cons of getting cosmetic surgery?

5. What are some of the positive and negative aspects of feminist approaches to ethics? How might a feminist approach be used to guide men as well as women in certain health care professions? What does a power-focused feminist approach offer that a care-focused feminist approach does not?

Cases

1. A retired patient comes into a clinic for an eye examination. His ophthalmologist discovers that his poor vision fails to meet minimum criteria for a driver's license in Alabama. There is no hope for his vision to improve. Should the physician report this patient to the highway department? When the physician expresses his concern to the patient, the patient moans, "But doctor, I only drive during the daytime, and to places that I am familiar

with . . . the store, church, the hospital. You may as well kill me and my spouse if you take away my license."

a. Which principle should be paramount in this case, in your estimation? Autonomy? Beneficence? Nonmaleficence? Justice?

b. If you were the physician, how would you help this patient?

2. Consider the following real-life case:
In 1980 Mr. Arato was diagnosed with kidney failure. He underwent surgery in July, 1980, to remove the kidney. The surgeon "detected a tumor on the 'tail' or distal portion of Mr. Arato's pancreas," received consent from Mrs. Arato to operate on the pancreas, and proceeded to remove the affected parts of the pancreas as well as the spleen and the failed kidney . Postoperative examination of the removed sections of the pancreas revealed they were malignant and so Mr. Arato was referred to oncologists. Upon visiting the oncologists, Mr. Arato filled out a questionnaire stating that he " 'wish[ed] to be told the truth about [his] condition' ". The oncologists discussed the usefulness of chemotherapy for pancreatic cancer with the Aratos and recommended Mr. Arato try it. But they did not disclose to the Aratos that, no matter what treatment was employed, patients with advanced pancreatic cancer were likely to live only a short amount of time. Their lack of full disclosure was based on the fact that "Mr. Arato had exhibited great anxiety over his condition" and they did not want "to deprive [him] of any hope of cure." Mr. Arato consented to the chemotherapy. The treatment did not cure his cancer, however, and he died in 1981. Mr. Arato's wife and children sued all the physicians involved in Mr. Arato's case. Among other things, they claimed that Mr. Arato would not have chosen to submit to chemotherapy if he had known just how bad his prognosis was; that the physicians offered "false hope" to him; and that because of this "false hope" Mr. Arato did not put his financial affairs in order before his death, leading to losses by his family after his death.

Source: Honorable Justice Armand Arabian, "*Arato v. Avedon* (1993)." Darnell Law Office [March 31, 2004] *http://www.darnall.net/cases/arato.htm* [Accessed August 2, 2004].

a. Did the physicians act beneficently or maleficently when they decided to give Mr. Arato "false hope"?

b. Did the principle of justice play a role in this case? If so, how?

c. Did the physicians violate Mr. Arato's autonomy? If so, how?

Endnotes

1. Alasdair MacIntyre, *After Virtue* (Notre Dame, IN: University of Notre Dame Press, 1981), pp. 6–7.

2. Ibid., p. 9.

3. Ibid., p. 10.

4. Michael Boylan, *Basic Ethics* (Upper Saddle River, NJ: Prentice Hall, 2000), p. 27.

5. Ibid., p. 4.

6. Aristotle, "Nicomachean ethics," Book 1, Chapter 2, in: Richard McKeon (ed.), *The Basic Works of Aristotle* (New York: Random House, 1941), p. 936.

7. Jeremy Bentham, "Principles of morals and legislation," in: Jeremy Bentham (ed.), *The Utilitarians* (New York: Anchor Books, 1973).

8. John Stuart Mill, "Utilitarianism," in: Jeremy Bentham (ed.), *The Utilitarians* (New York: Anchor Books, 1973).

9. David Wasserman, "Killing Mary to save Jodie: conjoined twins and individual rights," *Philosophy & Public Policy Quarterly*, 21, no. 1 (Winter 2001): 9.

10. Ibid., p.14.

11. Immanuel Kant, *Groundwork of the Metaphysics of Morals* (tr.) H. J. Paton (New York: Harper & Row, 1956), pp. 74–75.

12. W. D. Ross, *The Right and The Good* (Oxford: Oxford University Press, 1930).

13. Aristotle, "Nicomachean ethics," in: W.D. Ross (ed.), *The Works of Aristotle Translated into English* (London: Oxford University Press, 1963).

14. Ibid.

15. Ibid.

16. Although Aristotle's virtue ethics has much to recommend it, what complicates its adoption as an ethical theory is that there are two kinds of Aristotelian virtue: intellectual and moral. Aristotle defined virtue generally as an activity of the soul (state of mind) that merits praise because it leads us to make "right" choices about what will contribute to our happiness. Intellectual virtues, such as practical wisdom (knowledge of how to secure the ends of human life) and intuitive reason (knowledge of the principles from which science proceeds), are a product of "teaching." We praise people who exhibit intellectual virtues because they able to *discern* those actions which will make them happy. In contrast, moral virtues such as courage, temperance, and justice are "a result of habit." We praise people who exhibit moral virtues because they are able to *perform*, almost spontaneously, those actions that do in fact make them happy.

17. American Medical Association, "Principles of medical ethics (1980)," in: Thomas A. Mappes and Jane S. Zembaty (eds.), *Biomedical Ethics*, 3rd ed. (New York: McGraw-Hill, 1991), p. 54.

18. Ronald Munson, *Intervention and Reflection: Basic Issues in Medical Ethics*, 6th ed. (Belmont, CA: Wadsworth/Thomson Learning, 2000), p. 26.

19. Leon R. Kass, *Toward a More Natural Science: Biology and Human Affairs* (New York: Free Press, 1985), p. 348.

20. Charles Siebert, "The cuts that go deeper," *New York Times Magazine*, 145, no. 50481 (July 7, 1996): 20.

21. George J. Annas, *The Rights of Patients* (Carbondale and Edwardsville, IL: Southern Illinois University Press, 1989), p. 2.

22. John Hospers, *Libertarianism: a Political Philosophy for Tomorrow* (Los Angeles: Nash, 1971), p. 12.

23. George J. Annas, *The Rights of Patients* (Carbondale and Edwardsville, IL: Southern Illinois University Press, 1989), p. 127.

24. John Rawls, *A Theory of Justice* (Cambridge, MA: Belknap Press, 1971), p. 83.

25. Ibid., p. 154.

26. Ibid., p. 83.

27. Ibid.

28. Carol Gilligan, *In a Different Voice* (Cambridge, MA: Harvard University Press, 1982).

29. Lawrence Kohlberg, "From is to ought: how to commit the naturalistic fallacy and get away with it in the study of moral development," in: T. Mischel (ed.), *Cognitive Development and Epistemology* (New York: Academic Press, 1974), pp. 164–165.

30. Carol Gilligan, "Moral orientation and moral development," in: Eva Feder Kittay and Diana T. Meyers (eds.), *Women and Moral Theory* (Totowa, NJ: Rowman & Littlefield, 1987), p. 25.

31. Alison M. Jaggar, "Feminist ethics," in: Lawrence Becker and Charlotte Becker (eds.), *Encyclopedia of Ethics* (New York: Garland, 1992), pp. 363–364.

32. Tom L. Beauchamp and James E. Childress, *Principles of Biomedical Ethics*, 4th ed. (New York: Oxford University Press, 1994), p. 38.

33. American Hospital Association, *Hospital Statistics* (Chicago: American Hospital Association, 1999).

34. Robert Pear, "Inept doctors seldom reported," *New York Times* (May 29, 2001): A2.

35. American Medical Association's Council on Ethical and Judicial Affairs, "Ethical issues in the growing AIDS crisis," *Journal of the American Medical Association*, 259 (1988): 1360–1361.

36. Raymond S. Edge and John Randall Groves, *Ethics of Health Care: a Guide for Clinical Practice* (Albany, NY: Delmar Publishers, 1999), p. 42.

37. Lonnie D. Kliever (ed.), *Dax's Case: Essays in Medical Ethics and Human Meaning* (Dallas: Southern Methodist University Press, 1989).

38. John Stuart Mill, in: Gertrude Himmelfarb (ed.), *On Liberty* (New York: Penguin Books, 1974), pp. 68–69.

39. American Hospital Association, "A patient's Bill of Rights," A statement affirmed by the AHA House of Delegation on February 6, 1973.

40. Gene Outka, "Social justice and equal access to health care," in: Robert M. Veatch and Roy Branson (eds.), *Ethics and Health Policy* (Cambridge: Ballinger Publishing Co., 1976).

41. Paul Freund, "Organ transplants: ethical and legal problems," in: Joel Feinberg and Hyman Gross (eds.), *Justice* (Belmont, CA: Dickenson Publishing Co., 1977), p. 184.

42. Tom L. Beauchamp and James E. Childress, *Principles of Biomedical Ethics*, 4th ed. (New York: Oxford University Press, 1994), p. 34.

43. Lisa Belkin, "The high cost of living," *New York Times Magazine* (January 31, 1993): 31–33, 44, 46, 56–57.

44. Ibid., p. 32.

45. Ibid., p. 44.

46. Ibid., p. 56.

chapter three

The Health Care Professional–Patient Relationship

I. INTRODUCTION

In the introduction to this book, we noted that health care professionals are a very diverse group of people with a wide variety of skills, and that the physician is no longer the sole pilot of the medical ship. Physicians may still find themselves leading, coordinating, or otherwise directing a health care team, but the team will probably not be content to simply obey orders anymore. On the contrary, depending on their particular professional identities and roles, nurses, social workers, physical and occupational therapists, health care administrators, and so forth will have their own ideas about how to balance the principles of nonmaleficence, beneficence, autonomy, and justice discussed in Chapter 2. Yet, for the most part, irrespective of their particular medical field, most health care professionals will share similar ideas about what it means to be a professional and how to relate properly to each other, their patients, and the institutions they serve.

II. THE PRACTICE–INSTITUTION RELATIONSHIP IN HEALTH CARE

Many people go through life working in occupations that provide them with ample paychecks but little in the way of personal satisfaction and social meaning. For them, a job is simply what one does to pay the bills, and Friday is met with exclamations of "Thank goodness, now I can do something I enjoy!" Interestingly, most committed professionals do not conceive of their work as a mere grind. Rather, they tend to view their work as a practice or calling to which they are dedicated and which energizes them. This positive view of work seems particularly pronounced among health care professionals who, despite the intrusions of managed care bureaucrats, the demands of sometimes unreasonable patients, and an overwhelming amount of information to master, still find it personally satisfying to use their healing skills for the good of humankind. Because the people whom they serve cannot always arrange for their bodies or psyches to break down during business hours, health care professionals are on call even when they are not officially at work. The task of healing is a 24-hour, 7-day-a-week responsibility for which health care professionals are accountable to a greater or lesser degree. Knowing this, health care professionals typically view their work as a mission.

In order to fully appreciate the idea of "work as mission," we need to better understand both what a practice is and what an institution is. According to philosopher Alasdair MacIntyre, a practice is a complex, cooperative human activity that has its own internal goods, satisfactions, and standards of excellence. For example, people who enter the practice of healing are attracted to the intellectual challenges it provides and the human relationships it creates; and they are willing to live up to its ideals as well as to obey its bottom-line rules. Comments MacIntyre:

> To enter into a practice is to accept the authority of those standards and the inadequacy of my own performance as judged by them. It is to subject my own attitude, choices, preferences and tastes to the standards which currently and partially define the practice. . . We have to learn to recognize what is due to whom; we have to be prepared to take whatever self-endangering risks are demanded along the way; and we have to listen carefully to what we are told about our own inadequacies and to reply with the same carefulness for the facts.[1]

MacIntyre's "take-home" message for health care professionals is that they have to be just, courageous, and honest people in order to become excellent healers. They must fulfill their obligations to their patients, colleagues, and profession; have the fortitude to work under conditions of uncertainty; and be self-reflective enough to realize their own and others' limits as healers. But, continues MacIntyre, no matter how good they are as healers, health care professionals cannot maintain their healing practice for long without the support of the institutions of medicine—institutions such as medical schools, hospitals, clinics, and laboratories. Yet, just because the practice–institution relationship is necessary, it does not mean it is problem-free. On the contrary, practices and institutions will inevitably get on each others' "nerves" because of the ways in which their priorities differ. As we just noted, the practice of healing is centrally concerned with satisfying the internal good of providing patients with quality care, and it is held together by the sealing cement of fundamentally cooperative human relationships, such as the health care professional–patient relationship. In contrast, the institutions of medicine are mainly focused on attaining external goods, such as high profits, and they are activated by the fragmentary fires of human competition. Thus, as MacIntyre sees it, if health care professionals do not want the practice of healing to become merely the business of medicine, they have to make sure that "the ideals and creativity" of their practice do not succumb to the "acquisitiveness" of medicine's institutions.[2]

III. MODELS OF THE HEALTH CARE
PROFESSIONAL–PATIENT RELATIONSHIP

Given that health care professionals increasingly find themselves working in institutions focused on the bottom line, their relationship to patients probably displays more conflict than it did a quarter of a century ago when the physician and patient often shared a long-term, one-on-one relationship, with the patient trusting the physician's expertise and authority. Today, as we have already noted, patients relate to a variety of health care professionals who enter and exit their lives in ways that defy predictability and undermine stability. For example, when my father was in a hospital and then a skilled nursing home recently, he was assigned to a health care team. Regrettably, my father's team members were continually changing, depending on who was on call, on vacation, running late, not answering messages, stressed out, sick, or just tired. Never once did my father's team gather together, and never once did they consult my father or me about the total "game plan" for my father. My overall impression was that too many cooks were stirring the broth and that my father's course of treatment had more to do with Medicare rules than anything else. In fact, it seemed as if the team was playing a game entitled "Beat-the-Medicare-Clock." They were trying to cram in as many tests and treatments as possible before my father, for lack of additional Medicare dollars, would be required to move out of the hospital into some other institution. My father kept muttering that he wished things were like they had been in the "old days" when your family doctor stuck with you through thick and thin. He wanted to relate to his health care professionals as persons, but they were so busy that they scarcely had time to consult with each other about his treatment, let alone with him or me. Interestingly, when I communicated my father's frustration to individual members of his health care team, they expressed their own unhappiness with the situation. Like my father, they wanted a more personal relationship with him, but felt overwhelmed by institutional demands. One nurse summed up the team's sentiments perfectly when she said, "This work is just too hard to do unless you know you have actually contributed to a patient's well-being and gotten to know him or her as a person, someway, somehow. But the 'powers that be' just don't seem to get it. All they seem to care about is money and whether we are knocking the rival hospital out of business. And then they wonder why so many of us 'burn out.'"

To be sure, this era is not the first time in human history that practice–institution tensions have troubled the health care professional–patient relationship. The "good old days," like all days, were somewhat bad. In fact, in the early 1970s, concerns about technology killing the heart and soul of medical practice were raised so routinely that philosopher Robert Veatch developed four, later five, models for the physician–patient relationship in particular. He labeled these models the engineering model, the priestly model, the collegial model, the contractual model, and the covenant model. He then urged physicians and other health care professionals to decide which of his proposed models was, on balance, the "ideal" model for a good health care professional–patient relationship.[3]

Veatch presented two of his models—the **engineering model** and the **priestly model**—as polar opposites. In general, health care engineers view themselves as skilled experts capable of running tests, performing surgeries, prescribing drugs, and otherwise treating disease. They tend not to view their patients as unique persons with fears and hopes, but as bodies in need of repair, approaching them in much the same way that auto mechanics approach broken-down autos. They tell the patient what the problem is and how they propose to fix it, focusing on the facts of the case and avoiding value-laden discussions such as whether it is a *good* idea, all things considered, to fix the problem ailing the patient.

In contrast to health care engineers, health care priests presume to be exceptionally insightful about the inner feelings of their patients. They claim they know not only how to treat their patients' ailments but also whether it is in the best interests of their patients to be so treated. In other words, because they are experts about medicine, health care priests start to think they are also experts about life and how it should be led. They encourage patients to confess their personal as well as medical secrets to them in an effort to provide care for patients' spirits and psyches as well as bodies.

Veatch's other models for the health care professional–patient relationship fall between the engineering and priestly models. In fact, the collegial, contractual, and covenant models are variations on a similar theme. The **collegial model** views the health care professional and the patient working together as full equals to codetermine what is best for the patient. The problem with this model is that health care professionals and patients are not really full equals. Knowledge is power, and the health care professional's expertise is something most patients lack. Moreover, collegial decision-making takes time. To be real partners, health care professionals and patients need to supplement the typical 10-to-15-minute rushed office visit with ongoing discussions; if health care professionals do not make time for phone calls or email correspondence, chances are that they and their patients will never become *bona fide* colleagues.

In contrast to the collegial model, the **contractual model** for the health care professional–patient relationship is more businesslike and less time-consuming. The health care professional simply offers the patient a range of medical goods and services, and then the patient decides whether he or she wants them. If so, the health care professional and patient enter into a contractual agreement, with both of them obligated to follow its terms. The weakness of this model is that most health care professionals and patients are not quite willing to regard their relationship as no more special than the one that exists between an auto salesperson and an auto purchaser.

Most likely, the lingering belief that the health care professional–patient relationship should be more than a business deal accounts for Veatch offering a fifth model for this relationship; namely, the **covenant model**. Unlike the contractual model, this model envisions the health care professional standing by the patient even if the patient can no longer pay the bills on time, or even if the patient has become increasingly infirm and grumpy. Because the covenant model recognizes the way in which patients remain dependent on health care professionals even when their "business deals" turn sour, it may represent an appropriate compromise between the collegial and contract models.

Although Veatch's models for the health care professional–patient relationship are remarkably complete, recently, Drs. Linda and Ezekiel Emanuel have offered a useful variation on them. According to the Emanuels, four alternative models for the health care professional–patient relationship vie for the endorsement of patients and health care professionals alike. They are the paternalistic model, the informative model, the interpretive model, and the deliberative model.[4] The **paternalistic model** is essentially Veatch's priestly model for the health care professional–patient relationship. The health care professional functions as a parent or guardian who presents selected information to the patient to get the patient to do what the health care professional thinks is best. In contrast to this model stands the **informative model**, similar to Veatch's engineering model. The health care professional serves as an information gatherer and technical specialist who provides the patient with as many facts as possible so the patient can determine what type of medical intervention best fits his or her own value system.

Like Veatch's collegial, contract, and covenant models, the Emanuels' next two models for the health care professional–patient relationship—the interpretive model and the deliberative model—are attempts to mediate between the paternalistic (priestly) model and the informative (engineering) model. Of these two models, the **interpretive model** remains squarely in the camp of patient autonomy. In this model, the health care professional serves as an advisor or counselor who wants to make sure that he or she is delivering to the patient the treatment the patient actually wants. Because too much as well as too little information can impede autonomy, and because patients frequently are not sure what they want, or do not want, in the way of treatment, the health care professional tries to elicit and understand the patient's values as fully as possible in order to recommend those treatments most likely to serve the patient's values. So if a patient with terminal cancer wants to live 6 months longer to witness the birth of her grandchild, then the health care professional will recommend to her those treatments most likely to stretch out her life.

More paternalistic in emphasis than the interpretive model is the Emmanuels' **deliberative model** for the health care professional–patient relationship. In this model the health care professional functions as a mentor who not only elicits and tries to understand the patient's values but also comments upon and, if necessary, criticizes them. So, for example, if a severely-diabetic single mother refuses to modify her high-carbohydrate, high-fat diet, the deliberative health care professional will strive to convince her that it is wrong for her to prefer chocolate candy to life itself, particularly if she has a child who needs her care and will be devastated if she dies. Whereas the interpretive health care professional seeks only to serve the patient's actual values, the deliberative health care professional aims to change these values when they clearly conflict with the value of an ongoing healthy life.

To determine whether the Emanuels' deliberative model is significantly different from the paternalistic model and a workable improvement on the interpretive model, it may be useful to consider the following hypothetical case:

Melissa was admitted to Saint Mary's Hospital after her college roommate, Nicole, returned from class and found her unconscious on the floor. Nicole called 911 and the medics found Melissa's heartbeat at 37 and estimated her weight to be around 70 pounds, an extremely low weight for a young woman of her height—approximately 5'5". Dr. Parker, the attending physician in the emergency room, examined Melissa, admitted her to the hospital, and ordered an intravenous line (IV) and a nasogastric feeding tube (NG) to treat Melissa's dehydration and emaciation. Upon regaining consciousness, Melissa became distressed about the IV line and the NG tube and demanded to see Dr. Parker.

Unlike Dr. Parker, some of the medical staff knew Melissa from previous admissions to the hospital. These admissions had been relatively frequent when Melissa was still a minor living with her parents. Melissa had been diagnosed with anorexia nervosa when she was 16, and over the past 6 years, virtually every treatment modality had been unsuccessfully tried on her. Since reaching age 18, Melissa had begun to rely nearly exclusively on psychotherapy, totally rejecting inpatient hospitalization and most forms of outpatient treatment.

Unaware of Melissa's long and unsuccessful struggle with anorexia, Dr. Parker arrived at Melissa's bedside with this prescription for her: another round of inpatient hospitalization. Melissa flatly refused, but countered with the offer of staying in the hospital until her weight hit 75 pounds. Melissa viewed this weight as acceptable for herself and one at which she functioned well enough to attain a 3.7 GPA last semester. She sought to reassure Dr. Parker, insisting that she had not meant to let her weight drop to 70 pounds. Rather, due to some particularly stressful recent factors in her life, the "beast" of anorexia had gotten the best of her, pushing her to eat less than usual and to exercise more. Unlike most anorexics Melissa typically consumed around 1,000 calories a day, which she had learned to burn off by engaging in approximately 2 hours of strenuous aerobic activity each day. Over the years, she learned how to hold her weight at 75 pounds without resorting to what she perceived as the extremes of other anorexics' behavior.

With Melissa's reference to the "beast" of anorexia, Dr. Parker reminded her of her medical record, which indicated several diagnoses of clinical depression. He added that he could not in good conscience agree to Melissa's proposal, since he very much doubted she was at all in control of her behavior. The "beast" of anorexia might strike again; and, in any event, 75 pounds—her preferred weight—was simply too low a weight to be viewed as anything other than very unhealthy, and probably life-imperiling. If Melissa refused to follow his orders, he would be forced to have her declared legally incompetent and mentally disordered so that he could commit her, against will, to the psychiatric unit of the hospital for inpatient treatment. He would then have her involuntarily committed to the mental ward of the hospital for inpatient treatment.

At this point in the conversation Melissa demanded that Dr. Parker consult with her psychiatrist, Dr. Larson. Within 15 minutes of Dr. Parker's call, Dr. Larson arrived on the scene. He took Dr. Parker aside and told him that, in his estimation, Melissa was competent and that she was not any more "mentally disordered" than many other people for whom a sound body and mind are a low priority. Over the last 2 years, Melissa had indeed maintained her weight at 75 pounds, and if Dr. Parker let Melissa have her way, she would probably return to her holding weight of 75 pounds and continue living as well as could be expected on her own terms.

Dr. Parker could not believe his ears. Viewing Dr. Larson as part of Melissa's problem, he did not attempt to mask his hostility. He said that he was going to ask for an immediate health care ethics committee consult. He reasoned this would be the first step to securing a court order to have Melissa involuntarily committed for inpatient hospitalization. Dr. Larson told him that this was a mistake, and he would resist him every step of the way. Hearing the commotion, Melissa pulled the NG tube out of her nose, the IV line out of her arm, and made an attempt to push out of her bed. Then, feeling weak, she fainted and was put back in bed. Dr. Parker ordered that she be restrained and that the NG tube and IV line be reinserted. Dr. Larson stormed out, as Dr. Parker dialed the number for the healthcare ethics committee.[5]

Reflecting on Melissa's case and the Emanuels' deliberative model for the health care professional–patient relationship, it appears that neither Dr. Parker nor Dr. Larson (at least on this occasion) tried to deliberate with Melissa, although, interestingly, Melissa tried to deliberate with Dr. Parker by offering to get her weight back up to 75 pounds. Not willing to seriously entertain Melissa's offer to him or to rethink his own values, Dr. Parker decided to act in a manifestly paternalistic manner, trying to force Melissa to do what he judged to be in her best interest. The fact that Melissa had managed to live well enough or her own terms for quite a long time made no difference to him. In contrast, Dr. Larson acted in an interpretive manner, stressing that Melissa's way of living, however unhealthy, was nonetheless her chosen way of living and that there probably was no use trying to convince her otherwise. Better to accept Melissa on her own terms than to try to break her will, he insisted.

Perhaps a third physician, a truly deliberative physician, could have established a different relationship with Melissa and persuaded her to voluntarily enter treatment yet again. But in cases like Melissa's one suspects that deliberation has been tried, only to fail repeatedly. On balance, it would seem that Dr. Larson did less overall harm to Melissa than Dr. Parker did. He seemed to respect Melissa's powers of self-judgment more than Dr. Parker did.

IV. Meeting the Demands of Competence and Care in the Health Care Professional–Patient Relationship

As difficult as it is for health care professionals to appropriately weigh competing ethical principles in cases like Melissa's, it is even more difficult for them to fully meet the basic demands of their profession—**competence** and **care**. Minimally, health care professionals have to be competent; that is, they have to have the knowledge and skills to treat their patients safely and effectively. For all practical purposes, if a health care professional has graduated an accredited school and is licensed or certified by appropriate authorities, then he or she is probably competent to practice medicine. But this fact does not mean that all health care professionals are equally talented or equally in command of their respective fields. Some health care professionals are exceptionally gifted, but others are simply average. Therefore, it is important for health care professionals to be honest enough (see Section II) to acknowledge to themselves and others the limits of their knowledge and to ask more able colleagues for their help when a patient's problems prove puzzling, perplexing, or overwhelming. In addition, health care professionals need to be honest enough to admit to themselves and others if they become impaired and therefore unable to provide competent care to their patients. Due to the stress and strain of their work, some health care professionals may become addicted to alcohol or to one or more of the drugs they use to treat patients, or they may start to lose their mental acumen and/or physical stamina. When such competence-undermining situations arise, health care professionals have an obligation to get treatment for their condition, and if treatment cannot help them, to retire from practice.

Sadly, not all impaired health care professionals are honest enough to stop treating patients when they should, putting their colleagues in the uncomfortable position of having to blow the whistle on them. Because a "whistle-blowing" incident may seriously harm the whistle-blower (who may be shunned as an interfering busybody) as well the impaired health care professional (who may lose status, prestige, or even livelihood subsequent to the whistle-blowing), it should be avoided if at all possible. Raymond S. Edge and John Randall Groves offer the following guidelines to a nurse, for example, who must decide whether or not to tell hospital authorities that a neurosurgeon with an "alcohol problem" may be imperiling patients' lives:

(1) The wrongdoing in question is grave and has created, or is likely to create, serious harm.

(2) The professional who is contemplating blowing the whistle has appropriate information and is competent to make a judgment about the wrongdoing.

(3) The professional has consulted others to confirm their information and judgment.

(4) All other internal resources to resolve the problem have been exhausted.

(5) There is a good likelihood that the whistle-blowing will serve a useful purpose.

(6) The harm created by the whistle-blowing is less than the harm done by a continuation of the wrongdoing.[6]

Unless the nurse understands the intricacies of neurosurgery, is sure the surgeon is an alcoholic, has talked to the surgeon about the problem, and has gotten trusted colleagues to offer treatment options to the surgeon, the nurse had best think twice before playing "hero." However, if the nurse has followed guidelines one through six above and concluded that the surgeon is indeed risking patients' lives, then the nurse should indeed blow the whistle. Unless patients can trust their health care professionals to police each other, patients are not likely to forgive them when mistakes are made, or to understand that medicine sometimes fails to help people not because health care professionals are at fault but simply because medicine's powers are limited.

Being a competent health care professional is not the equivalent of being a caring health care professional, however. To be caring, the health care professional must do more than effectively treat patients. He or she must also try to care about the patient as a person with particular hopes, dreams, fears, and desires. A caring health care professional is well aware of the distinction between treating a disease on the one hand and healing a patient on the other—that is, helping the patient come to terms with the meaning of the disease in and for his or her life. Comments Paul Samuels, M.D.:

> . . . I work hard at keeping up with the latest developments. I want to be technically first rate. After all, that's what patients need. But that is only the mechanical aspect of care. I feel what really counts is the human aspect. That is both a lot tougher and a lot more rewarding. It is a great privilege being a healer. Entering patients' worlds and listening to their pain, helping them make sense of their suffering, helping them to cope with the burden of disease—all that is what makes my life rewarding. . . [7]

Because the idea of being a fully caring health care professional defies easy definition, it may be best to proceed by way of further examples. In her essay, "Travels in the Valley of the Shadow," Joanne Lynn, M.D. recounts how she came to understand the difference between providing *competent* health care to a patient on one hand and providing *caring* health care on the other. She relates the following personal anecdote:

> As a neophyte physician for home care service, I went to see an octogenarian couple at home; Mr. Phillips with Alzheimer's type dementia had forgotten how to swallow. This I knew how to treat. I installed a feeding tube, gave instructions, and left feeling quite good about my skills. On the next day, I received a frantic call from the home care nurse. Mrs. Phillips had called nearly incoherent and crying and the nurse wanted me to come along to reevaluate what had nearly become a crisis situation.
>
> Mrs. Phillips met us at the door and kept repeating that she loved Bill very much and would do almost anything that helped him, but that she had not been able to do what I had asked. It took awhile to understand whether anything was technically difficult or whether there had been some adverse occurrence, like aspiration or vomiting. Nothing of that sort was the problem. Mrs. Phillips finally pulled herself together enough to look at me directly and say, "I just can't tie him down to our bed." Suddenly I saw the situation from her perspective. This man with whom she had lived for sixty years and whom she had tended during nearly a decade of mental decline was not really my "problem of nutrition and hydration" but her husband, lover, and spouse. Tying him down was not a mechanical solution to the problem of keeping a feeding tube in place, but a deeply offensive abuse.
>
> In the discussion that followed, I also realized that taking him from home in order to place a gastrostomy tube was hard to justify for his benefit and contrary to the preference of his wife. Seeing him—and her—in their home made it easier to see the impropriety of intervention. Letting him live as well as he had been living for as long as possible seemed the best course. He died at home some two months later. The only assistance needed from the "health care system" was an aide to help with a bath most days and occasional visits from and phone calls to the home care nurse. It makes me shudder to think how often we caregivers inflict terrible suffering as we thoughtlessly pursue correction of a physiological abnormality.[8]

Because Dr. Lynn took the time to get to see Mr. Phillips through Mrs. Phillips' eyes, she realized that although a gastrostomy tube was the standard of care in cases like his, the best way to care for Mr. Phillips was actually to let Mrs. Phillips spoon-feed him. Although Mr. Phillips would die a bit sooner without artificial food and hydration, he would die in a way befitting the husband, lover, and spouse he had always been.

Urged to view the Dr. Lynns of the medical world as ideal caregivers, some health care professionals will immediately protest that they simply do not have the time to get to know their patients as persons, or that their specialty— say, trauma—demands that they treat patients as quickly as possible. Although such protests may at times be justified, they do not always, or necessarily, serve as an excuse for not trying to put care back into health care. According to reporter Nancy Shute, many health care professionals, particularly primary care physicians are finding ways "to bring back the empathy and personal attention epitomized by TV doctor Marcus Welby."[9]

Some physicians are trying to improve patients' access to them by going into low-overhead, solo practice. They see fewer patients, but offset the accompanying loss of income by doing everything "from answering the phone to giving shots to filling out insurance forms"[10] themselves.

Other physicians are trying something equally daring. They are seeing patients in groups. Invented by clinical psychologist Edward Noffsinger in 1996, the "drop-in group medical appointment"[11] seems to have two advantages. First, it permits physicians to treat patients more efficiently by not having to repeat to patient after patient the same facts about chronic diseases such as depression, diabetes, high blood pressure, asthma, and arthritis. Second, and just as importantly, the group medical appointment lets patients spend not just a few minutes but an hour or more with their physician. It also gives patients opportunities to compare notes, to counsel and console each other, and to realize that their problems are not unique to them.

Still other physicians are trying to increase contact with patients by encouraging them to use email for questions, prescriptions, and the like. Although email medicine may become quite popular in the future when millions of aging, computer-savvy baby boomers and Gen-Xers need an increasing amount of health care, at present it remains controversial among older physicians in particular. They doubt physicians can forge close relationships with patients they seldom see in person.[12]

V. RESPECTING THE RIGHTS OF PATIENTS IN THE HEALTH CARE PROFESSIONAL–PATIENT RELATIONSHIP

So far we have focused on health care professionals' responsibilities to patients without once mentioning patients' rights. In recent years, however, patients' Bills of Rights have been promulgated in virtually every health care institution. In fact, upon admission to a hospital or a skilled nursing home, patients immediately receive a list of their rights. Some of these lists are quite short and general. Others include such rights as "the right to examine and receive an explanation of [their] bill regardless of source of payment,"[13] a right that is of growing importance as more patients are sent home with bills that promise to bankrupt them. Still others include such rights as the right to be given sufficient pain medication,[14] a right that patients increasingly invoke as they realize they need not suffer in silence. But irrespective of their differences, almost every list of patients' rights includes some reference to patients' right to (1) confidentiality and privacy; (2) truthfulness, veracity, and full disclosure; and (3) informed consent. Thus, it is particularly important to discuss these three patients' rights in detail.

A. Confidentiality and Privacy

In a society that seems to take delight in knowing everyone's intimate secrets, it is no wonder that patients demand as a matter of right that health care professionals keep private their personal information. The importance of confidentiality goes back to the time of Hippocrates. The Hippocratic Oath required health care professionals to keep to themselves what they saw or heard in the course of treatment or even "outside of treatment in regard to the life of men [sic]."[15] Currently, the importance of confidentiality is highlighted in law as well as in most health care professional codes. One of the main reasons for maintaining confidentiality is that when patients present themselves for treatment, they must reveal to health care professionals many things about their physical and mental weaknesses, some of them embarrassing, others disgusting. If health care professionals routinely communicated such sensitive patient information to third parties, patients would lose trust in health care professionals and think twice about candidly sharing their medical problems with them. As a result, health care professionals would be deprived of the information they need in order to provide quality care to patients. Thus, it is essential that health care professionals put a premium on confidentiality.

There are exceptions to confidentiality, however. The law requires health care professionals to report suspected cases of both child and elder abuse and negligence. So, too, does it require them to report poisonings, industrial accidents, communicable diseases, gunshot or knife wounds, and narcotic use. In addition, health care professionals are instructed to breach confidentiality in order to protect the welfare of an individual or the community. For example, if a patient tells his psychiatrist that he is going to kill someone, and the psychiatrist has good reason to think her patient is capable of such violence, then the psychiatrist has a duty to institute involuntary civil commitment procedures, inform relevant authorities, and/or directly warn those at risk of harm. Similarly, if a patient tests positive for HIV/AIDS and the physician knows the patient has no intention of telling his or her spouse about the diagnosis, then the physician has a duty to warn the unsuspecting spouse directly or indirectly (with the help of public health officials, for example).

Deciding when to breach confidentiality is no easy matter, however, and it is likely to become a larger problem in the future because of our increased ability to screen for genetic diseases in particular. Genetic counselors wonder how to handle patients who refuse to share certain kinds of genetic information with family members and friends. For example, should or should not a genetic counselor remain silent when a 21-year-old man who tests positive for Huntington's Disease refuses to tell his fiancée, who very much wants children, about his condition? Does she or does she not have a right to know about her future husband's disease—a disease that will begin to manifest its devastating neurological symptoms in the prime of his life, and that may be inherited by one or more of his biological children? As we shall discuss at some length in Chapter 8, as more genetic information is amassed about people, patients have increasing concerns about this information remaining in their control.

One fact that makes it much more difficult to maintain patient confidentiality nowadays is the way in which patients' medical information is gathered, stored, and disseminated. Fifty years ago, approximately 90% of health care was delivered to patients by a solo practitioner assisted by a small staff—perhaps a nurse and a receptionist. Physicians typically stored their handwritten notes about patients' family histories, diagnoses, prognoses, and treatments in office file cabinets. There, they tended to gather dust. Today, more than 90% of patients' health care is delivered, as we have already noted, by large health care teams whose members seem to be in a permanent state of Heraclitean flux.[16] Health care professionals come and go depending on either the demands of their group's practice or the terms of their patients' managed care plans—"plans" that repeatedly switch patients willy nilly from one health care professional to another. As a consequence of this state of affairs, a veritable legion of health care administrators keep detailed records on patients, and the information they gather is typically stored electronically in so-called data warehouses.[17] Not only do health care professionals stake some claim to these records, so do health insurance administrators, employers, public health officials, lawyers, police authorities, and news reporters.[18] One might well wonder, then, as Dr. Mark Siegler has, whether the interests of third parties in patients' records, as well as the ascendancy of the large health care team approach to patient care, has not made confidentiality a "decrepit concept."[19] With so many people having access to information about patients for so many different reasons, is there really any point in perpetuating what Siegler views as the myth of confidentiality?

Rather than dismissing confidentiality as a myth, however, it may be preferable for health care professionals and patients to have a candid discussion about the contents of patients' medical records and with whom the information can be shared and for what reasons. Edge and Groves, for example, insist, "Policies must be designed to balance the right to legitimate personal privacy while not offsetting the institutional need to make necessary information quickly and easily available to those who have a legitimate claim to it."[20] Rather than trying to go back to the days when only one or a very few health care professionals had access to patients' medical information, they recommend the development of specific policies aimed at maintaining clear lines between proper and improper uses and misuses of patient information.

Edge and Randall's advice is good so far as it goes, but how would they assess a policy such as the **Health Insurance Portability and Accountability Act (HIPAA)**? Enacted by Congress in 1996, HIPAA had two initial goals. The first goal was simply "to ensure continuity of care and maintenance of insurance coverage while switching jobs and health plans."[21] The second, related goal was to limit health care professionals' disclosure of patient health care information to third parties, especially health care insurers who wanted the information for "improper purposes" like denying patients' coverage for preexisting health conditions. As HIPAA evolved during the period from 1996–2003, health care institutions realized that in order to avoid stiff criminal and civil penalties, they had to do several things. Specifically, they needed to get the patients' prior written consent for the release of their health information to third parties; to give patients better access to their own medical records and the opportunity to correct them; and to establish privacy-conscious business practices.[22]

Unfortunately, some health care institutions initially interpreted HIPAA too literally and became overly zealous in the campaign to prevent "Big Brother from knowing everything about everyone's medical condition."[23] For example, shortly after HIPAA's passage into law, my unconscious father was rushed to the hospital and admitted for treatment. When I phoned to find out my father's room number, no one would tell me because he had not specifically authorized disclosing his whereabouts to anyone. I had to drive down to the hospital and prove not only that I was my father's daughter but also that he would want me to know his whereabouts. Later, I went to see some of the hospital's administrators and convinced them that their interpretation of the letter of the HIPAA law was "over the top" in situations such as the one in which my unconscious father and I had found ourselves. I also persuaded them, as later official commentaries on HIPAA made clear, that the "minimum necessary exchange of information" clause in HIPAA was not meant to prevent members of health care teams from talking to each other in detail about a patient's condition. Nor was it meant to prevent them from consulting other health care professionals to assist in patients' care. Rather, it was meant to prevent thoughtless "elevator" conversations about patients and gossip sessions at church socials and the like. Laws such as HIPAA are a must in the kind of society in which we live, but they need to be tweaked when practical experience proves them to undermine rather than bolster patient care.

B. Truthfulness, Veracity, and Full Disclosure

As important as confidentiality is to the patient–health care professional relationship, it is not more important than truthfulness, veracity, and full disclosure. There are many reasons for endorsing the view that honesty is the best policy in the realm of health care, but two of them are of particular significance. First, patients expect a higher level of truthfulness from health care professionals than they demand from politicians, lawyers, and telephone solicitors, for example. Too much is at stake for patients to feel satisfied with less than a totally truthful health care professional. Second, in order to make good decisions about their actions and life plans, patients must know the truth about their health status. For example, if a physician tells me that I can count on living to a ripe old age, when he suspects that I will be dead before the year is out, he robs me of the opportunity to spend my remaining few days in the manner I feel is most meaningful.

Fortunately, U.S. health care professionals have gone from believing "the less said the better" to "the more said the better" where patients' diagnoses and prognoses are concerned. Robert Veatch et al. point out, "[i]n a study of physician attitudes, Donald Oken in 1962 found that eighty-eight percent of physicians would tend to withhold a diagnosis of cancer. In 1979, just seventeen years later, Dennis Novak repeated essentially the same study finding that ninety-eight percent of physicians would tend to disclose."[24] Moreover, physicians have moved from telling first the patient's family and then the patient the "bad news" about the patient's health status to immediately and directly discussing the patient's health status with the patient, even to the exclusion of family members.[25] As a result of major empirical studies as well as many years of clinical experience, health care professionals have become convinced that, at least in the United States, most patients want the whole truth and nothing but the truth about their medical condition.

Yet, despite the fact that patients view themselves as autonomous, competent adults who are able to handle bad medical news maturely, most patients agree with health care professionals that there may be legitimate exceptions to the full and truthful disclosure rule. For example, due to a lack of empirical studies and long clinical experience, it is not clear that patients in the early stages of Alzheimer's disease want to be told their diagnosis.[26] If patients with a family history for a disease like Huntington's disease can avoid knowing their destiny by not getting genetically screened for HD, why should patients in the early stages of Alzheimer's disease be forced to confront their fate just because a physician diagnoses the condition during an office visit? The fact that most people may want to know the bad news about themselves sooner rather than later does not mean all people have this desire. In fact, there are entire cultures in which giving patients their "death sentence" is viewed with horror. For example, Ruth Macklin points out that in some Native American Indian cultures, in particular the Navajo culture, people think that merely to speak about the possibility of death is somehow to cause death to happen. Therefore, many Navajos do not want to know their diagnosis and prognosis if it is a bad one, and their families and friends demand that health care professionals communicate only good news or hopeful news to the patient. In such circumstances, the culturally sensitive health care professional's best option is to reflect on Macklin's observation:

> . . . Navajos holding traditional beliefs can act autonomously only when they are not thinking in a negative way. If doctors tell them about bad contingencies, that will lead to negative thinking, which in their view will fail to maintain and restore health.[27]

Because the goal of both the health care professional and the patient is to maintain and restore health, the health care professional is obligated to share with the patient only those elements of the truth the patient wants. But to the degree the health care professional does not know the patient as a person, chances are that mistakes will be made: Too few or too many beans will be spilled.

C. Informed Consent

There are, as we have just noted, exceptions to the honesty-is-always-the-best-policy rule. Nonetheless, it is important to stress once again that most patients want to know the truth about their condition and if there is anything that can be done to improve it. They also want the power to accept or reject whatever remedy is proposed. Therefore, informed consent, typically defined "as the willing acceptance of a medical intervention by a patient after adequate disclosure by the physician of the nature of the intervention, its risk and benefits, as well as of alternatives with their risks and benefits,"[28] is one of the lynchpins of the health care professional–patient relationship.

Two phrases in the definition of informed consent are of particular significance, namely, "willing acceptance" and "adequate disclosure." In the United States, it is presumed that if a person is an adult, he or she is able to willingly accept or refuse medical interventions for himself or herself. *Bona fide* decision-makers have their own values and goals. In addition, they have the ability to understand information; to reason and deliberate about possible courses of action; and to communicate their decisions to others.[29] If an adult patient lacks one or more of the elements necessary for decision-making, health care professionals may challenge the patient's ability to give informed consent.

Determining whether a patient is incompetent can be quite easy or quite difficult in the clinical context. If a patient is in a persistent vegetative state or a deep coma, then clearly the patient is not a competent decision-maker. Similarly, if a patient is severely mentally retarded, in the late stages of Alzheimer's disease, in extreme pain, or in a hallucinatory state, the patient is in no position to make decisions and therefore incompetent. However, if a patient is mildly mentally retarded, in the early stages of Alzheimer's disease, under the influence of alcohol or narcotics, stressed out, or exhausted, then health care professionals may have difficulty determining whether the patient is capable of giving informed consent. In addition, health care professionals may have trouble distinguishing between truly incompetent patients on the one hand and patients who, in their estimation, are "bad" decision-makers on the other. The mere fact that a patient does not accept health care professionals' recommendations does not necessarily mean that that patient is incompetent. Rather, it may only mean that the patient is a quirky or eccentric person with unusual values or goals, or a religious person whose beliefs preclude certain kinds of medical treatments. Only if it is apparent that the patient cannot think for herself or himself, should health care professionals seek a surrogate decision-maker for the patient, that is, someone capable of making the decision the patient would make were he or she competent. Assessing whether a patient has the capacity to willingly consent to medical procedures is only half the informed-consent story, however. Disclosing enough information for decision-making purposes to a competent patient is, as we noted above, the other half. But what constitutes adequate information? Currently, the two main legal standards for disclosure are the customary practice standard and the reasonable patient standard. The **customary practice standard** requires health care professionals to disclose to patients the information reasonable health care professionals in their locale would disclose under the same or similar conditions. The advantage of this standard is that reasonable health care professionals are probably the best judges of what constitutes an appropriate disclosure of information to patients. The disadvantage of this approach is, however, that it is interpreted through the grid of local, state, or regional community standards. Reasonable health care professionals in one state may customarily be much more closemouthed with patients than reasonable health care professionals in another state, for example. Somehow, it does not seem fair that if a patient lives in New York City instead of Charlotte, North Carolina, he or she will be told more—or less—about the risks and benefits of a certain treatment or research experiment.

In contrast to the customary practice standard, the **reasonable patient standard** requires health care professionals to disclose to patients all the facts a reasonable patient anywhere would consider necessary to make a good treatment choice. The advantage of this second standard is clear. Whether patients live in North Carolina or New York, they have a right to the same information; reasonability does not depend on geography. Despite its major advantage, the reasonable patient standard is, like the customary practice standard, subject to multiple interpretations, a distinct disadvantage. Specifying the information to which reasonable patients anywhere are entitled is very difficult. Still, it is generally agreed that, no matter where they reside, reasonable patients would likely want the following kind of information before they consent to a recommended procedure or take a prescribed drug:

(1) A diagnosis and prognosis for their disease or disability

(2) The nature of the proposed treatment procedure(s) and drug(s) in terms nonexperts can comprehend

(3) The risks and hazards of the proposed treatment procedure(s) and/or drug(s)

(4) The probability that the proposed treatment procedure(s) and/or drug (s) will be successful

(5) Alternatives to the proposed treatment procedure(s) and/or drug(s) including no treatment

(6) Anticipated benefits of the proposed procedure(s) and/or drug(s) if any.[30]

Although he admits that "delineating the exact type of warning that a [health care professional] must provide in a particular case is virtually impossible because of the unlimited number of clinical circumstances that occur in every day practice,"[31] Louis Brunetti, a physician who is also a lawyer, nonetheless claims that it is not that difficult to imagine the kind of warnings reasonable patients typically want. He points out that people want to know whether a proposed treatment procedure and/or drug is therapeutic or experimental, and whether it will require recovery time. In addition, they want to know the magnitude, probability, and duration of the significant risks associated with a proposed treatment procedure or drug. Finally, people want to know their treatment options, including the alternative of doing nothing. Asked which significant risks health care professionals should disclose to reasonable patients, Brunetti offers the following two thumb rules: (1) disclose the risks, if the *probability* of the harm is high (even though the *severity* of the harm is low); and (2) disclose the risks, if the *severity* of the harm is high (even though the *probability* of the harm is low).[32]

Some of Brunetti's most interesting specifications of the standard elements of informed consent are related to communicating the probability that the proposed treatment will be successful and/or beneficial to patients. As he sees it, reasonable patients typically want to know what the health care professional views as a successful treatment so that they can decide whether, in their estimation, they agree. For example, a surgeon may proclaim an organ transplantation a major success, but the patient may view it as a failure if he or she has to live life in a diminished state thereafter. In addition, Brunetti insists that, with respect to anticipated benefits, reasonable patients usually want to know not only the magnitude of the benefit but also its duration and probability. So, for example, imagine that a woman goes to a cosmetic surgeon for a facelift. Given the risks and hazards, to say nothing of the expense of this unnecessary medical treatment, she probably will want a realistic idea of how she will look after the facelift and how long its beautifying effects will last. Told that the surgery will not make her 50-year-old face look 20 but 40 at best, and that it will have to be repeated every 3 to 5 years or so, the woman may decide that the pain of the procedure is not worth the gain.

Sadly, some health care professionals try to meet the two legal standards for disclosure of information to patients in a minimalistic, bureaucratic fashion. Protesting that they are too busy to discuss at length every plus and minus of every possible treatment for patients, they give the patient a detailed form on which is printed all the information a "reasonable" patient needs and more. They then ask the patient to read the form (which is presumably written in an understandable way) and sign the form, if they agree with its terms. Put into such circumstances, most patients read the form quickly and even sign it on the spot, sometimes for no reason other than they do not want to hurt the health care professional's feelings.

But not all health care professionals think that meeting the customary practice and reasonable patient standards for disclosure of information to patients is an onerous, unnecessarily burdensome, excessively time-consuming task—on the contrary. They agree with Brunetti that informed consent should not be a formalistic "ritual" but an ongoing process that provides health care professionals with "an important opportunity . . . to improve communication with their patients."[33] These are the kind of health care professionals who schedule office visits with patients for the sole purpose of discussing their treatment options; send their patients home to discuss these options with family members and friends; encourage them to consult with other experts or to do their own research on their disease, if they are so inclined; and never let a patient sign a form unless they are confident that the patient really understands the information on it.

VI. CONCLUSION

Like all human relationships, the health care professional–patient relationship is context-dependent and person-specific. Some people rarely see health care professionals, and when they decide to do so have no interest in relating to the health care professional(s) on call. All they want is a "magic bullet" for their ailment so that they can go about their ordinary business. Other people, however, want a personal as well as a professional relationship with their healers. These are the kind of people who "doctor shop" if their finances, work schedule, access to transportation, and family responsibilities permit. They look for health care professionals whose treatment styles mesh with their medical needs. Similarly, health care professionals tend to sort themselves out into specialists or generalists, researchers or clinicians, engineers or priests depending on their human relationship skills and their own personal needs for human intimacy. And this is as it should be, provided that, irrespective of their personal styles, health care professionals always show respect for their patients as persons.

Respectful health care professionals can be trusted to keep their patients' secrets, to speak the truth to their patients, and to make sure patients fully understand and truly want this treatment recommended to them. In addition, respectful health care professionals remind themselves that each and every one of their patients—rich or poor, dirty or clean, beautiful or ugly, literate or illiterate, likable or hateful—is a person with a meaning and a destiny. It is no coincidence that the two codes of professional health care ethics with the longest traditions in the United States both begin with the concept of respect. The American Medical Association begins its Principles of Medical Ethics with the statement, "A physician shall be dedicated to providing competent medical care, with compassion and respect for human dignity and rights"[34] and the American Nurses Association begins its Code of

Ethics for Nurses with the statement, "The nurse, in all professional relationships, practices with compassion and respect for inherent dignity, worth, and considerations of social or economic status, personal attributes, or the nature of health problems."[35] Respect is the absolute bedrock for a good health care professional–patient relationship, whereas intimacy is a matter of feasibility and desirability on the part of both health care professionals and patients.

Discussion Questions

1. When it comes to your own health care, how much in the way of competency and personal care do you want from health care professionals? How much competency are you willing to sacrifice for more in the way of personal care? How much personal care are you willing to sacrifice for more in the way of competency? Describe the kind of health care professional you want to take care of you.

2. List and explain situations where confidentiality must be maintained and where exceptions may be made.

3. Who owns a patient's records? Who should have access to them? Would you be willing to share your medical records? Are you in favor of all medical information—including genetic information—being stored in a computerized information system so that health care professionals have easy access to it when you need treatment? How can society protect you from people who do not need this information to treat you?

4. Should law enforcement officials have immediate access to one's medical records
   a. in all hospitals and doctors offices?
   b. in drug treatment centers?
   c. in government-funded health care arenas?

5. Who decides if a patient is competent? By what criteria is this decision made? How would you go about deciding whether someone is competent?

6. Should health care professionals be required to tell patients if they have had impairment problems in the past? If they are currently being treated for an impairment problem?

Case Studies

1. Janice is a 45-year-old woman with chronic myelogenous leukemia, who has shown interest in having as much information about her condition as is necessary to make decisions concerning future treatment. Her physician tells her that response rates to chemotherapy are good and that recent studies suggests more than 70% of patients have survival rates of 10 years or more. The remaining 30% of patients die within 10 years. What Janice's physician fails to tell her is that preliminary studies indicate that approximately

12% of the long-term survivors get either pancreatic cancer or a coagulation disorder that leads to secondary complications and systemic compromise. In a discussion of Janice's case during a staff meeting, her physician justifies his withholding of information on the grounds that this knowledge might unduly alarm her and cause her to refuse treatment, which in turn will spoil her chance for long-term survival. He also argues that because the research is not conclusive and 12% is a low figure, he is not morally obligated to communicate the risk. After all, her physician says, health care professionals do not have the time to inform every patient about every risk to which they might be subject.

a. Does Janice have a right to the information the physician is withholding?
b. Is the physician's refusal to disclose complete information to Janice justified by his concern over how she will respond to the information? By his supposed lack of time to communicate every conceivable treatment risk to Janice?
c. Does the physician violate his duty to "do no harm" in this case? Why or why not?

2. Lincoln is a 21-year-old college student, who lives at home to control expenses. His parents bring him into Mid-Town Urgent Care with extreme fatigue and lethargy as well as dizziness and giddiness. Laboratory examinations show a 1.79 red blood cell count, hemoglobin of 3.4, and hematocrit of 10.4, all of which indicate severe anemia due to hemorrhaging. The staff physician recommends a transfusion of two units of whole blood, which Lincoln is hesitant to accept on the grounds that he adheres to the beliefs of Jehovah's Witnesses. When the physician and nursing staff explain to him that if he does not accept the transfusion he will die within hours, he seems on the verge of accepting the transfusion after all and asks to consult with his parents. Before a decision is reached, Lincoln loses consciousness. The parents' response is that because acceptance of the transfusion will compromise Lincoln's soul, it should not be administered.

a. Has the medical staff met their obligation or should the physician go ahead and transfuse?
b. If the parents' wishes are followed, is it possible that Lincoln's autonomy may be violated?
c. If the parents refuse the transfusion, are they acting in their son's best interests?
d. If the parents agree to the transfusion, but upon awakening Lincoln expresses disgust and anger at both his parents and the medical staff, what would you as an ethicist discuss with Lincoln? With his parents? With the medical staff?

3. After arriving at an acute-care center, Julie complains of a fever of unknown origin and requests an antibiotic. Her symptoms seem flu-like and the diagnosis is confirmed with a flu antibody test. The staff physician explains that antibiotics are useless against the flu because influenza is a viral

infection and antibiotics only act against bacterial infections. Julie rejects the physician's explanation and insists on an antibiotic in addition to the physician's recommendations of rest and fluids. The physician considers writing the prescription because the antibiotic will do no immediate harm and may improve Julie's psychological state. Yet, the physician is well aware that the overuse of antibiotics makes it more likely that Julie will develop antibiotic resistant bacteria over time.

a. Should Julie's request be honored?

b. Is it appropriate for physicians to offer treatments whose sole purpose is to provide psychological comfort, when that comfort is based on a false belief and misunderstanding?

c. If Julie's physician does not write the prescription, has the physician met her or his moral obligations to her?

d. How might a placebo, which Julie falsely believes is an antibiotic, be used in this situation? Is this an ethical option?

Endnotes

1. Alasdair MacIntyre, *After Virtue* (Notre Dame, IN: University of Notre Dame Press, 1981), pp. 177–178.

2. Ibid., p. 181.

3. Robert M. Veatch, *A Theory of Medical Ethics* (New York: Basic Books, 1981).

4. Ezekiel Emanuel and Linda Emanuel, "Four models of physician–patient relationship," *Journal of American Medical Association*, 267, no. 16 (April 22, 1992): 2221–2226.

5. The case of Melissa is a hypothetical case based on information provided to me by several physicians specializing in eating disorders.

6. Raymond S. Edge and John Randall Groves, *The Ethics of Health Care: a Guide for Clinical Practices*, 2nd ed. (Albany, NY: Delmar Publishers, Inc., 1999), p. 94.

7. Quoted in Arthur Kleinman, *The Illness Narratives: Suffering, Healing and the Human Condition* (New York: Basic Books, Inc., 1988), p. 213.

8. Joanne Lynn, "Travels in the valley of the shadow," in: Howard Spiro, Mary G. McCren Curnen, Enid Peschel, and Deborah St. James (eds.), *Empathy and the Practice of Medicine* (New Haven, CT: Yale University Press, 1993), pp. 43–44.

9. Nancy Shute, "That old-time medicine," *U.S. News & World Report* (April 22, 2002): 56.

10. Ibid., p. 57.

11. Ibid., p. 58.

12. Ibid., p. 60.

13. American Hospital Association, "A patient's Bill of Rights" (Chicago: American Hospital Association, 1975).

14. George Annas, *The Rights of Patients*, 2nd ed. (Carbondale and Edwardsville, IL: Southern Illinois University Press, 1989), p. 263.

15. Hippocrates, "Hippocratic Oath," in: G.E.R. Lloyd (ed.), *Hippocratic Writings* (Harmond Sworth, Middlesex: Penguin, 1978), p. 67.

16. Victor Fuchs, *Who Shall Live?* (New York: Basic Books, 1974), p. 56.

17. Marc D. Hiller, "Computers, medical records, and the right to privacy," *Journal of Health Politics, Policy and Law*, 6, no. 3 (Fall, 1981): 463–487.

18. Raymond S. Edge and John Randall Groves, *The Ethics of Health Care: a Guide for Clinical Practices*, 2nd ed. (Albany, NY: Delmar Publishers, Inc., 1999), p. 76.

19. Mark Siegler, "Confidentiality in medicine—a decrepit concept," *New England Journal of Medicine*, 307 (1982): 1518–1521.

20. Raymond S. Edge and John Randall Groves, *Ethics of Health Care: a Guide for Clinical Practice*, 2nd ed. (Albany, NY: Delmar Publishers, Inc.), p. 70.

21. "Privacy regs complicate communication for care," *Medical Ethics Advisor*, 19, no. 10 (October 2003): 116.

22. Ibid., p. 117.

23. "New privacy rules mean new requirements," *Medical Ethics Advisor*, 17, no. 3 (March 2001): 31–32.

24. Robert M. Veatch et al., "Bioethics," in: *Ethics Applied* , 3rd ed. (Boston: Pearson Education, 2000), p. 209.

25. American Medical Association, "Principles of medical ethics (1847, 1957, 1980, 1990)," in: Wanda Teays and Laura Purdy (eds.), *Bioethics, Justice and Health Care* (Belmont, CA: Wadsworth, 2001), pp. 177–180.

26. Margaret A. Drickamer, and Mark S. Lachs, "Should patients with Alzheimer's Disease be told their diagnosis?" *The New England Journal of Medicine*, 326, no. 14 (April 2, 1992): 947–951.

27. Ruth Macklin, *Against Relativism* (New York: Oxford University Press, 1999), p. 121.

28. Albert R. Jonsen, Mark Siegler, and William J. Winslade, *Clinical Ethics*, 5th ed. (New York: McGraw-Hill, 2002), p. 55.

29. Louis L. Brunetti, "Informed consent," in: Louis L. Brunetti and Lance K. Stell (eds.), *A Physician's Guide to the Legal and Ethical Aspects of Patient Care* (Charlotte, NC: Carolinas Medical Center, 1994), p. 3.54.

30. Ibid., p. 3.47.

31. Ibid.

32. Ibid., p. 3.49.

33. Ibid.

34. American Medical Association House of Delegates, *Principles of Medical Ethics*, Adopted June 17, 2001.

35. American Nurses Association House of Delegates, *Code of Ethics for Nurses*, Adopted 2001.

chapter four

Biological Givens or Social Constructions?

I. INTRODUCTION

Not only are we interested in matters related to health and disease, we seem preoccupied and obsessed by them. Newspapers flood our collective consciousness with the latest medical news, and several health care professionals even have their own radio shows, which almost always feature call-ins from people suffering from one or another disease syndrome or addiction. In addition, popular television programs focus on emergency room crises, sometimes providing us with the opportunity to view actual operations performed in living color. Nothing is left to our imagination, as skilled teams of health care professionals transplant hearts, resection bowels, and amputate limbs right in front of our eyes. No matter where we go or with whom we speak, the conversation gradually drifts towards health-related topics. What ails you? What diet are you on, low-fat or low-carbohydrate? What exercise regimen are you following? What prescription drugs are you taking? Have you had your annual physical examination yet? Are you taking good care of yourself? Seemingly, the concepts of health and disease have nearly replaced those of good and evil, and our value as human beings is increasingly judged in terms of our health status.

II. GOALS OF HEALTH CARE

Our growing desire to first achieve and then maintain an optimal health status probably accounts for our willingness to spend a markedly high percentage of our Gross National Product (GNP) on health care. According to the World Health Organization, the United States spent more than any other nation—1.4 trillion dollars in the year 2000—on maintaining or improving the health status of its citizens.[1] Currently, there are probably more hospitals, nursing homes, pharmacies, spas, and fitness centers in the United States than there are churches, synagogues, and other houses of worship. Yet, despite our fixation on health, we remain unsure about the primary, essential, and/or legitimate goals of health care.

A. The Prolongation of Life

Most of us think that an important purpose of health care is the prolongation of life. We reason that if this were not the case, we would not rush people to emergency rooms, get them on lists for organ transplants, or put them on high-tech life-support systems. Nor would we be striving to increase the length of the average life span. Nevertheless, few people seem to value life for life's sake, viewing as ill-advised, for example, a decision to aggressively treat a minimally conscious octogenarian suffering from a painful, terminal disease.

Yet even if it is not the mission of health care to prolong life no matter what, it still may be the mission of health care to enable people to live high-quality lives as long as possible—say for ninety, one-hundred, or even more years—and to keep people as vigorous as possible as long as possible. In fact, some people believe that health care professionals should fight against aging and death and help their patients achieve something akin to corporeal immortality here on earth. Others vociferously disagree, however. As they see it, the attempt to live forever is a blatant affront to God's natural law which mandates the degeneration, decomposition, and death of every instance of organic life. Certainly, if "death shall be no more" became the official motto of health care professionals, religious authorities would probably raise their voices in protest. Most religions apparently require death, if for no other reason than that death is the condition of entry into a spiritual life, purportedly better than earthly life. Thus, it is at least debatable whether the elimination of death should be viewed as the overriding aim of health care.

B. Alleviation of Pain and Suffering

Another purpose of health care is the alleviation of pain and suffering. But this goal of health care is also limited. To be sure, health care professionals need to become better providers of palliative care. Morphine and other opiates should be made available to patients who would otherwise twist and writhe in pain, hour after hour. But there comes a point when the price of adequate pain relief is consciousness itself. Indeed, the only way to free some patients from pain is to put them into a state of terminal coma or deep sleep until the actual moment of death arrives.[2] But given that patients in terminal comas are, for all practical purposes, already dead, why not just kill them with a lethal injection? Then their death would be official sooner rather than later. Are there really good reasons to think such an action would be less compatible with health care professionals' caring mission than putting patients into terminal comas?

Moreover, even if it were possible for health care professionals to alleviate most patients' pain without putting them into a terminal coma or killing them, an important question would remain; namely, should health care professionals attempt to assuage not only patients' physiological pains but also their psychological and spiritual pains, their sufferings? The answer to this last question would seem to be a resounding "yes." If they are able, health care professionals should spare patients unnecessary suffering by providing them with psychological counseling and, if wanted, spiritual support. With the help of skilled psychiatrists, counselors, and faith leaders (for example, ministers, priests, and rabbis), most suffering patients can cope with the fears, anxieties, stresses, strains, tensions, and frustrations that inevitably accompany the processes of human degeneration, decomposition, disintegration, and dying. But *most* patients are not *all* patients. There are some patients whose sufferings are so great that there is no way to console them. They experience their existence as a living hell. In such circumstances, what is the health care professional's role? If death is the only way to end a patient's emotional suffering or existential angst, is it the duty of the health care professional to help that patient die as quickly as possible? If so, what becomes of religious ideals such as redemptive suffering, or philosophical ideals such as coming to terms with human finitude and courageously struggling on, even when a profound sense of meaninglessness gnaws at the core of one's sense of self? Will health care really be better if, in the name of eradicating all human suffering as well as pain, health care professionals assume near-godly roles?[3]

C. Promotion of Health and Prevention of Disease

Yet another goal of health care is promoting health and preventing disease, and providing patients with significant opportunities to participate responsibly in their own health care. This view of health care's function switches the focus from health care professionals fighting death to health care professionals helping people live life as fully as possible. It also highlights the ways in which preventive medicine is a prophylactic for curative medicine. To the extent that health care professionals help people become and stay healthy, they avoid having to treat, oftentimes very aggressively, patients with diseases that could have been avoided.

Particularly significant about a preventive view of health care is the way in which it intersects with so-called **public health initiatives**. Traditionally, the main objectives of public health programs have been controlling communicable diseases, particularly airborne ones and sexually transmitted ones; maintaining the safety of water and food supplies as well as sanitation systems; providing timely responses to natural disasters such as hurricanes, tornadoes, floods, droughts, and fires; and, most recently, addressing the threat of bioterrorism. In addition, public health officials have focused on health-enhancing educational efforts. Not only do public health officials warn the public about the health risks of certain types of sexual activities, addictive behaviors, and aggressive drives, they also encourage the public to take care of themselves by eating nutritious food, getting enough sleep, and visiting health care professionals on a regular basis.

The value of educating the public about the relationship between lifestyle choices and health status is hard to overemphasize. In a recent study reported by Michael Wines in *The New York Times*, researchers contrasted the health status of people in two cities located within 2 hours of each other: Pitkyarsanta, Russia and Joensu, Finland. They discovered that, despite nearly identical environmental conditions and genetic profiles in Pitkyarsanta and Joensu, the health status of the people in these two cities was very different. Indeed, men in Joensu typically lived 15 years longer than men in Pitkyarsanta did, and women in Joensu typically lived 7 years longer than women in Pitkyarsanta did.[4]

Puzzled by the health-status disparities they uncovered, the researchers hypothesized that lifestyle choices were the cause of the Russians' bad health and the Finns' good health, respectively. The collapse of the old Soviet Union had left Russians jobless, bored, poor, demoralized, and primed to seek comfort in fatty foods, vodka, cigarettes, and other addictive substances.[5] In contrast, the Finns were the picture of health for a variety of reasons over and beyond the booming state of their economy. Concerned about the poor health status of its population a quarter-century ago, the Finnish government had, at that time, undertaken several large scale public health initiatives to improve it. Chief among these initiatives was the North Karelian Project, a sustained effort to help Finns change their lifestyles in order to reduce their high risk for heart disease, in particular. Finnish public health officials produced thousands of posters that depicted the bad effects of butter and cigarettes on the heart and lungs. In addition, they convinced public officials to ban smoking in public and to subsidize farmers who agreed to grow berries on their farmlands rather than to graze dairy cows.[6] Unlike cream and butter, blueberries and raspberries do not clog arteries with cholesterol.

The effects of these simple, low-cost public health initiatives on Finns' health status were sizable. In North Karelian cities such as Joensu, deaths related to heart disease and lung cancer were decreased by nearly 70% in just 25 years, and life expectancy increased by almost 8 years for men and 6 years for women. When Russian public health officials decided to test the Finns' recipe for success in Russia, Finnish public health officials offered to help them. Together, the Russians and Finns organized health fairs; gave lectures on the harmful effects of excessive eating, drinking, and smoking; and sponsored contests, including one that awarded Russians who were able to stop smoking for at least one month an all-expenses-paid trip to Finland!

Regrettably, these joint Finnish–Russian public health initiatives did not have the same success in Pitkyarsanta as they had had in Joensu. Both

Finnish and Russian public health officials attributed the disappointing outcome to Russia's overall national malaise. Perceptively, one Finnish physician observed, "People are not willing to change their life styles when they have to struggle to survive."[7] In other words, when people are without work and other purposeful life-activities, it is very difficult to wean them permanently from creature comforts. Thus, no matter how much effort is made to educate Russians about the pluses of a healthy life style, their overall health status is not likely to improve dramatically unless Russia's social and economic problems are solved. It is hard to want to take good care of oneself if one is without a meaningful future.

Of course, Russia is not the only nation that can, other things being equal, learn valuable lessons from Finnish public health initiatives. Despite excellent economic and social conditions, too many Americans nonetheless drink, smoke, and eat excessively. Public health officials in the United States speculate that Americans fail to take personal responsibility for maintaining their own health status because they are overly reliant on so-called miracle cures. The current attitude among many Americans seems to be "eat, drink, and be merry," for tomorrow the health care gurus will have a pill or a non-invasive treatment to make the consequences of one's indulgences go away. The reality, however, is that an ounce of prevention is still worth at least a pound of cure. Americans will continue to die younger and sicker than they should, so long as they continue to rely too much on curative medicine and not enough on preventive medicine. Obesity is a case in point. Despite the fact that study after study shows that overweight and obese people are more likely to have diabetes, hypertension, and heart disease, restaurants continue to supersize meal portions and Americans continue to snack on high-calorie foods as they sit in front of their computer screens or television sets. They reason that some day researchers will develop a pill that melts away fat, and literally enables them to have their cake and eat it too. For now, if they get too fat, there is always stomach-stapling and jaw-wiring.

III. The Concepts of Health and Disease

Understanding the concepts of health and disease, the dueling dyad that underpins health care, is no easy matter since both these concepts are variably defined. Paradoxically, health is not necessarily the absence of disease, disability, or defect, because many persons with diseases, disabilities, or defects are quite healthy. For example, although persons with the gene for Huntington's disease will eventually manifest the symptoms of this degenerative neurological condition, they will be able to lead healthy lives during the 40 or 50 years that they remain symptom-free. Similarly, people who cannot see or hear, or who have had a limb amputated are often very healthy. In fact, some people who have had limbs amputated are competitive athletes, and most people who are unable to hear or see nonetheless lead active personal and professional lives.

But if health is other than, or more than, the absence of disease, disability, or defect, then precisely what is health and why should we care about its definition? Perhaps the most important reason to care about the definition of health—and disease, defect, or disability—is that the definitions of terms affect us in many ways, some of them highly significant.[8] For example, if we accept the World Health Organization's (WHO) definition of health as "a state of complete physical, mental and social well-being and not merely the absence of disease or infirmity,"[9] then most people probably are somewhat unhealthy. After all, many individuals experience down-in-the-dumps days that fall short of clinical depression but are nonetheless de-energizing and even demoralizing. Should health care professionals provide these "unhappy campers" with ample supplies of Prozac or some other antidepressant? If so, it would seem that the business of health care professionals is to make everyone not simply healthy but also happy, because, if we think about it, it makes just as much sense to define *happiness* as "a state of complete physical, mental, and social well-being" as it does to define *health* with these same words. Either the WHO definition of health is too inclusive, or there is no difference, in our society at least, between happiness and health.

A. Nonnormative View of Disease and Health

Careful reflection on definitions of health—such as the WHO definition of health offered above—has led to two basic interpretations of health and its correlate, disease, namely, the **nonnormative** view and the **normative** view. According to bioethicist Arthur Caplan, the nonnormative view of disease and health claims that because all biological organisms, including human beings, are the product of a purposeful and organized biological evolution, health is best understood as the functioning of a biological organism in conformity with its natural design.[10] Thus, no matter how healthy I think I am or feel I am, I am diseased if my kidneys fail to remove toxic buildups from my blood; if my heart does not pump enough blood to my organs or tissues; if my legs or arms are not able to move; or if I feel compelled to shoplift, gamble, or drink excessively. To be sure, an individual with kidney disease may refuse to view himself as having health problems, working as hard as he worked before beginning a regimen of kidney dialysis. In contrast, another individual with the same degree of renal disease may want to view himself as a very unhealthy man, entitled to much pampering.

Defenders of the nonnormative view of health and disease claim that differences in individuals' reactions to having a disease, as in the example above, rest on a distinction between disease and illness. Whereas disease is purportedly an objective state of affairs, illness is supposedly a subjective state of affairs. For example, epilepsy is a malfunction of the neurological system, whether its victim experiences it as a blessing bestowed by the gods (the traditional Laotian term for epilepsy is "the spirit catches you and then you fall down"), or a life-threatening condition that can cause considerable personal embarrassment or trauma.[11]

A variant of the view that disease is some sort of organic malfunction, says Caplan, is the notion that health is species-typical functioning and that disease is a deviation from species-typical functioning. If most people have a certain blood pressure, cholesterol level, or white blood cell count, then statistically significant departures from the typical condition are probable candidates for the label, "disease."[12] Among health care professionals, physicians seem particularly fond of a statistical view of health, and it is this view of health that may account for much of the weighing, measuring, and testing that occurs in physicians' offices. Despite the common sense appeal of this view, there is at least one problem with it. Just because a person deviates from a mean in a statistically significant way does not necessarily indicate that he or she is diseased. For example, Olympic athletes are not viewed as diseased because they can run faster or jump higher than most people. Similarly, people whose IQs (intelligence quotients) or EQs (emotionality quotients) are extraordinarily high are viewed as anything but diseased. Instead, they are viewed enviously as uncommonly blessed individuals. Finally, people whose overall health status is excellent, but who weigh 20%–25% less or more than what is supposedly ideal for species-typical functioning, are not diseased even if their bodies are aesthetically displeasing—that is, too thin or too fat.

B. Normative View of Disease and Health

Unlike proponents of the nonnormative view of health and disease, proponents of the normative view of health and disease insist that value claims are part of the meaning of health and disease. In other words, no matter how many facts we know about the functioning of a particular organ or system of organs, a deviation upward or downward from species-typical or species-average functioning will count as a disease only if people regard the deviation as a *disvalue*—something to be avoided.[13] For example, consider the debate that has swirled around homosexuality. Is it a sexual preference, a life-style choice, a sin, or a disease to be treated on account of its statistical deviation from the mean of heterosexuality? Originally classified as a disease by the American Psychiatric Association (APA), homosexuality was declassified as a medical problem by that same group in 1980.[14] Was this change in classification due to some new biological facts that had been discovered about homosexuality—for example, that homosexuals are far more numerous than previously thought, or that most individuals are bisexual? Or, instead, was the APA's declassification of homosexuality as a medical problem the result of its growing conviction that society should be equally accepting of individuals, whether they have a same-sex sexual preference or an opposite-sex sexual preference? In the estimation of normativists, the answer to such questions is clear: labeling or not labeling homosexuality a disease is not a factual decision but a value-laden one.

The normative view of health or disease seems quite plausible. Most societies have routinely defined diseases as states of affair that had little to do with lack of species-typical functioning and much to do with behaviors and personalities they found offensive or inappropriate. For example, subsequent to the Civil War in the United States, the birth rate plunged. According to historians Carroll Smith-Rosenberg and Charles Rosenberg, the drop could not have come at a worse time. The Civil War had decimated the American male population, and there was a real need for couples to have as many babies as possible. Speculating that women's growing reluctance to be little more than baby-makers was the result of "imbalances" in women's reproductive systems, physicians conveniently discovered two new female diseases: neurathenia and hysteria. Young women who manifested "neurotic" or "hysterical" symptoms such as irritability, aches and pains, lassitude, and nervousness, and who did not seem to want children, were confined to their bedrooms for a rest cure. The rationale for a "treatment" that included no intellectual or social stimulation was that the body is a closed system, possessing only a limited amount of energy and that "energy expended in one area was necessarily removed from another."[15] Bluntly put, a girl's "brain and ovary could not develop at the same time."[16] A choice had to be made, and, in this case, nineteenth-century U.S. society clearly chose the female ovary over the female brain. Commented the regents of the University of Wisconsin in 1877:

> . . . it is better that the future matrons of the state should be without a University training than that it should be produced at the fearful expense of ruined health; better that the future mothers of the state should be robust, hearty, healthy women, than that, by over study, they entail upon their descendants the germs of disease.[17]

Fortunately, the sexist views expressed in this quote no longer prevail in the United States. Few, if any, physicians and university regents in the United States would dare suggest that women's brains are to take second place to women's ovaries, or that a woman who chooses to divert all her energies to academic studies is diseased. With changes U.S. views about women's nature and function has come the disappearance or redefinition of many nineteenth-century female "diseases."

Another point that bolsters the normative understanding of health and disease is the fact that what counts as a disease varies from culture to culture. In the United States, epilepsy is a recognized, neurological disease that is managed with pharmaceutical drugs. In Laos, at least among the Hmong people, epilepsy (*qaug dab peg*) is not so much regarded a disease as a sign that one is "fit for divine office."[18] Indeed, Hmong epileptics often become shamans. Their condition is a sacred calling they cannot refuse; for if they reject their spiritual destiny, they will die. Among the Hmong, epilepsy must remain, to some degree, unmanageable. It is not a condition human beings should seek to bring under total control.

A final argument that bolsters the view that disease and health are normative is that, within a culture, people often disagree about whether someone is healthy or diseased. For example, many U.S. health care professionals insist that female gymnasts' low body-fat levels, enlarged hearts, weakened bones, spotty or absent menstrual cycles, and stressed muscles indicate a lack of health. In contrast, U.S. sports trainers, managers, and many of the women who suffer from all of the conditions just described insist that female gymnasts are very healthy. They reason that a person who can perform the way female gymnasts do, and exercise as long and hard as they do, has to be healthy. Otherwise they could not keep pushing their bodies the way they do. The question then becomes, who has the story right? Is a 70-pound, 5-foot, 13-year-old female gymnast healthy or diseased? Does there or does there not come a time when certain facts about one's physiology trump any belief one may have about being healthy? Who decides what is too thin for a gymnast—a health care professional, a parent, a coach, or the gymnast herself? Even if health is a combination of facts and values, is it more about facts or is it more about values?

Perhaps some of the answers to the questions raised above may be found in the following excerpt from *Little Girls in Pretty Boxes*, a journalistic account of elite female gymnasts and figure skaters. Joan Ryan notes:

> Our national obsession with weight, our glorification of thinness, have gone completely unchecked in gymnastics and figure skating. The cultural forces that have produced extravagantly bony fashion models have taken their toll on gymnasts and skaters already insecure about their bodies. Not surprisingly, eating disorders are common in both sports, and in gymnastics they're rampant.[19]

Although normativists believe that the definition of a disease usually depends on the individual's and culture's distinct values, they do not deny that there are some states of body and mind that virtually everyone values or, alternatively, disvalues. According to Caplan, values such as "life is preferable to death, ability is preferable to disability, and pleasure is more desirable than pain"[20] are fairly universal. In other words, even if diverse individuals and cultures sometimes disagree about whether a certain physical, mental, and even spiritual condition is desirable, they do not always disagree with each other's assessments. For example, it is very unlikely that anyone anywhere thinks it is better to have AIDS than not to have it. Thus, so long as it is possible to achieve some level of consensus about values as well as facts,

Caplan thinks we should define disease as a "'dysfunction' that is 'disvalued' in terms of both human goals and the design of the human body and the human mind, to the extent to which this can be known."[21]

Adding credence to the view that we all share certain basic assumptions about desirable states of body and mind is the role that ideas such as balance or moderation play in peoples' understanding of health. For example, the fundamental principles in Traditional Chinese Medicine (TCM) are the interdependent concepts of Yin and Yang. The universe is maintained by the interaction between these two interdependent opposites, each providing the other with meaning. Yin is associated with qualities such as cold, stillness, passivity, darkness, and potentiality. Yang is linked to qualities such as heat, movement, light, activity, brightness, and actuality. Illness is an imbalance in Yin and Yang's interaction; health is achieved by those individuals who are able to balance between their Yin and Yang qualities. In Ayurvedic medicine, the traditional medicine of India, great stress is put on determining one's dominant body and spirit type and then prescribing a certain diet, sleep, and exercise program tailored to keep the particular individual's whole self operating in a harmonious way. Finally, in Western biomedicine, behavior disorders and many addictions are increasingly viewed as the product of people's inability to live moderately. In the United States, for example, many people oscillate between a life of excesses on the one hand and a life of deprivations on the other. It is either feast—too much emotion and sensual gratification—or famine—too little emotion and sensual gratification.

IV. THE CONCEPTS OF WELLNESS AND ILLNESS

Closely related to the concepts of health and disease are the concepts of **illness** and **wellness**. Although there is usually a correlation between being healthy and feeling well on the one hand and being diseased and feeling ill on the other, there are exceptions to this general rule, particularly with respect to the disease–illness correlation. Significantly, most health care professionals are less interested in *defining* disease and health than in making people *feel* less ill and more well.

One exception to the disease-and-illness-go-together rule is the hypochondriac. The hypochondriac may feel ill even though there is no objective evidence that he or she suffers from a disease. According to Dr. Arthur Kleinmann:

> Hypochondriasis creates a reversal of the archetypal medical relationship in which the patient complains of illness and the physician diagnoses disease. Rather, in hypochondriasis the patient complains of disease ("I fear that I have cancer of the throat"; "I'm convinced I'm dying of heart disease"; "I know,

I just know I've got an autoimmune disease"), and the doctor can confirm only illness.[22]

Although health care professionals are fairly good judges about which of their patients are hypochondriacs, they are not infallible judges. Because diagnosis is as much an art as a science, and because even the best tests yield false positives and negatives, thoughtful health care professionals are generally hesitant to pigeonhole a patient as a definite hypochondriac. Comments Dr. Kleinmann: "the hypochondriac's doubt has an exact complement in that of the practitioner, who knows at heart that, in spite of trying to convince the hypochondriac to the contrary, he can never be completely certain himself that the patient doesn't have a disease."[23]

Another exception to the disease–illness rule is the patient who feels fine only to discover that he or she is suffering from a disease, indeed a fatal disease. For example, a friend of mine, who looked like one of the male models in a fitness magazine, went for his annual physical. His blood tests revealed a rare, almost always fatal, blood cancer. My friend was dead within 6 months of this finding. One day he was pumping iron in the weight room; the next thing we knew, he was on his death bed. Similarly, one Wednesday morning, my 29-year-old son was enjoying his life. He phoned me from his office that he was on the verge of closing his first big business deal and that he was on the way out of his office for lunch with a new friend. Two hours later a hospital official phoned me. My son, whose health status I never questioned, had had a heart attack and was undergoing emergency surgery. One year later, I still find it difficult to believe that my "healthy" son actually is very diseased.

Fortunately, most diseased people feel ill and most people who feel ill are diseased. Were this not the case, health care professionals would have even a harder time diagnosing and treating patients than they do now. Health care professionals use patients' reports of illness to confirm or, in some instances test, results. To be sure, determining the cause(s) of a patient's illness is no easy task, particularly when the patient's report of illness is sketchy, hard to understand, and full of exaggerations or minimizations or when the health care professional has little time for conversation and/or few interpretive skills. Unless the health care professional and patient both engage actively in diagnosing the patient's disease, however, diagnostic mistakes will be made and the treatments prescribed will not be as good or particularized as they should be.

A. The Illness Experience

Although it is challenging for health care professionals to change their diagnoses, prognoses, and treatment recommendations as a patient's disease evolves, it is vital that they do so. Precisely because medicine is an art as well as a science, health care professionals have to develop their interpretive skills as well as analytic skills. In other words, health care professionals have to take the time to listen to patients' stories of sickness. It is not enough for them to look at patients' test results.

In order to help us better understand the patient's illness experience, Kleinmann asks us to imagine three patients: (1) an adolescent quadriplegic; (2) a business executive who hides his asthma from his professional colleagues but not his family; and (3) a young woman recovering from a disfiguring mastectomy. The adolescent quadriplegic experiences his illness as a trap from which he cannot escape and which requires constant monitoring and treatment; the asthmatic business executive views his illness as a condition that forces him to lead two lives: a professional life, in which he musters all his energies to project strength and health, and a personal life, in which he lets go and exposes himself as vulnerable and out of control; and the recovering cancer patient experiences her situation as a bodily mutilation made worse by the threat of her disease recurring and further ravaging her body. As Kleinmann sees it, health care professionals cannot truly help any of these individuals unless they first ask themselves, "What does my patient's disease *mean* to him or her? How does it *feel* to him or her?"[24]

Kleinmann claims that illness has at least five meanings. First, illness has a **biological meaning**. It is, after all, rooted in disease, experienced in the form of symptoms, and reported to others in a variety of ways. Whereas some people have a rich sickness vocabulary and are able to describe their aches and pains at length, other people cannot find the words to express what they are feeling, where, or how. For example, I grew up in a working-class household. From childhood on, it was made clear to me that I did not have time to get sick and that unless I came down with the bubonic plague or worse, I was not really sick. Rather, I was just complaining unnecessarily. My parents called such complaining "belly-aching." I am not sure why. As a result of this hardline approach to illness, I learned how to tolerate and ignore a great deal of discomfort and even pain. Moreover, to this day, I am unable to answer questions such as "Where does it hurt?" and "What kind of pain is it?" In contrast, my husband grew up in a household where family members were encouraged to describe every conceivable ache and pain, no matter how small, in detail. As a result of his experiences, my husband can distinguish between all sorts of pains. Moreover, he is enormously interested in his bodily functions, continually commenting on how this or that part of his body feels and whether his feelings warrant a day in bed, or not.

Over and beyond its biological meaning, says Kleinmann, illness has a **cultural meaning**. It is not an accident that certain diseases and symptoms dominate a society's consciousness, while others are ignored. For example, breast cancer, heart disease, prostate cancer, eating disorders, attention deficit disorder, and chronic fatigue syndrome are some of the diseases most often discussed in the United States. Interestingly, each of these diseases is somehow related either to a preoccupation with physical beauty and sexual performance, or to an inability to withstand the stresses and strains of contemporary American life. In addition, some of these diseases seem connected to America's wealth (anorexia, bulimia, and obesity are rare in famine-ridden societies), while others seem linked to America's "twenty-four–seven" lifestyle.

A third illness meaning is **personal**, according to Kleinmann. For example, a flare-up of diabetes may act, he says, like a sponge, "soak[ing] up personal and social significance from the world of the sick person."[25] The sores that will not heal on a diabetic man's legs may signal impeding amputation and dependency on a family that is already angry at dad for not taking better care of himself. Hooked up to a bag of IV antibiotics, the diabetic man becomes focused on whether the sore on his leg is getting better, staying the same, or getting worse. He knows that unless the antibiotic treatment works, his life may never be the same again. Thoughts of the beginning of the end begin to interrupt the diabetic man's sleep as he wonders what life in a wheelchair may be like.

A fourth illness meaning, says Kleinmann, is **social**; that is, the effect a patient's illness has on family, friends, and coworkers, as they collectively and individually deal with the management of his or her illness. For example, when my ailing, 86-year-old mother-in-law came to live in an apartment close to where my husband and I live, I did not anticipate just how much our lives would change. For over a 2-year period, we focused on my mother-in-law's household needs, meals, medications, adjustment problems, depressions, hip replacements, and lapses of memory. Most difficult for my husband was the eventual need to find a nursing home for his mother. It broke my husband's heart (and mine too) to watch a fiercely independent women submit to a daily schedule shaped not by her desires but by others' convenience. When she died, our emotions were profoundly mixed. On the one hand, we wanted her back; but on the other, we were happy for her. No longer would she suffer, and at last she would be free.

The final and fifth meaning of illness is **moral**. Illness teaches us lessons about life's ultimate meanings. Kleinmann comments, "Change, caprice, and chaos, experienced in the body, challenge what order we are led to believe—need to believe—exists. Disability and death force us to reconsider lives and our world."[26] Such reflections, disturbing as they are, may be illness's primary gift to us. They offer us the opportunity to set our lives in order, to come to terms with the meaning of our destiny, and to make ourselves whole. In short, entering into the process of our death may be our best chance to heal ourselves from what really ails us.

B. The Wellness Experience

Of course, people do not always feel ill. Oftentimes they feel well, particularly if they are not suffering from any acute or chronic disease, their bodies and minds are operating at peak levels, and their relationships at home and at work are strong and supportive. Although he chooses to label as "health" what I mean by **wellness**, I nonetheless think Leon Kass, M.D.'s definition of health is helpful here:

> ... Health is a natural standard or norm—not a moral norm, not a 'value' as opposed to a 'fact' not an obligation—a state of being that reveals itself in activity as a standard of bodily excellence or fitness, relative to each species and to some extent to individuals, recognizable if not definable, and to some extent attainable.[27]

Confessing that he cannot describe in sufficient detail a healthy (well) human being, Kass instead offers us a full description of a healthy (well) *squirrel!* He claims:

> ... [The ideally functioning squirrel] is a bushy-tailed fellow who looks and acts like a squirrel; who leaps through the trees with great daring; who gathers, buries, covers but later uncovers and recovers his acorns; who perches out on a limb cracking his nuts, sniffing the air for smells of danger, alert, cautious, with his tail beating rhythmically, who chatters and plays and courts and mates, and rears his [sic] young in large improbable-looking homes at the tops of trees; who fights with vigor and forages with cunning; who shows spiritedness, even anger, and more prudence than many human beings.[28]

To be sure, squirrels (even squirrels like this one) are not human beings. Still Kass's description of a healthy squirrel, with the obvious transpositions into human terms, is not that different from a description of a healthy human being in the prime of life.

V. Conclusion

No discussion of health and disease, or wellness and illness, would be complete without a detailed discussion of the difference between curing and healing, first alluded to in Chapter 3. Whereas curing has to do with eliminating the symptoms of a disease, healing has to do with understanding and, ultimately, accepting one's discomfort, distress, and diminishment as an opportunity for self-transformation. Unlike curing, which focuses on the disease itself, healing stresses the cause of the disease and how one's mind and spirit can help one's body deal with disease. Curing targets a disease as the enemy and encourages the patient to follow health care professionals' orders. In contrast, healing focuses on the restoration of balance and harmony within the patient and prompts the patient to assume some responsibility for getting better. Finally, curing is an interruption in living one's life. The patient has to stop everything and focus on getting well. Life is put on hold. In contrast, healing is the process of balancing the forces inside oneself against the forces outside. "It is," according to Dr. Andrew Weil, "a state of resilience that allows one [sic] to move through the world and not get thrown off balance."[29]

Dr. Sherwin Nuland eloquently articulates a further difference between healing and curing. In moving detail, he tells the story of his close friend, Bob, who decided to prepare for death rather than prolonging his poor-quality life with yet another experimental cancer treatment. In particular, Nuland recalls the last Christmas party his friend hosted:

> Bob made it all work that evening. He had Carolyn [his wife] turn the rheostats down so that his guests would not see the full depth of his jaundice in the dimmed light. At dinner, he sat at the head of the happy, noisy table and pretended to eat, although he was long past being able to take sufficient food to get proper nourishment. Every two hours during the course of the long evening, he agonizingly dragged himself into the kitchen so that Carolyn might give him a shot of morphine to control his pain. When all the guests had said their goodbyes—so many friends of long years and decades never to be seen again—Bob was back in bed, Carolyn asked him how the evening had been. To this day, she remembers his exact words: 'Perhaps one of the best Christmases I ever had.'[30]

Later when Nuland visited his friend's grave, he realized just how well a very diseased person can be. Before he died, his friend Bob had arranged to have the following epitaph engraved on his footstone: "And it was always said of him that he knew how to keep Christmas well." Although there was no way to cure Bob's cancer, Bob used his cancer as the opportunity to heal himself—to transform himself into the kind of person who can "*keep Christmas well*" no matter what.

Interestingly, Eastern traditions of medicine have put more emphasis on the role of the environment, the holistic nature of care, and the concepts of health and wellness than Western traditions, which have focused on the role of science, the curative nature of medicine, and the concepts of disease and illness. In this connection, Raymond S. Edge and John Randall Groves have observed that the great practitioners of traditional Chinese medicine strove to keep their patients well rather than waiting for them to be laid low with disease. Similarly, the best practitioners of Ayurvedic medicine, the traditional medicine of India, used the "natural strength" of patients to maintain and promote their well being, including their emotional and spiritual well being.[31] Wellness is much more than the possession of a sound body and mind, in many Eastern medical traditions. Rather, having proper self-respect and self-esteem, meaningful work, right relationships with people, and realistic ideals about one's vulnerabilities and ultimate demise are the necessary conditions for human wellness.

Discussion Questions

1. What are the three major purposes of health care? Provide examples.
2. Compare and contrast *pain* and *suffering*. Describe a pain experience you have had. Describe a suffering experience you have had. Was it easier or harder for you to control your pain than your suffering? Should a physician provide deadly narcotics to a terminal cancer patient whose pain cannot be controlled? Should a physician provide deadly narcotics to a clinically depressed patient who has been depressed for five or more years and whose mental sufferings are tremendous?
3. Define health. Define disease. Would an 80-year-old person define these terms differently than a 40-year-old person or a 20-year-old person? Would someone from India or Germany define health and disease the same way as someone from the United States?
4. Compare and contrast curative medicine and preventive medicine. Which form of medicine do you think is most important? Which form of medicine do you rely upon the most?
5. Are eating disorders culturally constructed or natural diseases? Is menopause a disease? Why or why not? Is aging a disease? Why or why not?
6. Define illness and contrast it with disease. Describe someone you know who has been ill. When they were ill how did your relationship with them change?
7. Compare and contrast the normative interpretation of health and the nonnormative interpretation of health. Provide examples to illustrate the relevant similarities and dissimilarities.
8. Is health becoming the supreme value in the United States? Are Americans too obsessed about their health? Why or why not? How many pleasures are you willing to deprive yourself of in order to be healthy?
9. Define and give examples of public health initiatives. Discuss the expanding role of public health initiatives and your reactions to them.
10. Should a person be operated on only when they have a "'dysfunction' that is 'disvalued' in terms of both human goals and the design of the human body and human mind?" How might this prevent elective surgeries and procedures? How might this affect the cost of health care and the cost of insurance? What might a distinction between function and value tell us about the need for, perhaps, a nose job that is carried out not because of a need but a desire to look a certain way?
11. Describe the characteristics of a health care professional who interprets and diagnoses their patients' diseases correctly.

Case Studies

1. Judy is a 74-year-old woman who lives alone, but receives assistance from some friendly neighbors. Her physician admits her to a hospital in order to treat her severe anemia resulting from gastric ulceration. Upon release from the hospital, Judy experiences bouts of confusion and memory loss. Her children, who live at a distance from her, want her to move into an

assisted living center where her needs can be better met. When not in a confused state, Judy repeatedly expresses her awareness of the risks she faces. Nonetheless, she expresses a desire to remain at home, claiming that she will suffer less at home.

a. Discuss the options in this case from the perspective of alleviating pain and suffering.

b. Is Judy's confusion and memory loss an illness? If so, discuss the levels of "meaning" Judy's illness has for herself and others.

c. Discuss this case in terms of wellness. What options do Judy and her family have? Can Judy ever be well again? What would count as well for a person in Judy's situation?

2. Dr. Berkeley, a primary care physician, works for a managed care organization that requires prior approval for diagnostic services and treatment. In many cases, medically indicated care has been denied to one of his patients because the individual did not meet the statistical profile the managed care company uses to establish criteria for health/disease/illness. Dr. Berkeley is outraged, but realizes that he will lose significant income if he breaks his contract with the managed care organization, or if they disenrol him from their list of physicians.

a. Discuss the pros and cons of using nonnormative standards of health and disease in this case. Do the same with respect to using normative standards.

b. Is it unethical for the physician to compromise patient care in order to stay enrolled in the managed care organization?

3. One morning, Ra Mi Tatasuwa waded with her two infant children into the ocean with one purpose only: to kill herself and them. Ra Mi could no longer tolerate life. Lifeguards spotted her and realized what she was planning. But they were unable to rescue either infant, both of whom drowned. However, Ra Mi survived, angry that she had been rescued: "If they understood my humiliation and suffering, then they would have let me die, typical Americans!!!"

Born and raised in Japan to be a dutiful wife and mother, Ra Mi had learned 3 days before her suicide attempt that her husband had a mistress for several years. To Ra Mi's way of thinking, she had failed as a wife and mother. Tormented by her sense of being worthless, she felt that only death could erase the disappointment she, and presumably also her children, had been to her husband, their father. For her, continuing life would be shameful. By committing suicide, she would do the honorable thing, according to Japanese tradition.

a. Is it ever right to commit suicide because one feels like a total failure? Was Ra Mi justified to take her children with her as she walked into death? Were they failures too?

b. Is the loss of one's meaning in life a disease? Is it an illness?

c. If Ra Mi was a woman from the United States, would it be "honorable" for her to commit suicide under the same circumstances? Whose view of suicide is actually right? The traditional Japanese view? The contemporary U.S. view? Some other "universal" view?

4. Odell Russ was diagnosed with both basal and squamous cell cancer when he was 43 years old. Now at 72, the cancer has reached a state where the left side of his neck will need to be removed and a skin flap from his back will need to be grafted in place on his neck. Without the surgery, physicians estimate that he will live only a few weeks and die a painful death. With the surgery, he can expect to live out his life with a few lifestyle modifications (no smoking and no alcohol). Odell rejects the idea because he does not wish to be disfigured and he does not want to change his lifestyle in any way whatsoever. His wife and daughter beg him to reconsider for their sake. The physicians involved are eager for a decision.

a. Discuss this case in terms of what Arthur Kleinmann calls an "illness experience."

b. How might Leon Kass's discussion of wellness assist Odell, his wife, and his daughter to reach a decision about what to do?

c. Is Odell making an irrational decision? Is it an immoral decision?

Endnotes

1. *World Health Report 2000* (Geneva, Switzerland: WHO Library, 2000), p. 200.
2. John D. Loeser, "Pain: an overview," *Lancet* (May 8, 1999): 1607–1609.
3. Howard Brody, *Stories of Sickness* (New Haven: Yale University Press, 1987), pp. 29–36.
4. Michael Wines, "Ailing Russia lives a tough life that's getting shorter," *New York Times* (December 3, 2000): 1, 19.
5. Ibid., p. 19.
6. Ibid.
7. Ibid.
8. Carolyn Crane Cutilli, "Health literacy: what you need to know," *Orthopaedic Nursing*, 24, no. 3 (May/June 2005): 227.
9. Preamble to the Constitution of the World Health Organization. Adopted by the International Health Conference held in New York from 19 June to 22 July 1946, and signed on 22 July 1946 by the representatives of sixty-one States; *Official Records of World Health Organization*, no. 2, p. 100.
10. Arthur L. Caplan, "The concepts of health, illness, and disease," in: Robert M. Veatch (ed.), *Medical Ethics* (Sudbury, MA: Jones and Bartlett Publishers, 1977), p. 66.

11. Anne Fadiman, *The Spirit Catches You and You Fall Down* (New York: Farrar, Straus and Giroux, 1997), p. 21.

12. Arthur L. Caplan, "The concepts of health, illness, and disease," in: Robert M. Veatch (ed.), *Medical Ethics* (Sudbury, MA: Jones and Bartlett Publishers, 1977), p. 67.

13. Ibid.

14. American Psychological Association, *Diagnostic and Statistic Manual of Mental Disorders III* (Washington, D.C.: APA, 1980).

15. Carroll Smith-Rosenberg and Charles Rosenberg, "The female animal: medical and biological views of woman and her role in nineteenth-century America," in: Arthur L. Caplan, H. Tristram Engelhardt, Jr., and James J. McCartney (eds.), *Concepts of Health and Disease* (Reading, MA: Addison-Wesley Publishing Co., 1981), p. 288.

16. Ibid.

17. Board of Regents, University of Wisconsin, *Annual Report for the Year Ending, September 30, 1877* (Madison, 1877), p. 45.

18. Anne Fadiman, *The Spirit Catches You and You Fall Down* (New York: Farrar, Straus and Giroux, 1997), p. 21.

19. Joan Ryan, *Little Girls in Pretty Boxes* (New York: Time Warner, 1995), p. 9.

20. Arthur L. Caplan, "The concepts of health, illness, and disease," in: Robert M. Veatch (ed.), *Medical Ethics* (Sudbury, MA: Jones and Bartlett Publishers, 1977), p. 71.

21. Ibid.

22. Arthur Kleinmann, *The Illness Narratives: Suffering, Healing and the Human Condition* (New York: Basic Books Inc., 1988), p. 195.

23. Ibid., pp. 196–197.

24. Ibid., p. 8.

25. Ibid., p. 31.

26. Ibid., p. 55.

27. Leon R. Kass, *Toward a More Natural Science: Biology and Human Affairs* (New York: Macmillan, 1985), p. 173.

28. Ibid.

29. Jeanette Leardi, "Integrative medicine expert Dr. Andrew Weil is bringing to Charlotte his message of holistic healing," *Charlotte Observer* (November 10, 2003): 1E.

30. Sherwin Nuland, *How We Die* (New York: A. A. Knopp, 1994).

31. Raymond S. Edge and John Randall Groves, *Ethics of Health Care* (New York: Delmar Publishers, 1999), pp. 239–249.

chapter five

Biomedical and Behavioral Research

I. INTRODUCTION

Biomedical and behavioral research has increased exponentially over the last few decades. So too has our concern about the ethical conduct of research studies on human subjects. On the one hand, scientific research has led to the development of surgical techniques, pharmaceutical products, and preventive strategies that have substantially ameliorated, managed, prevented, or even eliminated some of the diseases and disabilities human beings most dread. On the other hand, scientific research has harmed as well as benefited human beings. Most of us are familiar with both World War II Nazi "medical" experiments on Jews, Gypsies, and Slavic peoples in particular,[1] and the World War II Japanese "medical" experiments on Chinese prisoners of war in Manchuria.[2] Thousands of imprisoned human beings were harmed and in some instances killed by scientists, researchers, and physicians who flagrantly violated the Hippocratic injunction, "Do no harm." In addition, most of us have heard about the infamous Tuskegee Syphilis Study. Carried out by the U.S. Public Health Service, this 40-year-long "study in nature" (1932–1972) recorded the course of untreated syphilis among 412 African-American men. They were kept ignorant of the true purpose of the study. Worse, the men were not treated for their disease when effective treatment (penicillin) became available, lest their access to treatment interfere with the study's results.[3]

Regrettably, the Tuskegee Syphilis Study is not the only sad chapter in the annals of U.S. medical history. Other sad chapters include the Willowbrook Hepatitis Experiment on mentally retarded children in a New York State school;[4] the Brooklyn Jewish Chronic Disease Hospital Case, in which elderly patients in poor health were injected with cancer cells, apparently without their informed consent;[5] the U.S. Cold War Radiation Experiments on some very vulnerable populations including pregnant women, prison inmates, mentally retarded children, and terminally ill cancer patients;[6] animal-to-human organ transplants (xenotransplants);[7] and other questionable transplant procedures using mechanical devices such as Barney Clark's artificial heart hooked permanently to an energy supply the size of a large refrigerator.[8]

II. Differences between Biomedical and Behavioral Research

According to Robert J. Levine, **biomedical research** aims to alleviate pain and suffering and/or to promote health and prevent disease.[9] Typically, biomedical researchers seek treatment and ideally cures for diseases such as cancer, diabetes, and osteoporosis.[10] However, they also seek remedies for biologically based mental abnormalities and addictions such as bipolar disease and alcoholism, respectively.[11]

In contrast to biomedical research, **behavioral research** is not focused on the physical or organic underpinnings of human disease, but rather on the psychological and sociological ramifications of human disease. In the main, behavioral researchers are more interested in understanding *how* alcoholics behave than in determining whether the causes of alcoholism are primarily genetic or mainly environmental. In addition, behavioral researchers are interested in how individuals' race, class, gender, age, religion, and sexual orientation affect their decisions, attitudes, and actions. Among the topics they most frequently address are human sexuality, aggression, and learning.

III. Brief History of Biomedical and Behavioral Research Regulation

Because biomedical and behavioral research can harm research subjects, systems have been established to regulate research on people. The major impetus for research regulations in the United States and throughout the world has its roots in the post–World War II Nuremberg trials of Nazi physicians who, as noted above, conducted experiments on non-consenting concentration camp prisoners, most of them Jewish. In 1947, an international tribune found 15 of these physicians guilty of "war crimes and crimes against humanity."[12] The type of "medical research" these physicians performed on human beings was, for the most part, nothing other than torture. Some of their "experiments" consisted in injecting people with various poisons and bacteria and then watching them die; others consisted of subjecting people to very high or very low atmospheric pressures and temperatures to see how long they could survive. None of the people who served as subjects for these experiments freely volunteered their bodies for such abuse. They were coerced to do so, with their only other option being immediate death in a gas chamber.

Shocked and deeply troubled by what had happened in Nazi Germany under the label of scientific research, the world community joined together in 1949 to sign a code for proper research ethics known as the **Nuremberg Code**. The lynchpin of this code was its provision that unless an individual voluntarily consents to participate in a medical experiment, he or she may not be used as a research subject. In addition to setting forth the essential requirements for voluntary consent, namely (1) the capacity to consent, (2) freedom from coercion, and (3) comprehension of the risks and benefits of the research, the Nuremberg Code articulated several other provisions for ethical research on human subjects. Researchers had to show that their experiments offered a favorable risk–benefit ratio to subjects, were appropriately designed, and permitted subjects to withdraw at any time.[13] Perhaps the most stringent requirement of the Nuremberg Code, as originally formulated, was its rule that prisoners, children, and patients in mental institutions should not be used as research subjects.

As biomedical and behavioral research began to burgeon, the research community realized that the Nuremberg Code needed to be supplemented. In 1964 the World Medical Association set forth additional recommendations to guide health care professionals involved in biomedical research on human subjects. Usually referred to as the **Helsinki Declaration**, this document, which has been amended several times, emphasizes that the interests of the research subject should always be given greater weight than those of society, and that every research subject in a study should get, not a placebo, but either the best current method of treatment or the experimental method of treatment.[14]

In addition to adopting the Nuremberg Code and the Declaration of Helsinki, both of which are international in scope, many nations have articulated their own ethical codes for research. For example, in 1974, the U.S. Congress passed the National Research Act. This act established a National Commission for the Protection of Human Subjects of Biomedical and Behavioral Research that met between 1974 and 1978. The outcome of these meetings was the **Belmont Report**, a document that identified three basic ethical principles for human subjects research: (1) respect for persons, (2) beneficence, and (3) justice.[15] This report also clarified the distinction between "practice" and "research." The term "practice," said the commissioners, "refers to interventions that are designed solely to enhance the well-being of an individual patient or client and that have a reasonable expectation of success."[16] In contrast, the term "research" "designates an activity designed to test a hypothesis, permit conclusions to be drawn, and thereby to develop or contribute to generalized knowledge (expressed, for example, in theories, principles, and statements of relationships)."[17] Whereas practice is intrinsically therapeutic, research is most often nontherapeutic. Confusion of goals sometimes sets in when an individual is both a patient and a research subject, or both a clinician and a researcher.

In addition to establishing the National Commission, the National Research Act of 1974 established the rudiments of a system of **Institutional Review Boards (IRBs)** to regulate federally funded research involving human subjects. An IRB is typically composed of an interdisciplinary group of social and natural scientists, one or more nonscientific members (preferably with ethics expertise), and at least one local community member who is not affiliated with the institution in which the IRB is housed. The task of an IRB is to review its institution's research protocols. Studies that are maximally risky and minimally beneficial to subjects and/or society are typically rejected, together with studies that violate subjects' autonomy and privacy.[18]

Institutional review boards are meant to safeguard research subjects' best interests without unnecessarily impeding the flow of scientific research. Sometimes IRBs get too vigilant. They require so much protection for subjects, that they unnecessarily restrict researchers' studies. At other times, however, IRBs get too slack. Overwhelmed by a large volume of lengthy protocols they cannot carefully process, and/or are biased in favor of researchers' interests, they support risky studies. For example, an IRB-approved study at the University of Pennsylvania recently resulted in the death of an 18-year-old subject in a Phase One safety trial for gene therapy. The dead teen's family filed a wrongful death claim, but their grievance was ultimately settled out of court for a substantial amount of money. The family alleged that, among other things, the researchers involved in the study failed to disclose their considerable financial links to the company whose product was being tested.[19]

IV. ETHICAL ISSUES IN BIOMEDICAL BEHAVIORAL RESEARCH

A. Biomedical Research Study Design

In order to correctly identify the ethical issues inherent in biomedical research, we must first understand the design of a standard, four-phase biomedical research study on an **investigational new drug (IND)**, for example. In phase one of the study, researchers determine how safe the IND is. If the IND proves to be safe, researchers begin phase two of the study. In phase two, researchers give the IND to a relatively small number of patients with the targeted disease to determine whether the IND is effective. In phase three of the study, researchers conduct a **randomized clinical trial (RCT)** of the IND on a large number of patients who have the targeted disease. The purpose of the RCT is to conclusively establish that the IND is at least as good as and, hopefully, better than one of the **established effective** drugs for the targeted disease. Finally, in phase four of the study, marketing companies typically take responsibility to monitor whether the IND has any unanticipated, deleterious side effects.[20]

Of the four phases of a standard biomedical research study, phase three—the RCT—has attracted the most ethical controversy. In an RCT, researchers typically divide subjects into two groups: one receives the IND and the other receives an established effective drug, that is, a drug that the medical profession regards as the best or one of the equally best available treatments for the targeted disease. If there is no established effective drug for the disease, one group of subjects receives the IND and the other receives a **placebo**, that is, a substance which is typically identical in appearance to the IND and may even have side effects similar to it, but is not expected to have any pharmacological effect on the condition being treated. Sometimes researchers design a study that involves three groups: the first receives the IND; the second, an established effective drug; and the third a placebo.

Importantly, most RCTs are **double-blind**. Neither the researchers nor the subjects know which drug, if any, the subject is receiving. When subjects plead to be placed in the IND group, researchers tell them that, at this stage of the research study, they do not know whether the IND, the established drug(s), or the placebo is the best treatment for the targeted disease. In other words, the researchers claim to be in a state of **equipoise** between the IND and alternatives to it. Therefore, subjects should not feel cheated or short-changed if they are assigned to the established effective treatment group or the placebo group instead of the IND group. If, however, it is possible for a subject to secure the IND without participating in the research study, researchers should let the subject know such an option exists. On occasion, physicians provide patients with an IND, permitting them to use the drug "off-label"—that is, for the purpose of treating diseases or conditions not mentioned on the label.[21]

One of the most difficult ethical decisions to make about a research study is the decision to stop it before it has been completed. Suppose that three-quarters of the way through a study it seems that the IND is far superior to the established effective drug and/or the placebo. Should the study be stopped immediately and all subjects be given the IND? Although health care ethicists may think the answer to this question is obvious, further reflection suggests that it is not. If the experiment is not carried through to its planned end, the researchers may not know for sure that the IND is indeed the drug of choice. In the novel *Arrowsmith*, Dr. Martin Arrowsmith, the protagonist, halts a research study intended to determine the efficacy of an experimental vaccine for a virulent plague. When it becomes clear to him that the vaccine is a lifesaver, he decides to inoculate everyone enrolled in the research study with the vaccine. Hailed a hero by the people whom he saves from death, Dr. Arrowsmith is nonetheless condemned by the scientific establishment as a renegade who has ruined an important research study. Another experiment will be required before "Science" can ascertain that the vaccine, rather than some other cause, actually cured the infected people.[22]

Fortunately, researchers in the present world of scientific studies are usually spared Dr. Arrowsmith's fate. Currently, there is wide consensus that a study should be terminated if (1) there is statistically significant, largely agreed upon evidence that the IND is the treatment of choice and (2) the research subjects in the control group(s) have a life-threatening condition or a condition that is very painful or debilitating. Although "Science" may feel cheated, researchers' primary duty is not toward "Science" but toward the human subjects in their studies.

B. Benefits versus Risks of Biomedical Research

Most biomedical research studies are not therapeutic. They do not directly benefit the individuals who enroll in them. Yet a high percentage of research subjects believe, almost as a matter of faith, that somehow or other their health will be better after the study than before. Therefore, researchers should make efforts to dash research subjects' unwarranted hopes. Comments Alexander Capron:

> A patient's emotional ties to the physician, his or her need for treatment (especially when conventional methods have proven effective), and the human tendency to overrate the benefits and underestimate the risks of a research technique, justify setting higher requirements for consent and imposing additional safeguards when therapy is combined with experimentation, lest investigators even unwittingly expose consenting patients to unreasonable risks.[23] Better to scare an individual out of participating in a study than to enroll him or her in it with false hopes.

V. ETHICAL ISSUES IN BEHAVIORAL RESEARCH

A. Behavioral Research Design

As in biomedical research, design plays an important role in determining the ethical parameters as well as scientific credibility of behavioral research. According to Herbert C. Kelman, most behavioral research falls into one of three categories.[24] Kelman's first category is **experimental manipulation** in a laboratory setting. Behavioral researchers create a set of psychological conditions in a controlled environment and observe their effects on subjects' attitudes, decisions, and/or actions. For example, in one study, Stanley Milgram wished to determine whether certain kinds of psychological pressure cause people to obey authority figures blindly. He got subjects to deliver what they thought were painful electric shocks to individuals whom they assumed were also genuinely participating in the study. However, the recipients of the bogus shocks were not really study participants but individuals hired by Milgram to feign signs of pain.[25] In a variant of this type of experimental manipulation, behavioral researchers ask subjects to play roles, as if they were actors in a theater production. Regrettably, such role-playing occasionally runs afoul, as it did when researchers asked subjects to play the roles of prison guards and inmates, respectively. The subjects played their roles too well, and began to actually exhibit the kind of aggressive, violent, and cruel behavior that occurs in real prisons. The researchers had to abruptly terminate the study because the subjects got entirely out of hand.[26]

Kelman's second category of behavioral research is **questioning respondents**. Researchers ask subjects about their values, habits, beliefs, dreams, aspirations, experiences, and so on. They use polls, market research, personal interviews, questionnaires, and tests (aptitude, achievement, and personality) to ensure the scientific reliability of the answers they receive to their questions. Such research is not without its own ethical problems, however. For example, in one study, a survey was administered to high school students to assess their knowledge about HIV-AIDS prevention. The students were asked whether they were sexually active, what types of sexual experience they had had (oral, vaginal, or anal intercourse), and the sex(es) of their partners. As a result of the students' participation in the survey, some parents discovered that their children routinely engaged in sexual activity, including homosexual activity in some cases. In addition, some students discovered they were at personal and considerable risk for developing HIV-AIDS. Depending on how parents and students responded to the information they received, some students who participated in the study were substantially harmed.[27]

Observation of targeted populations, such as members of a specific profession, sub-culture, or counter-culture, is Kelman's third category of behavioral research. Observation becomes ethically problematic when researchers observe a targeted population without informing them that they are being watched. For example, in one controversial case, a researcher conducted a study of gay men's sexual activities in public restrooms. He presented himself as a homosexual and volunteered to serve as their "watch queen," alerting them to the presence of the police in the area. During his period of service as "watch queen," the researcher recorded identifying information about the men having sex in the restrooms and then used it to track them down for interviews regarding their background and family life (which, by the way, was sometimes *heterosexual* family life). Only at that time did the subjects realize that, unbeknownst to them, they had been "participating" in a research study. Unfortunately, in published reports of the study, the detail was such that the identity of some of the subjects, including some with wives and children, was unintentionally disclosed.[28]

B. Benefits versus Risks of Behavioral Research

As we just noted, some behavioral research, including research that looks innocuous on the surface, may actually have quite harmful consequences for subjects without in any way benefiting them. For example, Kelman describes a study in which researchers told elementary school teachers that one group of children were intellectually gifted, but that another group were not. In reality, both groups of children were roughly equivalent in intelligence. The aim of the study was to determine the effects of self-fulfilling prophecies on both the children's and teachers' behavior. As it so happened, the children in the supposedly gifted experimental group made significantly greater gains in IQ than the children in the supposedly nongifted control group. The researchers hypothesized that the children in the experimental group did better than the children in the control group for two reasons: (1) the teachers, expecting them to do well, cued them towards success and (2) the children, encouraged to think of themselves as smart, focused on their studies. But to the degree that the researchers' hypothesis was correct, the children in the supposedly nongifted central group were harmed. Had the teachers made a fuss over how smart they were, they might have thought better of themselves and done just as well as the children in the supposedly gifted experimental group.[29]

As bad as it is to misrepresent subjects' true intellectual abilities to themselves and others, it is even worse to cause them to dislike/hate themselves. Realizing that some behavioral researchers tread on thin ice, as Milgram did in his controversial obedience-to-authority study, Kelman admonishes his colleagues to help their subjects "work through their [negative research experiences]."[30] In addition, he warns his colleagues, ". . . the stresses, anxieties, self-discoveries, or experiences of rejection [conceivably] created in an experiment, a depth interview or a self-analytic group discussion might [even] induce psychotic reactions in vulnerable individuals."[31] To cause a research subject to literally "crackup" is not "just one of those things." On the contrary, it is to have caused major harm, perhaps irreparable harm to a fellow human being. Like biomedical researchers, behavioral researchers must ask themselves whether their studies are truly worth the risks they pose to some subjects. Some studies are best not done.

VI. ETHICAL AND LEGAL ISSUES IN INFORMED CONSENT

Precisely because so many biomedical and behavioral studies promise no direct therapeutic benefits to subjects, while putting them at some risk, it is especially important to secure individuals' **informed consent** before enrolling them in a study. In general, the requirements for informed consent in the nontherapeutic research setting are the same as the ones in the therapeutic clinical setting. The subject must be able to understand the consequences of giving consent and be free from any kind of pressure or coercion that would render his or her consent involuntary. In addition, the researcher must not only provide the subject with enough information to give meaningful consent but also make a concerted effort to help the subject understand the provided information.[32]

A. Information Issues

Although informed consent forms are far from uniform, they typically require an explanation of the purpose(s) of the research, the expected duration of the research, a full description of the procedures involved, and a disclosure of the research design. Researchers must be sure subjects understand both the **risks** and the **benefits** to which they will be exposed. Are the risks large or small? Are they likely or unlikely? Are they physical or emotional? Is there any chance that the subject's very life may be threatened? Similarly, are the benefits to subjects *direct*, such as a cure for their disease? Or, are they simply *collateral* (good health care during the study) or *aspirational* (helping fellow sufferers down the line)?[33] Although subjects may be willing to expose themselves to small risks for collateral or aspirational benefits, they may not be willing to expose themselves to large risks unless a direct benefit is likely.

As important as it is for researchers to disclose to subjects the risks and benefits of participation in a research study is for them to disclose to subjects appropriate **alternative procedures** or courses of treatment. In particular, researchers should discuss with subjects the alternative of nonparticipation in the study. For example, in the case of patients suffering from an advanced form of cancer, biomedical researchers should make it clear to subjects that palliative care may be a better option for them than an experimental regime of virulent, energy-sapping drugs. Similarly, in studies like Milgram's obedience study, behavioral researchers should make clear to subjects that a study may bring out previously suppressed, highly unflattering aspects of their personality or character.

Researchers also need to disclose to subjects whether information gleaned about them will remain entirely **anonymous** or simply **confidential**. Information is anonymous when no identifying information appears directly on subjects' records, and only researchers are able to link subjects' identities to their records. It is confidential when identifying material appears on patients' records, but only researchers have access to it. Anonymity or confidentiality is very important to subjects who wish to keep private their participation in certain studies like HIV-AIDS, clinical depression, aggression, and eating disorder studies. It is also of importance to subjects who have concerns about employers, insurers, or even family members and friends finding out about their condition and then penalizing them in some way because of it.

Not only do subjects need to be guaranteed privacy, they also need to be **compensated** for participating in the study, especially if the study site is located at a place that is inconvenient for them to reach or they have to spend long hours at the study site. As it stands, subjects may be monetarily compensated for loss of time and/or wages. They may also be given small gifts or sums of money as tokens of thanks or incentives to participate in a study. However, researchers are not permitted to use large material rewards as a means to weaken individuals' free will so that they enroll in studies they would otherwise avoid.[34]

Related to the matter of compensation for study participation is the matter of **financial liability** in the event of an adverse effect to a subject. The reigning view is that nonnegligent researchers and institutions should incur no financial liability, provided the subjects in the study participated in an informed and willing manner. Because of this policy (not always made crystal clear to subjects), lawyer George Annas recommends that subjects should not participate in a study unless they are promised subsidized medical care for study harms to them.[35] Another possibility, less taxing on researchers and institutions than Annas's recommendation, is to provide an adequate health care insurance policy to subjects who do not already have one.

Finally, researchers need to inform subjects that they will not lose one or more of their benefits simply because they **refuse** to participate in a study or want to **withdraw** from it. For example, patients, who are being treated for a disease with an established effective therapy, may fear that unless they agree to participate in a research study, the quality of their present care will begin to spiral downwards. Researchers should reassure these patients that their quality of care will remain constant whether they choose (1) not to participate in the study; (2) to participate in the study for its full duration; or (3) to participate in the study for only part of its duration. Similarly, people who rely on social programs for the necessities of life should be reassured that if they refuse to participate in a study, they will not lose their benefits. For example, if researchers want to study the behavior of residents in a shelter for battered women, they should make it clear to potential subjects that whether they decide to enroll in the study or not, they will be permitted to stay at the shelter.

Depending on the complexity of a research experiment, communicating all this information to subjects can be challenging. Yet every attempt must be made to help subjects understand the pros and cons of participating in a biomedical or behavioral research study. Clear communication is particularly vital when subjects are minimally educated, with limited skills in English, or prone to errors in judgment because of life circumstances. Just to be on the safe side, researchers should compose their informed consent forms at approximately the eighth- through tenth-grade level, translating them into languages other than English whenever there is a need to do so.[36]

Although researchers typically take their duty to secure informed consent very seriously, they nonetheless point out that, for scientific reasons, some information may need to be temporarily hidden from subjects during the course of certain studies. For example, in the realm of biomedical research, an RCT can work only if the subjects do not know whether they have been assigned to the placebo group, the established-effective therapy group, or the experimental treatment group. Similarly, in the realm of behavioral research, some studies about people's attitudes, beliefs, habits, or activities cannot work if people know observations are being made about them. For example, if subjects know that their tendency to conform is being studied, many of them will struggle particularly hard to act in a nonconformist manner.

Acknowledging that, on occasion, researchers may need to be less than totally candid with subjects for some length of time, the authors of the Belmont Report formulated guidelines for exceptions to the **no-deception** rule in research studies. The guidelines are as follows:

> In all cases of research involving incomplete disclosure, such research is justified only if it is clear that (1) incomplete disclosure is truly necessary to accomplish the goals of the research, (2) there are no undisclosed risks to subjects that are more than minimal, and (3) there is an adequate plan for debriefing subjects, when appropriate and for dissemination of research results to them. Information about risks should never be withheld for the purpose of eliciting the cooperation of subjects, and truthful answers should always be given to direct questions about the research. Care should be taken to distinguish the cases in which disclosure would destroy or invalidate the research from cases in which disclosure would simply inconvenience the investigation.[37]

Clearly, exceptions to the no-deception rule are to be avoided as much as possible by researchers.

B. Competency Issues

For the most part, research subjects are competent adults who are able to understand and appreciate the relative risks and benefits of the study in which they have enrolled. Not all research subjects are competent adults, however. For example, researchers sometimes need to conduct studies on children in order to find cures for childhood diseases, or on decisionally impaired adults to find effective treatments for senile dementia, Alzheimer's disease, or serious mood disorders such as schizophrenia or bipolar disorder.

Because no one should harm children if at all possible, the federal government has developed strict regulations for research on children. In order to be permitted, a research study on children must ordinarily present "no greater than minimal risk to children enrolled in it."[38] A minimal risk is defined as one that a child "ordinarily encounter[s] in daily life or during the performance of routine physical or psychological examinations and tests."[39] Examples of minimal risks include surveys, noninvasive physiological monitoring, and obtaining blood and urine samples.

In some instances, research studies that present greater than minimal risk to children may be conducted. Specifically, more than minimally risky studies that offer the "prospect of direct benefit" or "contribute to the well-being" of children are sometimes permitted.[40] An example of such a study would be a study of a new leukemia drug that promises to put into remission children's leukemia. Less frequently, research studies that present more than minimal risk to children are permitted for altruistic reasons, but only if the increase over minimal risk is very small—a bit more than submitting to a blood test but far less than submitting to a spinal tap.[41] So, for example, a healthy child may be enrolled in an RCT for a new, life-saving drug even though the drug has, as a possible side effect, mild hiccups for a few minutes.

Whether risk to children is minimal or more than minimal and whether benefit to children is direct or indirect, it is children's surrogates, typically parents, who decide whether participation in a study is in the child's best interests; however, because researchers find it difficult to work with children who do not want to be in a study, and because it is important to treat children with respect, researchers usually require that children over the age of 7 **assent** to study participation.[42] When a child refuses to assent to study enrollment because of concerns about the discomfort, pain, or boredom involved in the study, researchers typically discuss the situation with the surrogate(s) to determine whether, all things considered, study enrollment is truly in the child's best interests.

Unlike children, who are by definition "children" if they fall below a certain chronological age (generally 18 or 21), decisionally impaired persons are a more difficult group of people to identify. Adil Shamoo and Felix A. Khin-Maung-Gyi note that there are two types of decisional impairment. One type is characterized by the fact that "cognitive impairment is the primary manifestation of disease,"[43] as in the case of Alzheimer's disease and senile dementia. The other type is characterized by the fact that "cognition is not central to the disease,"[44] as in the case of schizophrenia and bipolar disease. Whereas someone with advanced Alzheimer's disease is clearly incompetent, someone with schizophrenia may be competent depending on whether their disease is waxing or waning, and/or whether their disease is being treated with currently available drugs and talk therapy.

As might be expected, the more risky and less directly beneficial to subjects a research study is, the more important it is to ascertain that potential subjects are truly competent. In fact, there is growing consensus within the research community that when risk to a decisionally impaired person is greater than minimal, not researchers but "an independent, qualified professional [should] assess the potential subject's capacity to consent."[45] If the decisionally impaired person is deemed competent, researchers may proceed to directly enroll him or her in a study. In contrast, if the decisionally impaired person is deemed incompetent, researchers must seek a surrogate's or guardian's consent for study enrollment.

VII. PROTECTIONISM AND ACCESSIONISM IN BIOMEDICAL AND BEHAVIORAL RESEARCH

Discussing regulations for research on children and decisionally impaired adults sets the stage for discussing how, over the last 30 years, the federal government's policies on research have shifted in a variety of ways. As a result of a series of research scandals, the U.S. public was very suspicious about medical research throughout the 1970s.[46] Among the studies that most horrified the public was a 1950s study conducted at Willowbrook, a New York State institution for mentally retarded children. The purpose of the study was to better understand issues related to the transmission of the hepatitis virus, a virus that is often rampant at institutions like Willowbrook where staff members are not always able to prevent children from infecting each other. One of the aspects of the study that generated the most debate was the researchers' decision, as part of their study design, to deliberately infect healthy children with the hepatitis virus by feeding them a solution made from the feces of children with active hepatitis.[47] The researchers failed to secure adequate informed consent from the children's parents for this aspect of their study. To make matters worse, some of the institution's administrators may have indicated to parents that better rooms and care would be given to children who participated in the study.[48]

Other cases that outraged the U.S. public were the San Antonio Contraception Study and the Jewish Chronic Disease Studies. In the San Antonio Contraception Study, the subjects were predominantly indigent women who lacked health care insurance and typically got low-cost or free contraceptives from public clinics. Researchers randomly assigned half of the women at one clinic to a placebo group and the other half to an active contraceptive group without telling them that some of them would be receiving pills that had no power to prevent pregnancy. As might be expected, some of the women in the placebo group became pregnant, the precise state of affairs they had hoped to avoid.[49] In the Jewish Chronic Disease Studies the subjects were very sick, quite elderly, and often demented cancer patients. Intent on studying the role a compromised immune system plays in the progression of cancer, researchers went so far as to inject live cancer cells into the bloodstream of selected subjects. They justified their action on the grounds that the selected subjects only had a few weeks or days to live anyway.[50]

Subsequent to the unethical studies just described and other studies like them, the federal government issued strict guidelines for research conducted on vulnerable patient populations. So strict were these guidelines, however, that researchers, who had done excellent studies on vulnerable populations in the past, switched to doing research on less controversial populations. In fact, within short order, most researchers' preferred population for study was adult White men. But this new research focus was not without its own problems. Before long, the very populations meant to be benefited by strict guidelines for research became the unintended "victims" of studies conducted almost exclusively on adult White males. For example, drugs were developed on the basis of all-White adult male studies and then distributed to children, women, and non-White men, as if there were no differences between the bodies of children and adults, or between the bodies of men and women, or between the bodies of White and non-White people. Physicians then prescribed these drugs to children, women, and non-White patients without pausing to think that a drug designed as the result of a study on White adult men may not work well or at all in women's, children's, or non-White people's bodies. Spared from the risks of participating in RCTs, many women, children, and non-White people found themselves exposed to sometimes more serious risks in their physicians' offices.

As the U.S. public became aware of the ways in which *not* participating in research studies could harm them, enthusiasm for protectionism began to wane. Among the groups that led the charge for increased access to participation in research studies were women's health activists.[51] They convinced the U.S. Congressional Caucus for Women's Issues to commission a study on whether the Department of Health and Human Services (DHHS) was as interested in women's health concerns as men's. The results of the study were shocking. They established that the DHHS had no overall strategy regarding what information about women's health was needed, or how to get that information to the average woman.

Realizing that it was very important to rectify this state of affairs, the Congress immediately directed the National Institutes of Health (NIH) to create an Office of Research on Women's Health (ORWH). The goal of the office, established in September 1990, was threefold: (1) to promote women's participation in health research studies; (2) to ensure that NIH-supported research pays due attention to women's health issues; and (3) to increase the number of women in the biomedical and behavioral sciences. In April 1991, Dr. Bernadine Healy, the first woman to head the NIH, launched a nationwide $625 million **Women's Health Initiative (WHI)**, consisting of over 160,000 women aged 50 years to 79 years to investigate the causes and potential prevention of major diseases of women—particularly heart disease; cancers of the breast, colon, and rectum; and osteoporosis. Completed in 2005, the study did indeed reveal that certain diseases act differently in women than men.[52] So popular has research on women's health concerns become that some men's groups have recently complained that men's health concerns are being neglected by researchers.

Another group that fought to have better access to research studies were HIV-AIDS activists. Concerned about the manifest suffering of people with HIV-AIDS, these activists demanded that persons with HIV-AIDS be allowed to enroll in studies for anti-AIDS drugs, and that they be given these drugs subsequent to the study if there was any chance of ongoing benefit from them. AIDS Coalition to Unleash Power (ACT-UP) adopted the slogan "A Drug Trial is Health Care Too," and gradually convinced public authorities of the wisdom of their view. Despite the fact that researchers feared that some people with HIV-AIDS were too desperate for help to give fully informed consent to study participation, they enrolled them in their studies anyway. The researchers reasoned, as did the general public, that desperate circumstances sometimes warrant compromises with rigid regulations.[53]

Whether accessionism (that is, the movement to gain access to studies) continues to rule the research realm is doubtful, however. There seems to be a pendulum swing back and forth between **protectionism** on the one hand and **accessionism** on the other. The virtue of accessionism is that people who want to try promising drugs or treatments to save, lengthen, or improve their lives are permitted to do so. This virtue is offset by accessionism's vice, however. Deciding to enroll large numbers of vulnerable people in a study may weaken study safeguards. As a result, things may go wrong more often than they should, and serious harm may befall some research subjects. Before anyone has a chance to step back from the situation and calculate the true ratio of harm sustained and benefit received, the general public will become outraged and insist that the government do something to protect unsuspecting citizens from researchers who want to use them as guinea pigs. For some reason or another, Americans have a particularly hard time shaping a moderate position on biomedical and behavioral research.

VIII. Ongoing and Emerging Debates in Biomedical Research in the United States

Depending on their political and religious values, social and economic condition, level of technological development, and other contextual features, nations develop particular concerns about certain types of research. As we shall discuss below, U.S. researchers continue to have concerns about studying vulnerable populations, especially if they are poor, illiterate, and desperate for medical help, or living in developing nations where research is relatively unregulated and people cannot afford to buy the life-saving drugs that result from the studies conducted on them. In addition to this traditional concern, however, new issues have emerged within the U.S. research community.

Among these issues are continuing use of placeboes in studies; misconduct in research; funding of research; the politicization of research; and conflicts of interest in research.

A. Vulnerable Populations in Developing Nations

Of all the issues noted above, none is more emblematic of the world in which we live than research conducted in developing nations by research teams from developed nations. Even when researchers from developed nations collaborate with researchers in developing nations, the risk of exploiting research subjects, many of whom are poor, illiterate, and without health care, is high. That this should be the case does not surprise Solomon R. Benatar, M.D. He observes that the world in which research is conducted is an unjust world, a world in which 25% of people live in abject poverty. It is also a world in which the desire to make high profits on life-saving drugs and treatments leads researchers, and the institutions or corporations that support them, to developing nations, where "easy access to patients, reduced costs, and less stringent regulations—the 'research sweat shop' equivalent— prevails."[54] Thus, as Benatar sees it, international research documents such as the ones issued by the World Medical Association (WMA) and the Council for International Organizations of Medical Sciences (CIOMS) must be given as much force as possible. The principles of autonomy, beneficence, and justice must be honored by researchers, whether their research is conducted within or outside the United States.

Honoring the principle of autonomy presents major challenges for researchers in developing nations. The informed consent procedures typically used in developed nations, such as the United States, may not work well in developing nations because of cultural differences. For example, in some developing nations, decisions are made communally rather than individually; and in others, individuals may feel obligated to give or withhold consent to please elders, spouses, or their entire community. Particular problems may surface when consent needs to be secured from illiterate subjects or from subjects who are from populations with very different beliefs about causes of illness and little familiarity with biomedicine, let alone concepts such as randomization and the placebo effect. Still other problems may arise when subjects fear signing a consent form, worrying that doing so may result in unanticipated harm befalling them in the future. Therefore, in order to be sure subjects really understand and consent to being in a study, researchers may have to present information and document consent in some very novel ways. For example, researchers in one developing nation wrote an informed consent form that included the lines: "Although I as a doctor believe that the disease is caused by germs (i.e. a virus or bacterium), I understand that you

believe that it is caused by a demon. I respect the fact that you have this belief and I should like you to try this medicine to remove the disease. Removing the disease is more important to us both than whether we think it is
caused by germs or a demon."[55]

As important as it is for researchers to respect the autonomy of research
subjects in developing nations, it is equally important to benefit them or at
least do them no harm. After much debate, the Declaration of Helsinki was
revised in 2000 to include a paragraph, numbered twenty-nine, that read as
follows: "The benefits, risks, burdens and effectiveness of a new method
should be tested against those of the best current prophylactic diagnostic and
therapeutic methods. This does not exclude the use of [a] placebo, or no
treatment, in studies where no prophylactic, diagnostic, or therapeutic
method exists."[56] As revised, paragraph number twenty-nine seemed to condemn studies such as the one done on pregnant women with HIV in eleven
developing nations to see if perinatal transmission of HIV to their infants
could be prevented with a lower and less-expensive dose of **azidothymidine**
(AZT) than the dose of AZT viewed as the standard of care in the United
States. At present, clinicians treating pregnant U.S. women with HIV adhere
to the protocol of a study called the AIDS Clinical Trials Group (ACTG) 076
study. Protocol 076 requires pregnant women to take five AZT pills per day
for 12 weeks prior to delivering their infant; to submit to intravenous AZT
during delivery of their infant; and, finally, to take four AZT pills per day for
6 weeks after delivering their infant. If adhered to, Protocol 076 typically reduces mother-to-fetus transmission of HIV by 66%. It costs about U.S.
$800.00, a sum that far exceeds the amount of money average persons in
most developing nations make annually.

Realizing that most pregnant women with HIV in developing nations
could not afford to spend U.S. $800.00 to spare their infant HIV, researchers
decided to test a short regimen that used only about 10% of the AZT used in
the long 076 regimen for a cost of about U.S. $80.00. But instead of testing this
short, low-cost regimen against the long, high-cost 076 regimen, researchers
tested it against a placebo, thereby depriving some of their subjects of any
AZT benefits whatsoever. The researchers justified their decision to use a
placebo on the grounds that *no treatment* for pregnant women with HIV *was*
the "standard of care" in developing nations and that the research subjects
who got the placebo were not worse off for receiving it, because if they had
not participated in the study they would not have received AZT either. Fur-
thermore, stressed the researchers, the women in the study who did get the
low-dose, low-cost AZT regimen were better off than they would otherwise
have been. Some members of the research ethics community supported the
researchers' study as a realistic way to proceed in developing nations. But
others denounced it as a clear violation of the principle of beneficence, not
only because the women who received the placebo received no benefit but
also because, at a cost of about U.S. $80.00, the low dose AZT regimen was

still too expensive for most people in developing nations to purchase. Sadly, about U.S. $10.00 constitutes the annual per capita health care expenditure in the poorest of poor developing nations.[57]

Questions about the purported beneficence of some research studies conducted in developing nations intersect with questions related to justice. If researchers know that the drug or treatment that results from their study will be one that their research subjects cannot afford, do they have some sort of obligation to pressure pharmaceutical companies, for example, to provide the drug or treatment for free or at very low cost to these subjects? Additionally, do researchers have some sort of obligation to pressure governments in developing nations and/or the international community as a whole to subsidize relatively low cost drugs and treatments for people who cannot afford them?

Such questions are difficult to answer because the line between being just on the one hand and being charitable on the other is not always bright. Consider, for example, the very profitable pharmaceutical industry, with profit margins as high as 30%. Do highly successful drug companies have a social responsibility to provide low-cost or free drugs to former research subjects in developing nations? After all, it does seem unfair to use people as research subjects in studies that result in life-saving, enormously profitable drugs, only to deny them access to these drugs because they cannot afford to purchase them. Yet, if highly profitable drug companies routinely give away their products to poor people in developing nations, as Merck, the Gates Foundation, Bristol-Myers Squibb, and Pfizer have in some African nations stricken with HIV-AIDS,[58] how long can they remain highly profitable? Still, if only for prudential reasons, such as fear of being undersold by developers of cheap generic versions of their products, profitable drug companies may wish to provide a *reasonable* amount of their products *pro bono* to people threatened with life-imperiling diseases in developing nations.

B. Continuing Use of Placebos

As noted above, paragraph twenty-nine of the most recent version of the Helsinki Agreement condemns unnecessary placebo-controlled studies no matter where they occur. But the U.S. Food and Drug Administration (FDA) maintains that very few placebo-controlled studies are truly "unnecessary." In fact, the FDA "continues to demand and defend placebo controlled evidence of efficacy and safety for the development of new pharmaceuticals, even if effective therapy exists."[59] The FDA takes this position because it "confer[s] on placebo control, a stature that ranks it with double-blinding and randomization as a hall mark of good science."[60] In other words, the FDA maintains that the best way to conclusively prove the therapeutic and adverse effects of a product is to test it against literally nothing; that is, a placebo.

But not all research scientists agree with the FDA's position on the value of placebo-controlled studies, particularly when an IND is intended to benefit people with mental health problems such as epilepsy, schizophrenia, and dementia. As these FDA critics see it, where there is the moral will, there is a scientific way to prove the safety and efficacy of an IND without using a placebo control. Not to seek this scientific way is, in their estimation, not only scientifically lazy but also flatly unethical when effective treatments are available for patients. Karin B. Michels and Kenneth J. Rothman provide the specific examples of a recent placebo-controlled trial of an antiepileptic medication called oxcarbazepine. The study protocol called for 102 patients to be withdrawn from their usual antiepileptic medication. To become eligible for inclusion in the study, which randomized patients to receive either a placebo or the IND, a patient had to experience two to ten seizures during withdrawal. During the trial, patients were not to be returned to their old medication unless they experienced four seizures. Michels and Rothman note that a startling 89% of the patients on the placebo met this "premature exit criterion."[61] In their estimation, when *no* treatment (that is, a placebo) is manifestly *bad* treatment for research subjects, researchers must ask themselves whether their insistence on a placebo-controlled study is based on a desire to conduct the best study possible or, instead, on a desire to conduct a "relatively quick and inexpensive" study.[62]

C. Funding Research: The Private–Public Split

Money is, as we just suggested, the root of some of the "evils" that occur in research. Although the general public may not realize it, there are some differences between publicly funded research on the one hand and privately funded research on the other. Private sector research is supported by private foundations such as the Robert Wood Johnson Foundation, private corporations (most often large pharmaceutical companies), and "disease groups" such as the Juvenile Diabetes Research Foundation. In contrast, public sector research is supported by the Federal Government mainly through the National Institutes of Health (NIH), which are part of the Department of Health and Human Services (DHHS). Other government agencies, including the Center for Disease Control (CDC), the Agency for Health Care Research and Quality (AHRQ), the Department of Defense (DOD), and the Veterans Health Administration (VHA), also provide public funds for research.

The goals of publicly funded research are probably most clearly stated by the NIH. They are as follows:

(1) Foster creative discoveries, innovative research strategies, and their applications to advance the nation's ability to protect and improve health.

(2) Develop and improve the nation's ability to prevent disease.

(3) Improve medical and associated sciences with an eye on the nation's economic well-being to ensure a high return on the public's investment on research.

(4) Serve as a leader and promoter of the highest level of scientific integrity, public accountability, and social responsibility.[63]

The NIH and other government agencies spend much of their time setting research priorities and determining the scientific merit of the numerous study protocols submitted to them. Among their chief responsibilities is to ensure that only high caliber studies are granted funding.

Because of the importance of protecting the nation's health, and the many diseases and disabilities that afflict (or may afflict) U.S. citizens, setting research priorities is a complex task. One way to assess the Federal Government's current research priorities is simply to see which research initiatives or programs receive the bulk of NIH funds. In 2003, the top ten NIH fund receivers were (in billions of dollars): (1) clinical research (8.0), (2) prevention (6.9), (3) cancer (5.8), (4) brain disorders (4.8), (5) neurosciences (4.7), (6) women's health (4.1), (7) pediatrics (3.1), (8) AIDS (2.8), (9) behavioral/ social (2.6), and (10) cardiovascular (2.1). In addition, because of growing fears about bioterrorism—that is, terrorists using biological or chemical agents to infect the U.S. pubic with dread diseases such as anthrax—funding to prevent its horrific effects increased over 500% (U.S. $1.7 billion) from 2002 to 2003.[64]

Not surprisingly, neither all researchers nor all members of the general public approve of the Federal Government's priorities for research. They suspect that its setting of priorities is not scientific but political. For example, some critics claim that the reason the government spends as much money as it does on AIDS and women's health research is because gay and feminist activists have accused the government of discriminating against homosexuals and women in the past. Other critics note that because of debates about abortion in the United States, it is very difficult to get government funding for research on stem cells, embryos, and fetuses.

Because governmental research priorities may not mesh with researchers' priorities, and also because public funding for research, though seemingly high (about U.S. $25 billion),[65] is actually quite low, more researchers are entering the private sector. Some of them choose to work for nonprofit disease organizations whose mission is to find a cure for specific diseases such as multiple sclerosis, diabetes, and Alzheimer's disease. Others conduct research with funds from well-endowed nonprofit foundations like the Gates, Hughes, and Heinz Foundations, all of which have the philanthropic mission of improving the quality of life for humankind. Still others find employment in for-profit private organizations, most often pharmaceutical companies that are interested in their line of research. There, they may be joined by researchers who are motivated to work in the private sector not so much because of some special research project near and dear to their hearts but because there is so much money to be made in the private sector. In addition, the private sector has the advantage of being highly unregulated and free to espouse any line of politics it chooses. Thus, it is not surprising that most work on therapeutic and reproductive cloning is funded by private monies.

D. Conflicts of Interest

Discussing public versus private funding of research immediately brings into focus the subject of conflicts of interest in research. One type of conflict of interest is **moral**. Researchers may be asked, for example, to develop products that can be used for evil rather than good purposes. Interestingly, years ago philosopher Bernard Williams discussed a hypothetical case[66] that featured a researcher convincing himself that "doing wrong" was actually "doing right." The case centered on a biochemist with heavy family responsibilities who finds that the job market in his field is very limited. After extensive job searching, he is finally offered a job in a company that does research in chemical and biological warfare. Although the biochemist is, in principle, opposed to such research, his wife begs him to take the job for her sake and that of the children; it is a choice between this job, the welfare line, or marginal employment as a dishwasher. In the course of mulling over his options, the biochemist discovers that if he fails to take the research job, the company is likely to hire another candidate, a brilliant scientist who wants to make a major contribution to germ warfare. Gradually, the biochemist convinces himself to take the job, on the grounds that his rival is likely to commit worse wrongs than he would. He is doing the "right" thing by doing the "wrong" thing. Regrettably, the kind of reasoning in which Williams's biochemist engaged is not unknown in the actual world of science and may account for why some good people wind up doing some very bad things.

Another type of conflict of interest is **political**. For example, researchers who work for the Heritage Foundation, a conservative think tank which supports free-market competition in the realm of health care, may manipulate their data to prove that universal health care insurance would ruin the U.S. economy. Similarly, researchers who work for the Commonwealth Fund, a liberal think tank which supports universal health care insurance, may be tempted to contort their findings to prove that free-market competition in the realm of health care would end in millions of Americans being abandoned to die on the streets. Clearly, science is not always pure, because some scientists are willing to sacrifice scientific integrity in the name of a political cause.

Still another type of conflict of interest is **financial**. Increasingly, researchers are tempted to cut corners, fudge data, and otherwise compromise the scientific method for financial gain. In the past, most research was, as we noted above, funded by the government, and researchers were viewed as conducting research for the benefit of the public. But, as we have also observed, an increasing percentage of the research now conducted in the United States is privately funded. In fact, pharmaceutical companies subsidize over 60% of the total biomedical research and development funding in the United States.[67] These companies pay researchers far more money than they would be paid in the public sector. In addition to research monies and generous salaries, many researchers enter into patent and royalty agreements with corporate sponsors and are even given stock or equity interests in the companies for which they are studying products. As a result of such states of affair, there is heightened concern that, in order to satisfy commercial sponsors, researchers will gradually transform what once were scientific and scholarly endeavors, lauded for their objectivity, into "money-grubbing" corporate research. Critics are swift to cite, for example, studies such as a recent survey in which one-fifth of researchers confessed "to delaying publication of their results by more than six months at least once in the last three years to allow for patent application, protect their scientific lead, or to slow the dissemination of results that would hurt sales of their sponsor's product . . ."[68]

Whether researchers are able to resist the lure of high salaries and state-of-the-art laboratories remains to be seen. In any event, government agencies, such as the FDA, now require clinical investigators to disclose conflicts of interest when they submit an application to market a new human drug. Among these conflicts of interests are the ones highlighted by Adil E. Shamoo and Felix A. Khin-Maung-Gyi:

> (1) Equity interest in the sponsor or the study: ownership interest, stock options, and equity in publicly traded corporations that exceeds $50,000 per year.
>
> (2) Proprietary interest, such as patents, trademarks, copyrights, or licensing agreements.
>
> (3) Payment by the sponsor of the study exceeding $25,000 to the investigator and/or the investigator's institution to support the activities of the investigator.[69]

IX. CONCLUSION

The major problem with any discussion of biomedical and behavioral research ethics is that there are simply too many international as well as national issues and topics to discuss in any detail. Thus, it is vital to bring back any discussion of research ethics to the core ethical principles that ought to guide it. Recently, Drs. Ezekiel Emanuel, David Wendler, and Christine Grady have articulated seven requirements for *ethical* clinical research. Although the guidelines they outline are intended for those conducting clinical/ biomedical research rather than behavioral research, they can easily be modified to fit the behavioral research arena.

According to Emanuel et al., the criteria for determining whether a research trial is ethical are as follows:

(1) Social or scientific value

(2) Scientific validity

(3) Fair subject selection

(4) Favorable risk-benefit ratio

(5) Independent review

(6) Informed consent

(7) Respect for potential and enrolled subjects[70]

In an effort to show how these seven criteria can be operationalized, Emanuel et al. apply them to two real life cases. The first case they consider dates back over a decade. Researchers conducted a study on an IND that promised to effectively control the nausea and vomiting that typically accompanies chemotherapy. Rather than testing the IND against the standard drug that was used at the time—a drug that was somewhat helpful in controlling nausea and vomiting—the researchers tested the IND against a placebo. In Emanuel's estimation, the researchers were *wrong* to use the placebo because they violated at least three of the criteria for ethical research: social or scientific value, scientific validity, and favorable risk–benefit ratio. It was not valuable to compare the IND to a placebo because there was a better treatment with which to compare it; namely, the standard drug that was used at that time to control nausea and vomiting. Moreover, it was not scientifically valid for the researchers to use a placebo because they knew fully well that the placebo would not help relieve cancer patients' discomfort. Finally, the promised benefits of the study—a slightly more effective drug for nausea and vomiting—did not outweigh its considerable risks; namely, subjecting some patients (the ones getting the placebo) to possibly uncontrolled nausea and vomiting, which was not, as the researchers protested, just "a transitory discomfort that results in no permanent disability,"[71] but a state of affairs that ". . . frequently results in poor nutritional intake, metabolic derangements, deterioration of physical and mental condition, as well as the possible rejection of potentially beneficial treatment."[72]

The second case which Emanuel et al. considered focused on a research study conducted in several developing nations on a new anti–rotavirus diarrhea vaccine. Although randomized tests in developed nations had proved the vaccine's efficacy in preventing rotavirus diarrhea, the vaccine was nonetheless temporarily withdrawn from the U.S. market because it posed a one-in-ten-thousand risk of intussusception (a condition in which the intestines start digesting themselves). Given that only one in five million U.S.

children die from rotavirus diarrhea annually,[73] a one-in-ten-thousand risk of intussusception from the vaccine struck U.S. public health authorities as too much risk to impose on the U.S. public. The question then arose whether randomized tests of the slightly risky vaccine could proceed in developing nations where about one in 200 children (for a total of 600,000 children per annum) die from rotavirus diarrhea.[74]

In answering the question posed above, Emanuel et al. concluded that the requirements of social or scientific value, scientific validity, fair subject selection, and favorable risk–benefit ratio cumulatively justified testing the (unmodified) vaccine in developing nations. They noted, first, that it was more valuable to prevent hundreds of thousands of deaths in developing nations immediately with a slightly risky vaccine than to wait several years for a perfectly safe vaccine to be developed in the United States. Second, they stated it was scientifically valid to test the slightly risky vaccine against a placebo control in developing nations because there was, at the time, no alternative to the imperfect vaccine—it was either the imperfect vaccine or nothing. Third, they asserted it was fair to select as subjects for the study infants and children in developing nations because they were the population most at risk for rotavirus diarrhea. Fourth, they stressed that the risk–benefit ratio of the study was very favorable in developing nations, even though it was unfavorable in highly privileged nations such as the United States.

To be sure, it is possible to quibble with the way in which Emanuel et al. applied their criteria to the two cases they analyzed. Appeals to context—that is, to the different circumstances that obtain in developing and developed nations—may, after all, be used as a shield for unethical research by unethical researchers. Yet the fact remains that, in order to be of any use to reflective people, even the most universal elements of an abstract code of research ethics must "be adapted to the health, economic, cultural, and technological conditions in which clinical research is conducted."[75] Ethical theory needs to serve the fact of human diversity. To be sure, the dialogue between ethical theory and practice can often be tense. But from its stressful moments can be born decisions that make good moral sense to people no matter where they live, or how good or bad their material conditions may be.

Discussion Questions

1. In your estimation, is there anything wrong about using accurate scientific data that is secured in the course of a series of unethical experiments (think here of the Nazi "experiments" on World War II concentration camp prisoners)? Why or why not?
2. A major issue in biomedical and behavioral research involves balancing the public's need for protection against the individual patient's right to autonomy.

In your opinion, are U.S. research subjects today typically overprotected or underprotected? Provide specific examples to justify your opinion.

3. In the 1960s the U.S. government conducted experiments on the hallucinogenic drug, LSD. Researchers did not inform research subjects that taking LSD would expose their gametes (sex cells) to possible damage. In addition, researchers used information from the research subjects' data forms to track individuals thought to be "subversive."

   a. To what extent did the government have an obligation to inform the research subjects of possible genetic damage to their [future] offspring?
   b. When, if ever, should the information provided by research subjects be made available to interested agencies and/or authorities for nonmedical reasons?
   c. If some negative consequence occurs in a government-sponsored trial in which informed consent was obtained properly, to what degree should the government be held responsible?

Case Studies

1. In order to participate in certain clinical trials, research subjects need to meet certain requirements. For example, trials that involve INDs for treating pancreatic cancer require that participants (1) have the type of cancer studied; (2) be nonterminal patients; (3) have normal insulin levels and kidney functioning; and (4) be able to carry out everyday activities for the length of the trial. In addition, such trials require a certain number of research subjects in order to be deemed statistically valid. Imagine a trial for an IND meant to treat pancreatic cancer in which the researchers are three subjects short of their participant goal. If the next three willing subjects meet only three out of four of the inclusion criteria should researchers allow them to participate in the study anyway?

   a. If the researchers do allow the three individuals to participate, should they report the fact that these individuals did not meet all the criteria? Should the researchers' Institutional Review Board (IRB) approve their study despite the fact that it has three subjects that do not quite fit the study's stated requirements? After all, the three subjects almost fit the criteria and they are desperate to get into the study.
   b. If one or more of these three patients are health care professionals, is their desire to participate in the study in any way at odds with their responsibilities to the scientific enterprise?
   c. If the study involves a nontherapeutic intervention, would that make a difference as to what the researchers should do?

2. A randomized trial of teenagers (ages 14–16) was developed to study the dermatologic effects of a body wash designed to slow the development of acne. No risks were anticipated. All potential research subjects were

asked to obtain consent from their parents. However, some parents refused to give consent because of the possibility of unanticipated risks.

a.   If a child wants to participate in the study, should the child's wishes override the parents' refusal to grant consent?

b.   If a child was 17, would this make a difference as to granting consent? If the situation involved a child between the ages of 11–13, would your answer be different? Why or why not?

Endnotes

1. George J. Annas and Michael A. Grodin (eds.), *The Nazi Doctors and the Nuremberg Code: Human Rights in Human Experimentation* (New York: Oxford University Press, 1992).

2. R. Gemer, I. Powell, and B. Roling, "Japan's biological weapons: 1930–1945," *Bulletin of Atomic Science*, 37, no. 8 (1981): 43.

3. Tuskegee Syphilis Study, Ad Hoc Panel to the Department of Health, Education, and Welfare, *Final Report* (Washington, D.C.: Public Health Service, 1973).

4. S. E. Lederer and Michael A. Grodin, "Historical overview: pediatric experimentation," in: Michael A. Grodin and Leonard H. Glantz (eds.), *Children as Research Subjects: Science, Ethics, and Law* (New York: Oxford University Press, 1994).

5. Jonathan D. Moreno, "Goodbye to all that: the end of moderate protectionism in human subjects research," *Hastings Center Report*, 31, no. 3 (May–June 2001): 9–17.

6. Advisory Committee on Human Radiation Experiments, *The Human Radiation Experiments* (New York: Oxford University Press, 1996).

7. Thomasine Kimbrough Krishner and Raymond Belliotti, "Baby Fae: a beastly business," *Journal of Medical Ethics*, 2 (1985): 178–183.

8. Albert R. Jonsen, "The selection of patients," in: Margery Shaw (ed.), *After Barney Clark* (Austin: University of Texas Press, 1984), pp. 6–8.

9. Robert J. Levine, "Research, biomedical," in: Warren T. Reich (ed.), *Encyclopedia of Bioethics* (New York: Macmillan Press, 1995), pp. 1481–1492.

10. Norman Daniels, "Clarifying the concept of medical necessity," *Proceedings of the Group Health Initiative* (Washington, D.C.: Group Health Association of America, 1991), pp. 693–707.

11. Robert J. Levine, "Research, biomedical," in: Warren T. Reich (ed.), *Encyclopedia of Bioethics* (New York: Macmillan Press, 1995), p. 1483.

12. "Nuremberg code of ethics in medical research," *Trials of War Criminals before the Nuremberg Military Tribunals under Control Council Law*, 10, no. 2 (Washington, D.C.: U.S. Government Printing Office: 1948–1949), pp. 181–182.

13. Ibid.

14. World Medical Association (WMA), *Declaration of Helsinki: Ethical Principles for Medical Research Involving Human Subjects* (adopted 18th WMA General Assembly, Helsinki, Finland, June 1964; as amended October 2000).

15. National Commission for the Protection of Human Subjects of Biomedical and Behavioral Research, *The Belmont Report: Ethical Guidelines for the Protection of Human Subjects of Research* (Washington, D.C.: DHEW, 1978).

16. Ibid.

17. Ibid.

18. Robert J. Amdur and Liz Bankert, "The consent document," in: Robert J. Amdur (ed.), *Institutional Review Board Member Handbook* (Sudbury, MA: Jones and Bartlett Publishers, 2002), p. 49.

19. Paul Gelsinger, "Jesse's intent," *Guinea Pig Zero*, 8 (2000): 7–19.

20. Walter Glannon, *Biomedical Ethics* (New York: Oxford University Press, 2005), p. 50.

21. George J. Annas, *The Rights of Patients*, 2nd ed. (Carbondale and Edwardsville, IL: Southern Illinois University Press, 1989), p. 156.

22. Sinclair Lewis, *Arrowsmith* (New York: Grossett and Dunlap, 1925).

23. Alexander M. Capron, "Human experimentation," in: Robert Veatch (ed.), *Medical Ethics* (Boston: Jones and Bartlett Publishers, 1989), p. 144.

24. Herbert C. Kelman, "Research, behavioral," in: Warren T. Reich (ed.), *Encyclopedia of Bioethics* (New York: Macmillan Press, 1995), p. 1470.

25. Stanley Milgram, *Obedience to Authority: an Experiment View* (New York: Harper & Row, 1974).

26. Philip G. Zimbardo, Craig Haney, Curtis W. Banks, and David Jaffo, "The psychology of imprisonment: privation, power, and pathology," in: Zick Rubin (ed.), *Doing Unto Others: Joining Molding, Conforming, Helping, Loving* (Englewood Cliffs, NJ: Prentice-Hall, 1974), pp. 61–73.

27. S. R. Phillips, "Asking the sensitive question: the ethics of survey research and teen sex." *IRB*, 16, no. 6 (1994): 1–7.

28. Donald P. Warwick, "Tearoom trade: means and ends in social research," *Hastings Center Report*, 1, no. 1 (1973): 27–38.

29. Herbert C. Kelman, "Research, behavioral," in: Warren T. Reich (ed.), *Encyclopedia of Bioethics* (New York: Macmillan Press, 1995), p. 1475.

30. Ibid.

31. Ibid., p. 1474.

32. Thomas M. Garrett, Harold W. Baillie, and Rosellen M. Garrett, *Health Care Ethics, Principles, and Problems*, 4th ed. (Upper Saddle River, NJ: Prentice-Hall, Inc., 2001), p. 31.

33. Nancy M. P. King, "Defining and describing benefit appropriately in clinical trials," *The Journal of Law, Medicine & Ethics*, 28, no. 4 (Winter 2000): 333.

34. Adil E. Shamoo and Felix A. Khin-Maung-Gyi, *Ethics of the Use of Human Subjects in Research* (New York: Garland Science, 2002), p. 47.

35. George J. Annas, *The Rights of Patients*, 2nd ed. (Carbondale and Edwardsville, IL: Southern Illinois University Press, 1989), p. 156.

36. Robert J. Amdur and Liz Bankert, "The consent document," in: Robert J. Amdur and Liz Bankert (eds.), *Institutional Review Board Member Handbook* (Sudbury, MA: Jones and Bartlett Publishers, 2002), p. 51.

37. National Commission for the Protection of Human Subject of Biomedical and Behavioral Research, *The Belmont Report* (Washington, D.C.: Government Printing Office, 1978), p. 12.

38. Robert Nelson and Robert J. Amdur, "Research involving children," in: Robert J. Amdur (ed.), *Institutional Review Board Member Handbook* (Sudbury, MA: Jones and Bartlett Publishers, 2002), p. 175.

39. Ibid., p. 179.

40. Ibid., p. 175.

41. Ibid.

42. Ibid., p. 180.

43. Adil E. Shamoo and Felix A. Khin-Maung-Gyi, *Ethics of the Use of Human Subjects in Research* (New York: Garland Science, 2002), p. 80.

44. Ibid., p. 81.

45. Ibid., p. 80.

46. Anna Mastroianni and Jeffrey Kahn, "Swinging on the pendulum: shifting views of Justice in human subjects research," *Hastings Center Report*, 31, no. 3 (May–June 2001): 22.

47. Robert J. Amdur, "A brief history of the IRB system," in: Robert J. Amdur (ed.), *Institutional Review Board Member Handbook* (Sudbury, MA: Jones and Bartlett Publishers, 2002), p. 15.

48. University of California Fullerton, "The dark history of research," *http:// www.~ref.usc.edu/~renold/480wk3ethics.htm* [accessed May 29, 2005].

49. Robert J. Amdur, "A brief history of the IRB system," in: Robert J. Amdur (ed.), *Institutional Review Board Member Handbook* (Sudbury, MA: Jones and Bartlett Publishers, 2002), p. 15.

50. Ibid., p. 16.

51. Rebecca Dresser, "Wanted: single, White male for medical research," *The Hustings Center Report*, 22, no. 1 (January–February 1992): 26.

52. James H. Rubin, "Neglected women's health research wins funds," *The Philadelphia Inquirer* (March 31, 1993): A3.

53. Jonathan D. Moreno, "Goodbye to all that: the end of moderate protectionism in human subjects' research," *The Hastings Center Report*, 21, no. 3 (May–June 2001): 13.

54. Solomon R. Benatar, "Justice and medical research: a global perspective," *Bioethics*, 15, no. 4 (August 2001): 337.

55. Nuffield Council on Bioethics, "The ethics of research related to healthcare in developing nations," *www.nuffieldbioethics.org/publications/developingcountries/ rep0000000887.asp* [accessed May 29, 2005].

56. World Medical Association (WMA), *Declaration of Helsinki* (amended by the 52nd WMA General Assembly, Edinburgh, Scotland, October 2000, note 7).

57. Solomon R. Benatar, "Justice and medical research: a global perspective," *Bioethics*, 15, no. 4 (August 2001): 335.

58. David B. Resnik, "Developing drugs for the developing world: an economic, legal, moral, and political dilemma," *Bioethics*, no. 1 (May 2001): 24.

59. Karin B. Michels and Kenneth J. Rothman, "Update on unethical use of place-bos in randomized trials," *Bioethics*, 17, no. 2 (April 2003): 189–190.

60. *Cited in* Robert J. Amdur, "Placebo-controlled trials," in: Robert J. Amdur (ed.), *Institutional Review Board Member Handbook* (Sudbury, MA: Jones and Bartlett Publishers, 2002), p. 159.

61. Karin B. Michels and Kenneth J. Rothman, "Update on unethical use of place-bos in randomized trials," *Bioethics*, 17, no. 2 (April 2003): 191.

62. Ibid., p. 190.

63. *Cited in* Richard Saul Wurman, *Understanding Healthcare* (Newport, RI: Quad Graphics, 2004), p. 271.

64. Ibid.

65. Ibid., p. 270.

66. J. J. C. Smart and Bernard Williams, *Utilitarianism: For and Against* (New York: Cambridge University Press, 1973), pp. 97–99.

67. David B. Resnik, "Developing drugs for the developing world: an economic, legal, moral, and political dilemma," *Bioethics*, no. 1 (May 2001): 14.

68. Shannon Brownless, "Doctors without borders: why you cannot trust medical journals anymore," *The Washington Monthly* (April 2004): 40.

69. Adil E. Shamoo and Felix A. Khin-Maung-Gyi, *Ethics of the Use of Human Subjects in Research* (New York: Garland Science, 2002), p. 69.

70. Ezekiel J. Emanuel, David Wendler, and Christine Grady, "What makes clinical research ethical?" *Journal of American Medical Association*, 283, no. 20 (May 24/31, 2000): 2701.

71. Ibid., p. 2708.

72. Ibid., p. 2709.

73. Ibid.

74. Ibid., p. 2710.

75. Ibid., p. 2701.

chapter six

Abortion

I. INTRODUCTION

Abortion is one of the most hotly debated ethical, legal, and social issues of our time, so much so that most of us find it hard to believe that, until relatively recent times, abortion was not a topic of much interest to Americans. Although the Hippocratic Oath prohibits abortion—"I will give no deadly medicine to anyone if asked, nor suggest any such counsel; and in like manner I will not give a woman a remedy to produce abortion—"[1] many historians doubt that Hippocrates (460–377 B.C.E.) actually wrote this line. To support their position, they point out that Hippocrates did not believe fetuses were animated, ensouled, or otherwise formed into persons at the moment of conception, but only sometime thereafter—specifically, gestational day 30 for male fetuses and gestational day 42 for female fetuses. Later, the ancient Greek philosopher, Aristotle (384–322 B.C.E.), concurred with Hippocrates, with one adjustment: Male fetuses achieve animation or ensoulment at gestational day 40, whereas female fetuses achieve it at gestational day 90.[2]

Significantly, Aristotle's conception of ensoulment or animation served as the basis of Roman Catholics' view of the fetus from the thirteenth century until the latter half of the nineteenth century. Later, medieval theologian St. Thomas Aquinas (A.D. 1224–1274) claimed that although killing a male fetus before gestational day 40 or a female fetus before gestational day 90 was not homicide, doing so after these two respective days was. Still later, English common law coined the term "quickening" for Aristotle's and Aquinas's moment of ensoulment or animation. Abortion before quickening—the moment when the pregnant woman first feels movement in her womb—was not considered a crime at all, and abortion after quickening was considered a misdemeanor only.

Following England's lead, U.S. legal authorities put few restrictions on abortion until the 1840s or so. Reproductive matters were left to women's discretion, and pregnant women largely relied on midwives to help them terminate unwanted pregnancies. However, this arrangement abruptly ended in the middle of the nineteenth century when the U.S. birth rate dropped dramatically. Suddenly, reproductive matters were of public concern. Physicians in the newly constituted all-male American Medical

Association (AMA) noticed not only that midwives—some of them less medically skilled than they were—had cornered the market in obstetrics but also that the "wrong" kind of women were having abortions. Specifically, AMA members were troubled that native-born, Protestant, upper- and middle-class women were far more likely than immigrant, Catholic, lower- and working-class women to have abortions. They worried that soon "they"—the people with supposedly bad genes—would outnumber "us"—the people with supposedly good genes—and that something had to be done to stop this from happening.[3]

Because of their desire to regulate abortions for the reasons discussed above, the increasingly powerful AMA began to press legislators for strict pre-quickening as well as post-quickening abortion laws. When legislators asked physicians why they should change the legal *status quo*, physicians responded that gestation was a "continuous process" from the moment of conception onwards, and, therefore, that a day-old conceptus was no less a human being than a quickened fetus. So successful were physicians in their push for restrictive abortion laws that by 1910 every U.S. state prohibited abortion at any stage of gestation, making exceptions only for a limited range of abortions intended to save the very life of the pregnant woman.[4]

As one might suspect, restrictive abortion laws did not prevent abortions from being performed. Rather, such laws pushed abortions underground, where they were often performed in unsafe conditions by unskilled persons. It is estimated that in 1936 alone 500,000 underground abortions were performed in the United States and that in 1960 the number swelled to 1,200,000.[5] Alarmed by the high number of women who were turning up in emergency rooms subsequent to botched abortions, a new generation of progressive physicians began to press for reforms in abortion laws. In addition, newly formed feminist groups like the National Organization of Women (NOW) went further, demanding that abortion laws be repealed and not simply reformed. So successful were these 1960s physicians and feminists, that by 1968—5 years before the landmark abortion decision, *Roe v. Wade*—eighteen states had already passed quite permissive abortion laws.

II. ABORTION TYPES AND METHODS

Before addressing the ethical, legal, and social issues that emerge in today's abortion debate, it is important to understand the difference between a spontaneous abortion on the one hand and an induced abortion on the other. In addition, it is helpful to be familiar with a wide variety of abortion methods. Whereas some abortion methods are difficult to distinguish from contraceptives, others are clearly and obviously destructive of fetal life.

A. Abortion Types: Spontaneous Versus Induced

A **spontaneous abortion** or **miscarriage** occurs when the woman's body naturally rejects the fetus (the term I will ordinarily use throughout this chapter to denote human life throughout the gestational process). Spontaneous abortions end from 10% to 50% of all pregnancies.[6] Precisely because spontaneous abortions occur naturally, uncaused by human intervention, they are viewed as morally uncontroversial; however, depending on how late in the pregnancy the miscarriage occurs, and how much the child is wanted, parents may experience considerable grief when a pregnancy spontaneously ends in the fetus's death. Many hospitals now provide supportive services to parents mourning the loss of the child for whom they had hoped. Such bereavement services typically include rituals that resemble something akin to a private wake and burial for the miscarried fetus.

In contrast to a spontaneous abortion, an **induced abortion** is the product of deliberate human intervention or intention. Sometimes a woman seeks an abortion not because she does not want to be pregnant, but because she does not want to be pregnant with a particular kind of child—for example, one that will be born with a serious genetic disease, or one that is the "wrong" sex (that is, a female instead of a male or vice versa). This type of induced abortion is best referred to as a **selective abortion**. Another type of induced abortion is best referred to as a **therapeutic abortion**. Here the woman seeks the abortion not because she does not want to be pregnant, or pregnant with a particular kind of child, but because something is physically Babitha, to get meant right, the word physically needs to be inserted but because something is physically wrong with her. For example, she will almost certainly die if she continues the pregnancy, or her health will be severely compromised. Although some people classify abortions for reasons of rape or incest as therapeutic abortions, performed to save the mental health of the woman, it is probably more appropriate to view such abortions as selective abortions. The woman does not want a particular kind of child; namely, a child that is produced as the result of rape or incest. Finally, and far more typically, a woman may seek an abortion simply because she does not want to be pregnant now or at all. This type of induced abortion is best termed an **elective abortion**, and it is the kind of abortion to which most antiabortionists or pro-life activists are most opposed.

B. Abortion Methods

Before health care professionals began to assist women who wanted abortions, women either solicited help from other women, as we noted above, or self-aborted. Among the abortion methods some women used were wearing tight corsets, falling down intentionally, traumatizing the abdominal region, and ingesting lead, arsenic, phosphorous, apiol, and other toxic chemicals.[7] In addition, other women used abortion methods ranging from inserting coat hangers, knitting needles, and knives into the cervix to introducing dangerous soaps and pastes into the vagina and/or uterus.[8] Sometimes these primitive abortion methods succeeded without causing harm to the pregnant woman; often they did not. Fortunately, most women in the United States no longer self-abort or use clearly dangerous abortion methods. Instead they seek the services of trained health care professionals who select from a variety of generally safe surgical and chemical abortion methods.

1. Surgical Techniques for Abortion

Surgical abortion methods include vacuum aspiration (D&E), hysterontomy, hysterectomy, and the much debated, but rarely used, partial-birth abortion (D&X). Because late-term abortions are far more risky and controversial than early-term abortions, it is important to emphasize that, in the United States, most abortions are performed in the first trimester. That is, 90%–95% of abortions occur in the first 12 weeks of pregnancy; 5%–10% occur between 12 and 16 weeks; 4% between 16 and 20 weeks; and only 1.5% occur after 21 weeks.[9]

a. Vacuum Aspiration (D&E)

Introduced in the United States around 1967, **vacuum aspiration** or **dilation and evacuation (D&E)** is the most common form of surgical abortion for early-term pregnancies. The physician dilates the cervix and inserts a small plastic tube into the uterus to suction out the fetus. The procedure requires only local anesthesia, less than 20 minutes on the operating table, and a relatively short time in the recovery room afterwards. Complications are infrequent and most women tolerate its discomforts fairly well.

b. Hysterectomy and Hysterontomy

Hysterectomies and hysterontomies are major operations used for late-term abortions. A hysterontomy removes only the fetus from the woman's body, whereas a hysterectomy removes the woman's uterus as well. Health care professionals try to avoid these abortion methods for two reasons: (1) maternal complications often accompany them, and (2) a number of fetuses survive the procedures. Fetuses that survive an abortion procedure are given the same kind of care given to any live-born infant. As one can imagine, these live births are particularly traumatic both for the woman who wanted to terminate her pregnancy and for the health care professionals who tried to assist her. In addition, they often result in an infant who, because of its prematurity and relatively low birth weight, begins life with some significant health-related challenges.

c. Partial-Birth Abortions (D&X)

Used only in very late abortions and for very serious reasons, partial-birth abortion or dilation and extraction (D&X), which we will discuss at length later in this chapter, accounts for about 2,200 of the abortions performed annually in the United States.[10] The physician partially delivers the fetus, and then punctures the fetus's skull, suctions out the brain, and crushes the fetus's skull before completing the abortion procedure. Suffice it to say, that most health care professionals view partial-birth abortion as a method of last resort, relying on it only when there is no other way to safeguard the women's health and/or life.

2. Chemical Techniques for Abortion

Chemical techniques for abortion include the so-called emergency contraception pills, mifepristone (RU 486), and medical induction of uterine contractions by means of saline solution or prostaglandins. The oral methods are used early in the first trimester of pregnancy, whereas the uterine methods are used in the second trimester.

a. Emergency Contraception (EC)

Sometimes referred to as the morning-after pill, the emergency contraception (EC) method of abortion consists in taking a double dose of birth control pills within 72 hours of unprotected sex and then a second, single dose 12 hours later. Women with access to birth control pills and who know how emergency contraception works (it has not been adequately publicized until recently) can medicate themselves. In contrast, women who do not have a handy supply of birth control pills need to quickly find a health care professional willing to prescribe birth control pills for them. Because finding such a health care professional can be time consuming, advocates of family planning have lobbied for a form of emergency contraception called **Plan B** that would be available over the counter without a physician's prescription.

Oftentimes, advocates of family planning claim that because emergency contraception works either by preventing fertilization or by preventing implantation of the just-fertilized egg, it is not really an abortion method. However, opponents of abortion maintain that if emergency contraception destroys the fertilized egg, it is an abortion method and should not be untruthfully presented as a contraceptive method.[11] Largely because of the controversy between advocates of family planning on the one hand and opponents of abortion on the other, as well as concerns about teenage girls having easy access to emergency contraception (over one million teenage girls in the United States get pregnant each year),[12] the Food and Drug Administration (FDA) denied approval of over-the-counter sale of Plan B in 2003.[13]

b. RU-486 Mifepristone

RU-486 was developed by a French pharmaceutical company, Rousse 1-CLAF and has been used in France since 1988. It became available in the United States in September 2000 after a long and heated controversy between advocates of family planning and antiabortion lobbyists. Sometimes called the "abortion pill," RU-486, an antiprogestin which dislodges the fetus from the uterus, needs to be administered in the first 7 weeks of pregnancy.

An RU-486 abortion is a several-step procedure. First, the woman takes the pill. Two days later, she returns to the health care professionals who gave it to her. They inject her with mistroprostol, a contraction-inducing prostaglandin that helps her expel the fetus from her body in about 4 hours. During this period of time, the woman is monitored for hemorrhaging, or sent home to expel the fetus there. Two weeks later the woman returns to the health care professionals' office for a final checkup that usually goes well. Only about 2%–5% of women who use RU-486 fail to have a complete chemical abortion and require a surgical one instead.[14]

Interestingly, RU-486 has not proved to be very popular in the United States for at least four reasons. First, health care professionals who are morally opposed to abortion are no more likely to facilitate an RU-486 abortion than any other kind of abortion. Second, and just as importantly, health care professionals morally unopposed to abortion may still be unwilling to prescribe RU-486 to pregnant women. They fear being harassed by antiabortionists or losing their reputation and business. Apparently, such fears are not unjustified. In one recent case, for example, a physician gave RU-486 to an 18-year-old patient himself because his nursing staff refused to administer the drug to her. Later, one of his nurses resigned and soon word got around town that he was an "abortion doctor." The physician's minister started to pray publicly for his soul. Subsequently, the physician lost so many patients that his practice was seriously eroded.[15] Third, many women decide against RU-486 when they realize it is not an instant abortion that miraculously dissolves the fetus. On the contrary, many women experience an RU-486 abortion "like a miscarriage, where they have to confront the product of conception"[16] in the form of a large blood clot passed in the toilet. Fourth, and finally, many women decide against RU-486 because it typically costs more than a D&E and usually requires more time off from work than a D&E.

c. Saline Solution

Used between the 17th and 20th week of pregnancy, the saline solution method of abortion requires an injection of hypertonic saline (a solution more concentrated in salts than normal cellular fluid). The physician withdraws a small amount of amniotic fluid from the amniotic sac containing the fetus, and replaces it with a 20%–25% saline solution intended to kill the fetus within the uterus. Labor is induced, and the dead fetus is usually delivered in 24–72 hours.[17] Although a saline abortion is simpler and less expensive than most other *second*-trimester methods of abortion, it is still less safe and more expensive than most *first*-trimester methods of abortion. Moreover, because the woman actually goes through labor and delivery, she may be traumatized severely.

d. Prostaglandins

Currently, physicians use either an intra-amniotic injection or a vaginal suppository to induce a second-trimester prostaglandin abortion which, as in a saline abortion, triggers labor and delivery fairly rapidly. The negative side effects of a prostaglandin abortion include possible severe gastrointestinal symptoms and cervical lacerations. In addition, the woman is, as in the saline-solution method of abortion, faced with the physical and emotional difficulty of enduring the same labor and delivery process she would go through, were her aim to give birth to a live infant. Even more problematically, not only the pregnant woman but also the health care professional may be faced with the unexpected birth of a live infant. If the fetus is farther along in the gestational process than the health care professional estimated, it may survive the abortion procedure because prostaglandins do not have the same deadly effects on the fetus as saline solution does.

III. ETHICAL ISSUES IN ABORTION

In the first 15 years after the 1973 legalization of abortion in the United States, the number of abortions rose from 760,000 to a peak of 1,600,000 in 1988. Since then the number of abortions has remained relatively constant until recently when it has begun to decline. Among the reasons cited for the late 1990s and early 2000s drop in U.S. abortion rates are (1) better sex education; (2) more accessible and effective contraceptives; (3) increased lack of access to abortion services either because no abortion provider is available and/or because of lack of funding; (4) greater acceptance of single mothers; (5) higher rates of infertility; and (6) a less favorable attitude toward using abortion as a means of birth control.[18] Still, the total number of abortions performed in the United States remains relatively high, and the U.S. population continues to debate the morality of abortion. Although the details of the abortion debate have varied throughout the years, the two issues that continue to preoccupy most people for whom abortion is an issue are (1) the moral status of the fetus and (2) the needs, interests, and rights of the pregnant woman.

A. The Moral Status of the Fetus

The moral status of the fetus raises a fundamental question: Is the fetus a fully human person? According to philosopher Frederick Jaffee, this answer to this question largely depends on how it is phrased. If we ask, "When during gestation does human life begin?" our conclusions about abortion are likely to be different than if we ask instead, "When does a fetus become a person who merits protection equal to or greater than the woman in whose body it is located and without whose body it would cease to exist?"[19] Jaffe notes that the choice between these two ways of phrasing the abortion question is value-laden. Most people are much more concerned about killing a human person than about ending a human life that is not yet a person. Thus, it is not surprising that there are at least three positions on the moral status of the fetus: (1) the extreme conservative position; (2) the extreme liberal position; and (3) the moderate position(s).

1. The Extreme Conservative Position on Personhood

As far as extreme conservatives are concerned, there is no difference between human life on the one hand and human personhood on the other. In order to defend their view that a human fetus is, from the moment of conception onward, the moral equivalent of a human adult, extreme conservatives note that virtually everyone agrees that a newborn infant is a person. They then add the point that working backward in time from the moment of birth to the moment of fertilization, there is no magic moment at which a human life suddenly became a human person. Fetal development, like child development, is simply the gradual and continuous development of a human person who comes into existence at the moment of conception and is born 9 months later.

The extreme conservative position on personhood has serious moral and legal consequences. If developing members of the human species are persons from the moment of their conception onward, and if it is wrong to kill a person without adequate justification, then it is wrong to abort a fetus.

Possible exceptions for the moral rule against killing a fetus would be to save the mother's very life or to spare her the grave psychological trauma associated with bringing to term a child conceived as the result of an act of rape or incest; however, most extreme conservatives do not permit even these exceptions to the moral rule against killing the fetus. They argue that because the fetus is not an aggressor trying to kill the woman, but simply an innocent victim of the same unfortunate circumstances in which she finds herself, the woman is not justified to kill her fetus in self-defense. In addition, extreme conservatives insist that even though a victim of rape or incest may find it extremely difficult to carry her pregnancy to term—indeed, the process may result in her mental breakdown—her fetus is no less a person than the fetus of a child conceived as the result of consensual sexual intercourse, and therefore it is no less wrong to kill it.

2. The Extreme Liberal Position on Personhood Extreme

In contrast to extreme conservatives, extreme liberals claim that the fetus is merely a part of the woman's body until it is removed from it. In other words, until the moment of birth or sometime thereafter—perhaps as late as age two—the fetus/infant does not become a human person. Whatever the fetus is while it is in a woman's body, it is not the kind of entity that manifests consciousness, reasoning, self-determined activity, the ability to communicate with others, and the presence of a concept of self.

Like its extreme conservative counterpart, the extreme liberal view on personhood has dramatic moral and legal consequences. If, at all stages of its development, the fetus is merely a part of the woman's body, and if the woman has the right to control what happens to her body, then all abortions are justified. Morally, there would seem to be no difference between aborting a first-trimester fetus because the woman cannot sustain a life-imperiling pregnancy on the one hand and aborting a third-trimester fetus because the woman wants to fit into a tiny bikini bathing suit on the other. If the only right at stake is the woman's right to physical autonomy or bodily integrity, then abortion on demand is her moral as well as legal right.

3. Moderate Positions on Personhood

Seeking a middle-of-the-road position on abortion, moderates maintain that a 1-day-old fertilized egg is not a person in the same way a 40-year-old adult or even a 1-day old infant is. They also maintain that a fetus, especially a third-trimester one, is not simply part of a woman's body in the way her kidney is. Because they value both fetal and maternal rights, moderates typically permit a wide range of economically-, socially-, psychologically-, and/or personally motivated early abortions as well as all medically necessary abortions, late as well as early.

In their attempt to further specify why some abortions (for example, early ones) are more justifiable than others, moderates claim that **personhood** should be linked to some identifiable point between conception and birth. **Viability** is one of the points most frequently mentioned as the morally relevant magic moment at which a human life becomes a human person. But viability is not an entirely reliable index of personhood for at least two reasons. First, it is not clear that the ability to exist independently of all other persons' bodies is the characteristic that magically transforms a human life into a human person. At most, such an ability is a necessary condition of personhood, and perhaps not even that. Conjoined twins are regarded as two separate persons; yet, if surgery is out of the question, each one of their lives is dependent on the other's body. Second, and perhaps more importantly, viability has already fallen from 28 weeks to 24 weeks due to a variety of technological and medical advances,[20] and may fall much lower if researchers develop incubators or artificial placenta in which human fetuses can be sustained *ex utero* no matter how prematurely they are born.

Given, then, that viability is such an unstable criterion for personhood, some moderates have expressed the view that personhood does not have anything to do with such *accidental* matters as the fetus's location or its ability to live independently, but with such *essential* matters as whether the fetus is or is not a unique individual with the capacity for rationality. Among these moderates are Thomas A. Shannon and Allan B. Wolter, O.F.M. who claim that a fertilized egg must undergo three processes before it becomes a full-fledged person. First, the fertilized egg has to become genetically distinct; that is, it must add to the genetic information within its chromosomes such supplementary genetic information as is found in the maternal mitochondria and in the maternal or paternal genetic messages conveyed through RNA or protein signs.[21] Next, the genetically distinct fertilized egg, now about a week old and implanted in the womb, has to become a unique individual, singular rather than plural in number.[22] This occurs around the third week of embryonic development during a stage called gastrulation, after which the cells of the genetically distinct fertilized egg are no longer totipotent (that is, each capable of forming an entire organism on its own).[23] Finally, the genetically distinct, uniquely individual fertilized egg has to develop the capacity for rationality, a capacity that will emerge only when its nervous system is integrated enough to support the possibility of rational activity. Such integration can be marked at one of two points: (1) at organogenesis, the appearance of all major systems of the body occurring around week 8 of gestation or (2) at the development of the thalamus, which permits the full integration of the nervous system, occurring around week 20 of gestation.

Depending on whether a moderate views organogenesis or the development of the thalamus as the moment after which a genetically distinct, uniquely individual fertilized egg attains the capacity for rationality and therefore personhood, he or she will permit morally a lesser or greater range of abortions. If brain birth is thought to occur at 8 weeks, then only first-trimester abortions will be viewed as permissible. But if brain birth is thought to occur at 20 weeks, then most second-trimester as well as first-trimester abortions will be viewed as permissible. Because 91% of abortions take place before the 12th week of pregnancy, the second of these two views of personhood would arguably permit the vast majority of abortions.[24]

B. The Needs, Interests, and Rights of Pregnant Women

The abortion debate is about not only the moral status of the fetus but also the needs, interests, and rights of pregnant women. Women are not simply containers for fetuses. On the contrary, they are persons just as much as, if not more than, fetuses. Thus, one of the key questions to ask in the abortion debate is whether it "can . . . be moral, under any circumstances, to make a women bear a child against her will?"[25]

1. Right to Bodily Integrity

In reflecting on the issue of abortion, many commentators have noted that the fetus's purported **right to life** must be weighed against the pregnant woman's **right to bodily integrity** and **privacy**. Among the most forceful defenders of pregnant women's rights is philosopher Judith Jarvis Thomson. She claims "that the mother and the unborn child are not like two tenants in a small house which has, by an unfortunate mistake, been rented to both: the mother owns the house."[26] Thomson's point is that possessing the right to life does not automatically give one person the right to use another person's body in order to keep on living. For instance, a man in renal failure who needs dialysis in order to survive has no right to take a woman by force and plug himself into her so that he can use her kidneys as long as he needs them. Analogously, the fetus has no right to use the body of its mother, even if it cannot survive outside of it.[27]

Thomson admits that her analogy is imperfect. It fits cases of unwanted pregnancy after rape or the use of faulty contraceptives far better than cases of unwanted pregnancy after voluntary intercourse. If a woman permits a man in renal failure to use her kidneys for a specified number of months, during which time a strong relationship develops between them, she may come to owe that man continuing access to her body even though he has no strict right to use her body. A sudden decision on her part to break a relationship she willingly initiated would seem *prima facie* wrong. Analogously, if a woman becomes pregnant because she wants to have a child, it would seem *prima facie* wrong for her to abort the fetus—especially if she has been hosting it for several months.[28]

2. *Right to Privacy*

Assuming that Thomson is correct—that the right to life does not include the right to use someone else's body to support that life—and even assuming (as Thomson does not) that *all fetal extractions* are therefore justifiable, unnecessary *fetal extinctions* would not also be justified. Nevertheless, when a woman seeks an abortion, **fetal extinction** rather than **fetal extraction** is her goal. She simply does not want to procreate—to bring another life into the world—at that time. In this connection, it would seem that the central right for women seeking an abortion is the right to privacy (to procreate or not) rather than merely the right to bodily integrity. In other words, were an artificial womb developed, most women would probably not be content to have their unwanted fetus transferred from their womb into it. Fetal extraction would not relieve them of the burden of being biological mothers—that is, of knowing that somewhere in the world at large exists a person they chose not to rear, and who might feel rejected because of this fact.

3. *Right to a Full Human Life*

Departing from arguments that base women's right to have an abortion on women's more fundamental rights to bodily integrity and privacy, philosopher Alison Jaggar roots women's right to have an abortion on every person's "right to a full human life and to whatever means are necessary to achieve this,"[29] and on the principle that "decisions should be made by those, and only by those, who are importantly affected by them."[30] Jaggar reasons that unless an individual or a group is prepared to rear to adulthood the fetus they save from abortion, he, she, or they have no moral grounds for compelling a woman to continue a pregnancy she wishes to terminate. Because she is the one who probably will have the responsibility to rear the infant to adulthood if it is born, the decision to have or not to have the infant should be hers.

But what about the father, should he not have some say in the abortion decision? What if he is willing to raise the infant to adulthood? To questions such as these, Jaggar responds that we must focus not on the individual man who wants to have his baby, but on the fact that pregnancy generally affects women in ways that it cannot possibly affect men, and also on the fact that, in the United States and most other nations, motherhood is generally a more burdensome institution than fatherhood. As Jaggar explains:

> Biology, law, and social conditioning work together to ensure that most women's lives are totally changed as the result of the birth of a child while men can choose how much they wish to be involved. It is for this reason that the

potential mother rather than the potential father should have the ultimate responsibility for deciding whether or not an abortion should be performed. If conventions regarding the degree of parental responsibility assumed by the mother and by the father were to change or if the law prescribing paternal child support were to be enforced more rigorously, then perhaps the father should be required to share with the mother in making the decision. (He could never take over the decision completely, of course, because it is not his body which is involved). But in the present social situation, the right of the woman to decide if she should abort is not limited by any right of the father.[31]

Jaggar further notes that if the father has no right to interfere with a woman's decision to abort, then certainly members of the public at large have no right to interfere with her decision, because they will play no role in rearing the child they would force her to have.

IV. LEGAL ISSUES IN ABORTION

As we noted in the introduction to this chapter, even before the U.S. Supreme Court ruled that states may not prohibit all abortions, many states already had moved in the direction of permissive abortion laws. For example, in the mid-1960s, Colorado, North Carolina, and California swiftly enacted into law the American Law Institute's (ALI) 1962 proposal that all U.S. states decriminalize abortions performed (1) to save the life or to preserve the health of the woman; (2) to terminate a pregnancy due to rape or incest; or (3) to avoid the birth of a severely defective fetus.[32] In addition, around the same time, New York passed a law permitting abortions on demand during the first and second trimesters of pregnancy.[33] As a result of variations in states' laws, some women had access to abortions, whereas others did not. Thus, the time seemed ripe to move the abortion issue out of the states' total control and partly into the hands of the Federal Government, particularly the U.S. Supreme Court.

A. *Roe v. Wade*

The case that determined the constitutionality or unconstitutionality of a variety of state abortion laws was *Roe v. Wade* (1973). In a seven-to-two decision, the U.S. Supreme Court ruled that the right to privacy entails that:

1. During the first trimester of pregnancy, states may not enact laws to interfere with a woman's and physician's abortion decision.
2. During the second trimester of pregnancy, states may enact laws, but only in such instances as to preserve and protect maternal health.
3. During the third trimester of pregnancy, states may enact laws to protect the viable fetus, but only if such laws make exceptions for those instances in which the woman's life or health (physical or mental) are at risk.

4. States may not enact laws requiring all abortions to be performed in accredited hospitals, or to be approved by hospital committees or a second medical opinion, or to be performed only on state residents.[34]

For all practical purposes, it seemed that U.S. women had won the right to abortion on demand during the first and second trimesters of pregnancy.

B. Post-*Roe v. Wade* Abortion Legislation

Because many opponents of abortion were outraged by the *Roe v. Wade* decision, they sought ways to weaken its impact. They lobbied for (1) public-funding restrictions on abortion procedures; (2) third-party consent or notification requirements for abortion; and (3) strict regulations for abortion providers. Although such lobbying efforts were not entirely successful, by no means were they a complete failure.

1. *Public-Funding restrictions*

Opponents of abortion had some of their first successes undermining *Roe v. Wade* by persuading many state legislatures to fund only *medically necessary* abortions for women on Medicaid, the publicly funded health care insurance program for poor people. Advocates of abortion vociferously objected to such legislation for two basic reasons. First, in their estimation, such legislation discriminated against poor women, who unlike rich women could not pay out-of-pocket for wanted, *medically unnecessary*, purely elective abortions. Second, the term *medically necessary* is subject to a wide variety of interpretations. Whereas opponents of elective abortion may limit *medically necessary* abortions to those performed to save a pregnant woman's very life, advocates of elective abortion may classify any one of the following reasons as reason enough for a *medically necessary* abortion: (1) physical reasons such as phlebitis, varicose veins, cancer, diabetes, myoma of the uterus, urinary tract infections, intrauterine device in utero, ulcerative colitis, previous cesarean sections, anemia, malnutrition, hyperemesis, and obesity; (2) psychological reasons such as stress; (3) humane reasons such as nonreported pregnancies due to rape or incest; (4) age reasons; (5) therapeutic reasons such as fetal abnormality; and (6) emotional reasons.[35]

Despite all their efforts, however, advocates of public funds for *medically unnecessary* abortions lost their day in court. In *Maher v. Roe* (1977),[36] *Beal v. Roe* (1977),[37] and *Harris v. McRae* (1980),[38] the U.S. Supreme Court ruled that states have no constitutional obligation to fund *medically unnecessary* abortions. Currently, only 15 states fund *medically unnecessary* abortions. As these states see it, it is less costly for them to fund an elective abortion for a woman on Medicaid than to subsidize the basic needs (food, clothing, and shelter) of the child she would otherwise bring into the world. The rest of the states fund only abortions that are necessary to save pregnant women's very lives and/or that terminate a pregnancy due to rape or incest.[39]

2. *Consent and Notification Provisions*

Another way opponents of abortion sought to blunt the full impact of the *Roe v. Wade* case was through the so-called third-party consent or notification provisions, which permit the intervention either of parents or spouses into the abortion decision. On the one hand, proponents of this type of legislation argued that since the abortion decision is so difficult to make, it is in the best interests of women to involve their parents or husbands in the process. On the other hand, opponents of the same legislation counterargued that parents and spouses do not always have the same interests as their daughters and wives do. Specifically, not every parent is fully supportive of a child and not every husband is totally in agreement with his wife's values and decisions.

In cases such as *Planned Parenthood of Central Missouri v. DanForth* (1976),[40] the U.S. Supreme Court made it clear that neither *spousal notification* nor *spousal consent* was necessary for abortion even if the woman's spouse was the biological father of the fetus. However, the U.S. Supreme Court has upheld both *parental consent* and *parental notification* laws, but with the proviso that states provide a judicial bypass procedure for minors unable or unwilling to involve their parents. The court has justified its ruling in cases such as *Bellotti v. Baird* (1979),[41] *H.L. v. Matheson* (1980),[42] and *Hodgson v. Minnesota* (1990)[43] largely on the grounds that, unlike adults, minors generally are not capable of giving full informed consent to an abortion and need the help of their parents to make such a major decision. Currently, thirty-six states have *parental consent* and/or *notification laws*, although only twenty-five enforce them. In all, thirteen other states have no such laws. One state, Connecticut, also requires minors seeking abortion to receive counseling that includes a parent–child discussion about abortion.[44] Although proponents of consent and notification laws describe them as in women's best interest, opponents view these measures as an attempt to decrease women's access to abortion, starting with the most vulnerable participants—young and frightened teenagers and married women who fear angering, disappointing, or otherwise alienating their boyfriends or husbands.

3. *Restrictions on Abortion Providers and Procedures*

Opponents of abortion also have had some success limiting women's abortion rights by imposing ever more strict regulations on abortion providers. In particular, they had tried to use the informed consent process as an opportunity to disseminate pro-life views. They have also attempted, with mixed success, to regulate the place, time, and method of abortion. Finally, they have sought to intimidate women who want abortions and health care professionals who provide them in a variety of ways, ranging from heckling and name-calling to bombing clinics and shooting physicians in cold blood.

a. Informed Consent

Opponents of abortion initially focused on ways to make the informed consent process for abortions more burdensome. They demanded that health care professionals provide women seeking abortions with material about the ways in which having an abortion could conceivably harm them and/or their fetus. For example, in Ohio, opponents of abortion lobbied for legislation that required physicians to provide their patients with certain information, including literature that declares "the unborn child is a human life from the moment of conception."[45] The legislation also required women to consider this information for 24 hours before going through with the abortion.[46] Similarly, in Pennsylvania opponents of abortion lobbied for legislation requiring abortion providers to give to their patients state-supplied printed materials about the anatomical and physiological characteristics of the fetus throughout its development, the risks of having an abortion, and alternatives to abortion.[47] Significantly, opponents of abortion in Ohio and Pennsylvania won the day in their respective states. The legislation they favored was passed. However, Ohio's and Pennsylvania's informed consent laws for abortion were ruled unconstitutional by the U.S. Supreme Court. In *City of Akron v. Akron Center for Reproductive Health* (1983),[48] the Court ruled that a state must remain neutral with regard to a woman's choice between childbirth and abortion. In other words, a state may not provide women with information biased either in the direction of birth or in the direction of abortion. In the related case of *Thornburgh v. American College of Obstetricians and Gynecologists* (1986),[49] the Court underscored this point. Specifically, Justice Blackmun wrote that, far from helping a woman make an autonomous decision about whether to have an abortion, counseling biased in the direction of birth serves only to "confuse and punish" women considering abortion.

In recent years, however, the U.S. Supreme Court has reconsidered its support of neutral abortion counseling only. In *Planned Parenthood of Southeastern Pennsylvania v. Casey* (1992),[50] for example, the Court ruled that a state may "enact persuasive measures which favor childbirth over abortion,"[51] provided that those measures do not impose an "undue burden"[52] on a woman's right to choose abortion. Specifically, a state may, if it chooses, require a woman who wants an abortion to receive from the physician state-supplied information about the developmental stages of fetal life; the alternatives to abortion; the availability of public assistance for medical expenses associated with prenatal care, delivery, and neonatal care; and the legal obligations of the father of the child to assist in the support of her child. According to the Court, women seeking abortions do not have a right *not* to hear information about abortion that may trouble or disturb them in some way or another. No one who lives in a pluralistic, free society should expect to hear only the kind of information that comforts and consoles them.

To be sure, opponents of special informed consent laws for abortion do not agree with the *Casey* decision. They console themselves with the fact that even though states now will be able to disseminate more pro-life material at publicly funded abortion clinics, the federal government no longer will be able, as it was until quite recently, to prohibit the distribution and discussion of pro-choice material at federally funded family planning clinics that do not offer abortion services. Back in 1984, then President Ronald Reagan issued an order, often referred to as the "gag rule," which forbade anyone working in a federally funded family planning clinic to discuss with patients the possibility of having an abortion. The rule, which was upheld by the U.S. Supreme Court in *Rust v. Sullivan* (1991),[53] was subsequently rescinded by President William Clinton in a 1993 executive order. He said that the **gag rule** undermined both the doctrine of informed consent and the health care professional–patient relationship.[54] Almost immediately after his election in 2001, President George W. Bush reincarnated the gag rule, this time abroad, making family planning funds in developing nations contingent upon agreements not to promote abortion. Defenders of women's rights have decried this global gag rule as a "cruel, extremist policy" that has resulted in "more unintended pregnancies, more unsafe abortions, and more maternal and child deaths" in developing nations than before its promulgation.[55]

b. Place of Abortion

In addition to their efforts to impose special informed-consent requirements on abortion providers, opponents of abortion have sought to limit the number of places providing abortions. In the past, courts have ruled that *private*, sectarian hospitals may refuse to offer abortion services for reasons of institutional conscience. More recently, courts have also ruled that *public* hospitals, clinics, or other tax-supported health care facilities are under no constitutional requirement to perform *elective* abortions. For example, in *Webster v. Reproductive Health Services* (1989),[56] the U.S. Supreme Court upheld a Missouri law that restricted abortion in the following three ways:

1. Public employees, including physicians and nurses, are forbidden to perform an abortion, except when necessary to save a woman's life.
2. Public hospitals, clinics, or other tax-supported facilities cannot be used to perform abortions not necessary to save a woman's life, even if no public funds are involved.

3. Physicians are required to perform tests to determine the viability of a fetus, if they have reason to believe the woman has been pregnant for at least 20 weeks.[57]

Prevented by the *Webster* ruling from seeking an elective abortion at a public hospital or clinic, a Missouri woman may still seek an elective abortion at a private hospital or clinic; however, since many private hospitals and clinics receive public money or have contractual arrangements with state or local governments, they might also fall under the *Webster* ruling.

Further limiting the number of places that may offer abortions are statutes that impose certain standards of care on abortion providers. Although the U.S. Supreme Court ruled in *Turnock v. Ragsdale* (1992)[58] that a state may not require abortion clinics to maintain the same standards as full-care hospitals, a state may still set quite high standards of care for abortion clinics. Depending on how high these standards are set, however, a significant number of abortion clinics may have to close their doors.

c. Time of Abortion

In addition to regulating the place of abortion, opponents of abortion have attempted to regulate the time of abortion. Specifically, they have sought to impose a waiting period between the signing of an abortion consent form and the abortion itself. At first, the U.S. Supreme Court seemed to disfavor waiting periods,[59] but in more recent years, most notably in *Planned Parenthood v. Casey* (1992),[60] the Court ruled as constitutional waiting periods that do not "unduly burden" women. Specifically, it maintained that it is not unreasonable for a state to ask a woman seeking an abortion to wait 24 hours between the time she requests an abortion and the time she actually has it.[61]

To be sure, pro-choice advocates have claimed in reaction to the *Casey* case that for many women, particularly poor women, a 24-hour waiting period does constitute an undue burden. Specifically, lawyer Janet Benshoof has observed that at least in the state of Pennsylvania, in which the *Casey* case originated:

> ... most women ... will have to endure forty-eight-hour to two-week delays before they can obtain the health care they seek. Since women will be forced to travel to clinics twice, and many will have to pay for accommodations, perhaps lose two days of wages, and pay for child care, this requirement will effectively preclude many low-income women and women living in rural areas from obtaining abortions. Among American women seeking abortions, twenty-seven percent must travel at least eighty kilometers to reach a provider, eighteen percent travel between eighty and 160 kilometers, and nine percent travel more than 160 kilometers.[62]

Other opponents of waiting periods add that even if a woman lives close to an abortion clinic, it is unlikely she will be well served by being forced to reconsider a decision she has probably had a very difficult time making. If society's goal is truly to protect the best interests of women and not simply to make women feel guilty about their decision to abort, then abortion providers should be permitted to use the same kind of informed-consent procedures for an abortion that they use for other chemical or surgical procedures. In addition, they should be permitted to schedule an abortion procedure at a time that is mutually convenient for them and their patient.

d. Method of Abortion

Although opponents of abortion have had little success regulating the method of abortion in the past, recent trends indicate increased support for regulating the method of abortion used for viable fetuses. As we noted above, abortion providers typically use one of three abortion procedures in the second and third trimester of pregnancy: hysterectomy, the prostaglandin method, or the saline solution method. Less frequently, and usually toward the end of the third trimester, they may elect to use the method of intact dilation and extraction, often referred to as "partial-birth" abortion. Whereas hysterectomy and the prostaglandin method may result in the birth of a live fetus, the saline solution method, properly performed, and the partial-birth method ensure the death of the fetus.

Opponents of abortion claim that even if a woman has a right to a safe abortion, she does not necessarily have a right to an entirely effective abortion; that is, an abortion that necessarily results in the death of the fetus. In particular, opponents of abortion claim that if a fetus is clearly viable, it is particularly wrong to kill it when it has partially or totally emerged from its mother's womb. Supporters of women's procreative rights respond that the method of abortion to use is a matter for abortion providers to determine and, more controversially, that women seeking abortions are entitled to fetal extinction as well as to fetal extraction.

Significantly, **partial-birth abortion**, which we briefly described earlier in this chapter, has created heated debate inside as well as outside the medical community. In 1997, the American Medical Association (AMA) issued a report in which it was stated that partial-birth abortion methods may not be as safe as other late third-trimester methods of abortion, and that partial-birth abortions may cause pain to the fetus.[63] Agreeing with the AMA that partial-birth abortion is rarely, if ever, medically indicated, the American College of Obstetricians and Gynecologists (ACOG) nonetheless recommended that the procedure not be legally banned. The ACOG based its recommendation on the view that all abortion decisions should be made within the context of the patient–physician relationship, and there may be instances in which a partial-birth abortion is indeed necessary to save the mother's life.[64] In 2003, President George Bush signed into law the Partial Birth Abortion

Ban Act. One of the most controversial features of the legislation is that it permits a partial-birth abortion only if the woman's very life is at stake. Sparing the woman a substantial risk to her health is not enough to justify an exception to the no-partial-birth abortion ban. Critics of the new legislation speculate it will not be able to withstand constitutional scrutiny. As they see it, women's right to bodily integrity is sufficiently strong to permit the use of whatever abortion technique health care professionals deem necessary to safeguard their patients' health. At present the implementation of the Partial Birth Abortion Ban Act has been delayed because at least three states—New York, California, and Nebraska—have ruled it unconstitutional.[65]

e. Persuasive Words, Coercive Tactics, and Outright Violence

A final way antiabortionists seek to limit abortions is by protesting against them in violent as well as in nonviolent ways. Many abortion seekers are verbally harassed or even physically assaulted by antiabortionists. Abortion clinics in the United States are routinely vandalized; and over a hundred of them have been burned or bombed since the late 1970s. In some instances, clinic employees have been seriously harmed or even killed. In addition, three U.S. physicians were murdered between 1993 and 1998 solely because they performed abortions.[66] The first of these physicians, Dr. David Gunn, was shot in 1993 after leaving a Florida abortion clinic where he performed abortions once a week. Before being murdered, Dr. Gunn's picture had been posted on the kind of "WANTED" signs F.B.I. agents use to catch criminals and terrorists. The second physician, Dr. John Britton, was also shot at a Florida abortion clinic. Because his murderer, a former minister, shot Dr. Britton in the head, Dr. Britton's bulletproof vest provided him no protection. The third physician, Dr. Barnett Slepian, was shot and killed in the kitchen of his New York residence in front of his wife and children.[67] Appropriately, the penalties for these crimes generally have been severe, including an execution and several life sentences.[68]

In recent years, the Court has attempted to regulate the behavior of antiabortionists who protest at clinics, target abortion providers for murder, and/or harass women seeking abortion. Specifically, in *Madsen v. Women's Health Center* (1998),[69] the U.S. Supreme Court upheld most of a Florida injunction that created a 36-foot buffer zone outside of a reproductive health clinic, and prohibited antiabortionists from protesting so loudly that they could be heard inside the clinic during working hours; however, the Court invalidated other provisions of the Florida injunction on the grounds that they were unnecessary to serve the government's interest in letting citizens go about their business. Among these provisions was one that created a 300-foot ban on picketing outside the residences of clinic workers. In a similar case, *Schenck v. Pro-Choice Network* (1997),[70] the Court upheld most of a New York State buffer-zone injunction, including its provision allowing only two sidewalk counselors at a time to enter a fixed 15-foot buffer zone to talk to women in a nonthreatening way, but requiring them to "cease and desist" and "exit the zone if asked to do so."[71] Finally, in *Hill v. Colorado* (2000),[72] the Court upheld the constitutionality of a 100-foot "zone of separation." Abortion protesters are not permitted to knowingly approach within 8 feet of a nonconsenting person for the purpose of disseminating antiabortion materials or expressing antiabortion sentiments. Their free speech is limited in a small way so that citizens may have "unimpeded access" to health care facilities.

IV. CONCLUSION

Despite the intensity of antiabortion activity that ranges from legislative and judicial initiatives to harassing abortion seekers, bombing abortion clinics, and murdering abortion providers, a 1998 New York Times/CBS News poll revealed that 61% of Americans support unrestricted abortion during the first trimester, 15% during the second trimester, and 7% during the third trimester.[73] Poll results such as this one suggest that most Americans disfavor highly restrictive abortion laws, such as the ones in the Arab world, Latin America, Central Asia, and sub-Saharan Africa. For example, in Argentina, Kenya, Pakistan, Peru, Saudi Arabia, Spain, and Thailand, abortion is permitted only if the pregnancy is the result of rape or incest, the fetus is significantly defective, or the woman's life or health is at serious risk; in Brazil, it is permitted only in the case of rape or incest or to save the woman's life; and in Indonesia, Nigeria, the Philippines, and Somalia, it is permitted only to save the woman's life.[74] Likewise most Americans disfavor the highly permissive abortion laws that have been operative in Russia for years. In Russia, the standard mode of birth control is abortion. The average Russian woman will have four abortions in her reproductive years.[75] Americans do not like to see either women's interests in privacy and bodily integrity or fetuses' interests in life systematically ignored. On the contrary, most Americans want what is best for both women and fetuses and are self-described "middle-of-the-roaders."

Developing a workable middle-of-the-road policy on abortion might begin with the realization that, whether we are **pro-choice** (a term frequently used for people who espouse permissive abortion policies) or **pro-life** (a term frequently used for people who espouse restrictive abortion policies), most of us recognize that living successfully in a pluralistic society requires continual compromises, negotiations, and discussions on our part. Certainly, we can all agree that one way to de-escalate the abortion debate is to reduce women's need for abortions. Generous public and private monies should be available to women who wish to continue their pregnancies but feel unable to do so for any number of reasons. In this connection, philosopher Alison Jaggar has stressed:

> . . . [a] real choice about abortion requires that a woman should be able to opt to have her child, as well as to abort it. This means that the full right to life of the child must be guaranteed either by community aid to the mother who wishes to raise it by herself, or by the provision of alternative arrangements that do not put the child who is not raised by its own mother at any significant disadvantage.[76]

In addition, safe, effective, and affordable contraceptives should be made easily accessible to all adult women and adolescent girls who wish to use them. Indeed, there is considerable evidence for the view that better and more accessible contraceptives as well as more emphasis on sex education, abstinence and slogans like "Not me, Not Now" have already helped reduce the number of abortions in the United States.[77]

To be sure, because no program of contraception is likely to be anywhere near 100% effective, the abortion option will need to be available for the foreseeable future. Rethinking the *Roe v. Wade* ruling for the new millennium might begin with a move to make abortions before the 20th week of pregnancy not only accessible and affordable but acceptable. In particular, obstetricians and gynecologists should be encouraged to prescribe RU-486 and/or morning-after pills to their patients, and even to perform first-trimester surgical abortions in their offices, provided they have the proper training, staff, and equipment to do so. At present, only 3.8% of abortions are done in physician's offices.[78] The rest are done either in hospitals (10.1%) or in clinics (86.1%).[79] Moreover, many medical schools fail to teach abortion procedures or do so in a perfunctory manner.[80] On the whole, physicians want little, if anything, to do with abortion. Sometimes their reasons for avoiding abortions are personal. They themselves are opposed morally to abortion. But often their main reason for opting out of the "abortion business" is that they fear social disapproval, which, as we have noted, can include anything from lost income to death. No wonder, then, that in some areas of the United States, women cannot find an abortion provider.

In exchange for the permissive, non-stigmatizing, early-abortion policy articulated above, a somewhat more restrictive policy for abortions after 20 weeks might be in order. Although abortions after this point would still be permitted for *therapeutic* reasons (for example, when the continuation of the pregnancy endangers the woman's life or health, or when there is a strong possibility that the unborn child is suffering from a serious disease or condition considered incurable at the time of diagnosis), abortions would not be permitted for *nontherapeutic* reasons (for example, when a healthy woman simply decides late in her pregnancy that she does not want to be a mother after all). In addition, partial-birth abortions would not be permitted unless there was *no other way* to save the life or preserve the health of the woman.

Admittedly, it may not be possible to achieve the kind of consensus on abortion described above. But failure to craft an abortion policy that everyone is willing to endorse does not mean that pro-choice advocates and pro-life advocates cannot better appreciate each other's goodness. Pro-choice advocates need to remember that the first "antiabortionists" were not politically motivated groups (and certainly not terrorists) but service groups who wanted to help unwed mothers. Currently, there are at least 3,000 emergency pregnancy centers in the United States, 20% of which offer not merely counseling and emergency funds to pregnant women but also hospital coverage, housing, job training, and postnatal care. Such services give disadvantaged women the choice to continue a pregnancy, a choice that is no less important than the choice to terminate a pregnancy. Likewise, pro-life advocates need to realize that their opponents are not selfish, heartless baby-killers. On the contrary, most pro-choice advocates take the abortion decision very seriously. As they see it, when a woman has an abortion, she is less likely to be thinking about her right to choose than about the life that, for a variety of reasons, she feels unready or unable to bring into the world. Really believing, and not just saying, that good people are on both sides of the abortion debate may be the necessary condition for successfully resolving the abortion debate once and for all.

Discussion Questions

1. How might the abortion debate change if men had abortions too?
2. Given the disparity in the two extremes of the abortion debate, how would you go about rethinking the issue in terms of gaining a consensus?
3. Would you ever recommend to someone that she have an abortion? If so, for what reason(s) would you do so? If not, why not?
4. Do you consider yourself "pro-choice," "Antiabortion," or "Pro-life"?
5. Which is the worst kind of abortion in your estimation? Which is the best?
6. Do you know a woman/girl who has had an abortion? Has her abortion changed your view of her? Why or why not?
7. Should men have more say in the abortion decision? Why or why not?
8. How would you teach the abortion issue in a medical school? Are there differences between a physician refusing to perform an abortion and a physician refusing to participate in assisted suicide?

Case Studies

1. Nancy is a 35-year-old married librarian with a daughter who is 7 years old. Earlier, at the age of 18, she had an abortion during the first months of pregnancy. Now, at the age of 35, she finds herself pregnant again.

She is advised that her amniocentesis and alpha feta protein markers indicate that her child may be at risk of Down's Syndrome. Nancy finds the decision to abort difficult because she feels differently about abortion having previously gone through one. Although she still believes that women have a right to have an abortion, she no longer feels that abortion is right for her.

a. Can Nancy be consistent in believing that abortion is morally permissible for women in general but not for herself at this time?

b. Should Nancy's counselor urge her to have an abortion?

c. Should the father of the child (her husband) have a say in Nancy's decision?

d. Nancy's counselor asked her whether it would be more difficult for her to terminate the pregnancy or raise the child with complications of Down's Syndrome. If you were in Nancy's position, would this question be the most important one for you? If so, why would it be important? If not, which question is most important for you?

e. If abortion is tolerated socially, should there be a limit on the number and/or type of abortion a woman has? For example, would it make a difference if Nancy is in the second trimester when she learns of the amniocentesis results? How would such limits on abortion be defined and enforced without violating personal privacy?

2. President George W. Bush recently signed a law that would fine physicians for performing partial-birth abortions (except in cases where the mother's life is threatened) and remove government funding from any clinics that participate in this practice. Advocates of this policy hail it as needed protection for the rights of the unborn. Critics note that this is the first step in a new attempt to roll back the *Roe v. Wade* decision by targeting health care professionals.

a. Discuss this law in terms of the rights of the fetus versus the rights of the woman versus the rights of the physicians and clinics.

b. Is this law morally justifiable from the point of view of either of the two extreme positions on abortion? If so, is there any way for the "winner" and "loser" to find common ground and create a different law that would result in their both being winners?

c. What kind of support should be available for those who support abortion? For those who oppose abortion? What restrictions, if any, should there be on funding abortions?

3. In December of 2003, the U.S. Congress began a debate on whether or not to allow RU-486, the "abortion pill," to be sold over the counter. As Gina Kolata reported in various columns for the *New York Times* (December 12, 2003; September 24, 2003; September 25, 2002; July 19, 1996), RU-486 is the first of two pills that must be taken in order to induce an early-term abortion. The second pill, which dilates the cervix, may cause bacterial infection in

some pregnant women. In the case of Holly Patterson, a bacterial infection resulted in her death. Opponents to abortion stress the health risks of RU-486, particularly bleeding and infection. Proponents of women's right to choose argue that RU-486 is relatively safe when used under proper guidance.

a. What ethical as opposed to medical concerns may antiabortion groups have about over-the-counter sales of RU-486?

b. Is an RU-486 abortion less ethically problematic than a partial-birth abortion? Provide precise reasons for your answer.

c. If you were a physician, would you favor over-the-counter sales of RU-486? Why or why not?

Endnotes

1. Jean Gray Platt et al. (eds.), "Special project: survey of abortion law," *Arizona State Law Journal*, 67 (1980): 78.

2. Jeffrey Reiman, *Abortion and the Ways We Value Human Life* (Lanham, MD: Rowman and Littlefield, 1999), p. 22.

3. Ibid., p. 29.

4. Ibid.

5. Ibid., p. 31.

6. Harold D. Swanson, *Human Reproduction: Biology and Social Change* (New York: Oxford University Press, 1974), p. 244.

7. Marlene Dixon, *The Future of Women* (San Francisco: Synthesis Publication, 1983), p. 129.

8. Daniel Callahan, *Abortion: Law, Choice, and Morality* (New York: Macmillan, 1972), p. 34.

9. Michael C. Brannigan and Judith A. Boss, *Healthcare Ethics in a Diverse Society* (Mountain View, CA: Mayfield Publishing Company, 2002), p. 75.

10. Debra Rosenberg, "Chipping at Roe," *Newsweek Magazine* (March 17, 2003): 41.

11. Phillip Stubblefield, "Self-administered emergency contraception—a second chance," *New England Journal of Medicine*, 339, no. 1 (July 2, 1998): 41–42.

12. Gregory E. Pence, *Classic Cases in Medical Ethics* (Boston: McGraw Hill, 2004), p. 148.

13. Eleanor B. Schwarz, "Plan B—the FDA and emergency contraception," *New England Journal of Medicine*, 351, no. 10 (September 2, 2004): 1031.

14. Alice Lake, "The new French pill," *McCall's Magazine* (March, 1990): 62.

15. Nancy Gibbs, "The FDA gives women a new abortion choice. But will they choose it? And will doctors be willing to take the heat?" *Time Magazine* (October 2, 2000), *www.cnn.com/ALLPOLITICS/time/2000/10/09/pill.html+Nancy+Gibbs+FDA+Gives+Women+New+Abortion+Choice&hl=en* [accessed October 7, 2004].

16. Ibid., p. 46.

17. Irwin W. Sherman and Vila G. Sherman, *Biology: A Human Approach*, 3rd ed. (New York: Oxford University Press, 1983), p. 205.

18. "Experts try to explain declining abortion rate," *CQ Researcher*, 44 (November 28, 1997): 1038.

19. Frederick S. Jaffee, "Enacting religious beliefs in a pluralistic society," *Hastings Center Report*, 8, no. 4 (August, 1978): 14.

20. Daniel Callahan, "How technology is refraining the abortion debate," *Hastings Center Report*, 16, no. 1 (February 1986): 34.

21. Thomas A. Shannon and Allan B. Wolter, "Reflections on the moral status of the pre-embryo," *Theological Studies*, 61 (1990): 621.

22. Ibid.

23. Bruce M. Carlson, *Patten's Foundations of Embryology*, 5th ed. (New York: McGraw Hill, 1988), p. 23: "Within the fertilized ovum lies the capability to form an entire organism. In many vertebrates the individual cells resulting from the first few division after fertilization retain this capability. In the jargon of embryology, such cells are described as totipotent. As development continues, the cells gradually lose the ability to form all the types of cells that are found in the adult body."

24. Karen Gervais and Steven Miles, *RU-486: New Issues in the American Abortion Debate* (Minneapolis: Center for Biomedical Ethics, 1990), p. 13.

25. Ellen Willis, "Putting women back into the abortion debate," *Village Voice* (July 16, 1985): 15.

26. Judith Jarvis Thomson, "A defense of abortion," in: Richard Wasserstrom (ed.), *Today's Moral Problems*, 3rd ed. (New York: MacMillan, 1985), p. 425.

27. Ibid., pp. 420–421.

28. Ibid., p. 426.

29. Alison Jaggar, "Abortion and a woman's right to decide," in: Carol C. Gould and Marx W. Wartofsky (eds.), *Woman and Philosophy: Toward a Theory of Liberation* (New York: Putnam's, 1976), pp. 352–353.

30. Ibid.

31. Ibid, p. 353.

32. Dennis Henesi, "How debate over abortion evolved with changes in science and society," *New York Times* (July 4, 1989): 9.

33. Ibid.

34. *Roe v. Wade*, 410 U.S. (1973).

35. American Civil Liberties Report, *The Impact of the Hyde Amendment on Medically Necessary Abortions* (New York: October, 1978): 25–49.

36. *Maher v. Roe* 432 U.S. (1977).

37. *Beal v. Doe*, 432 U.S. (1977).

38. *Harris v. McRae*, 448 U.S. 297 (1980).

39. "Portraits of injustice," *Reproductive Freedom in the States* (New York: Center for Reproductive Law and Policy, February 25, 1995).

40. *Planned Parenthood of Central Missouri v. Danforth*, 428 U.S. 52 (1976).

41. *Bellotti v. Baird*, 443 U.S. 132 (1976).

42. *H. L. v. Matheson*, 450 U.S. 398 (1981).

43. *Hodgson v. Minnesota*, 497 U.S. 417 (1990).

44. "Restrictions on young women," *Reproductive Freedom in the States* (New York: Center for Reproductive Law and Policy, September 8, 1994).

45. *Akron, Ohio, Codified Ordinances*, chapter 1879, 1870.03 (1978).

46. Ibid.

47. *Thornburgh v. American College of Obstetricians and Gynecologists*, 476 U.S. 747 (1986).

48. *City of Akron v. Akron Center for Reproductive Health Services*, 462 U.S. 416 (1983).

49. *Thornburgh v. American College of Obstetricians and Gynecologists*, 476 U.S. 747 (1986).

50. *Planned Parenthood of Southeastern Pennsylvania v. Casey*, 505 U.S. 833 (1992).

51. Ibid.

52. Ibid.

53. *Rust v. Sullivan*, 500 U.S. 173 (1991).

54. Carole Joffe, "Fertility control: social issues," in: Warren T. Reich (ed.), *Encyclopedia of Bioethics* (New York: Simon and Schuster/Macmillian, 1995), p. 829.

55. Karen L. Baird, "Globalizing reproductive control: consequences of the 'Global gag rule,'" in: Rosemarie Tong, Anne Donchin, and Susan Dodds (eds.), *Linking Visions: Feminist Bioethics, Human Rights, and the Developing World* (Lanham, MD: Rowman and Littlefield, 2004).

56. *Webster v. Reproductive Health Services*, 492 U.S. 490 (1989).

57. Ronald Munson, *Intervention and Reflection: Basic Issues in Medical Ethics*, 6th ed. (Belmont, CA: Wadsworth, 2000), p. 69.

58. *Turnock v. Ragsdale*, 503 U.S. 916 (1992).

59. *Planned Parenthood Association of Kansas City v. Ashcroft*, 462 U.S. 476 (1983); *Simopoulous v. Virginia*, 462 U.S. 506 (1983); *City of Akron v. Akron Center for Reproductive Health*, 462 U.S. 416 (1983).

60. *Planned Parenthood of Southeastern Pennsylvania v. Casey*, 505 U.S. 833 (1992).

61. "The status of a woman's right to choose abortion," *Reproductive Freedom in the States* (New York: Center for Reproductive Law and Policy, September 8, 1994), p. 2.

62. Janet Benshoof, *"Planned Parenthood v. Casey*: the impact of the new undue burden standard on reproductive health care," *Trends in Health Care, Law, and Ethics*, 8, no. 3 (Summer 1993): 27.

63. Diane M. Granelli, "Medicine adds to debate on late-term abortion: abortion rights leaders urges end to 'half truth,'" *American Medical News*, 3 (March 1997): 28.

64. Cases from Gloria Feldt and Ralph Reed, "The abortion debate: opposing views on partial-birth abortion," *Cosmopolitan Magazine* (July 1997): 155–156.

65. "Nebraska judge finds partial-birth abortion ban act unconstitutional," *Women's Health Weekly* (September 30, 2004): 69.

66. Richard Kofp, Richard Conway Casey, and Phyllis Hamilton, "Round one for women's health," *New York Times* (September 13, 2004): A22.

67. "Abortion-related crime increased in 1997," *Providence Journal* (January 1998): F5.

68. Rick Jervis, "Execution of anti-abortionist creates fear of backlash," *Chicago Tribune* (August 31, 2003).

69. *Madsen v. Women's Health Center*, 512 U.S. 753 (1994).

70. *Schenck v. Pro-Choice Network,* 519 U.S. 357 (1997).

71. Ibid.

72. *Hill v. Colorado* 530 U.S. 703 (2000).

73. Barbara Weiss, *"Roe v. Wade* at 25: the tough questions linger," *Medical Economics,* 75 (August 10, 1998): 138.

74. "Expanding access to safe abortion: key policy issues," *Women's International Network News,* 19, no. 4 (Autumn 1993): 27.

75. Andrzej Kulczycki and Malcolm Potts, "Abortion and fertility regulation," *Lancet,* 347, no. 9016 (June 15, 1996): 1663.

76. Alison Jaggar, "Abortion and a woman's right to decide," in: Carol C. Gould and Marx W. Wartofsky (eds.), *Women and Philosophy: Toward a Theory of Liberation* (New York: Putnam's 1976), p. 357.

77. Elizabeth Hayt, "Surprise, mom: I'm against abortion," *The New York Times Sunday Styles* (March 30, 2003): Section 9 (10).

78. Taman Lewin, "Hurdles increase for many women seeking abortions," *New York Times* (March 15, 1992): 11.

79. Ibid.

80. Joan Beck, "Give doctors a 'choice' on abortion," *Charlotte Observer* (February 24, 1995): 9A.

chapter seven

Reproduction-Assisting Technologies: Donor Insemination, *In Vitro* Fertilization, and Beyond

I. INTRODUCTION

Although most people assume that when they decide to have a child, they will be able to do so, some of them may be sadly surprised. Indeed, in the United States, about one in nine married couples are infertile; that is, unable to achieve pregnancy within 1 year of unprotected intercourse.[1] Infertility rates vary with age and socioeconomic class. Largely due to the biological effects of aging, older women generally have higher rates of infertility than younger women; however, over the last quarter-century the infertility rate of young women, aged 20–24, has climbed from 4% to 11%. Part of the increase may be explained by rising rates of sexually transmitted diseases which, if left untreated, can cause infertility,[2] but a fair amount of the increase remains unexplained. In addition, the infertility rate of men, both younger and older, has also inched upward due to a variety of circumstances including substance abuse, the side effects of some routinely prescribed pharmaceuticals, and certain occupational hazards.[3]

Because so many people in the United States are infertile, a growing number of health care professionals are specializing in infertility or assisted-reproduction services. At present, about one million couples seek infertility services annually, and each year general practitioners, obstetrician-gynecologists, urologists, and endocrinologists see anywhere from 110,000 to 160,000 new cases.[4] The fact that the U.S. infertility services business is a four-billion-dollar a year industry, and that *in vitro* fertilization (IVF) procedures alone have increased 37% between 1995 and 1998, attests to just how much Americans want infertility services.[5]

As we shall see, infertility and assisted-reproduction services are a mixed blessing. When these technologies succeed, the beneficiaries are very happy, even ecstatic. There is nothing quite like bringing home a baby to a

137

nursery that prospective parents feared would remain empty forever; however, when these technologies fail—and they sometimes do—their users may become discouraged, even depressed. In some instances, they may simply refuse to believe that medicine cannot work a miracle for them, insisting that health care professionals keep trying to get them pregnant no matter what. Some people become so desperate for a baby that they let "baby hunger" consume their whole lives. Thus, there is a case to be made that, like any set of medical technologies, assisted-reproduction technologies should be used judiciously in order to avoid unnecessary emotional as well as economic costs.

II. TREATMENTS FOR INFERTILITY

For decades, treatments for infertility tended to focus primarily on women, as if infertility was strictly a "female" problem. However, statistics show that just about as many men as women have infertility problems. Specifically, 35% of infertility cases are due to a male factor, 35% to a female factor, 20% to a combined male and female factor, and 10% to unexplained causes.[6]

A. Routine Treatment

Most male infertility factors such as low sperm count, poor quality sperm, and minimally mobile sperm can be corrected by means of artificial insemination by husband (AIH). In AIH, a man's sperm are pooled from several semen samples, treated with a variety of substances to increase sperm volume and/or quality, and then directly inserted into the woman's uterus. In the event that a man has no sperm or suffers from a genetic disorder, the recommended course of action is artificial insemination by donor (AID). Recently, a new technique called intracytoplasmic sperm injection (ICSI) has been developed. So far, ICSI results have been very encouraging. In this type of artificial insemination, a man's sperm are examined microscopically. From the sample available to them, infertility specialists select a *single* sperm which they then directly inject into the egg cell. ICSI is successful 50%–60% of the time it is used, but it is quite expensive, particularly when it is preceded by a sperm integrity test and an intense antioxidant regimen to improve the likelihood of a man having at least one healthy sperm. In fact, costs can run as high as $20,000.[7]

Only after male factors for infertility are ruled out, do infertility specialists turn their attention to female factors, which, as a rule, are more difficult to treat than male factors. Among the female factors for infertility are a wide range of ovulatory disorders, tubal problems, cervical problems, and uterine abnormalities. Some of these factors can be remedied with surgery and others can be corrected with fertility drugs such as Clomid, Pergonal, or Fertinex which help women ovulate more eggs.

In the event that ordinary treatments for female infertility are unsuccessful, infertility specialists usually recommend a high-tech intervention such as *in vitro* fertilization (IVF). In this assisted-reproduction technique, eggs are removed from a woman's ovaries through a hollow needle, fertilized with sperm, and left to develop in a petri dish for about 2–3 days. One or more of the resulting young embryos are then transferred into the woman's uterus.

Approximately 24% of the women treated with IVF get pregnant. However, only about 78% of these women actually bring home a baby.[8] There are many variations on IVF, including gamete intrafallopian tube transfer (GIFT) and zygote intrafallopian tube transfer (ZIFT). The former technique allows fertilization to take place in the woman's body and, like the latter technique, has a slightly higher success rate than IVF. In the event a woman has no eggs or has diseased or otherwise damaged eggs, a donor's eggs or, more recently, just the cytoplasm of a donor's eggs may be used instead. Finally, in the event a woman cannot or will not carry a pregnancy to term, another woman, variously referred to as a surrogate mother or gestational mother, may agree to do so for her.

III. ETHICAL AND LEGAL DIMENSIONS OF DONOR INSEMINATION (DI)

A. Ethical Dimensions of Donor Insemination (DI)

As we noted above, there are two types of **artificial insemination (AI)**— **artificial insemination by husband** and **artificial insemination by donor**. Increasingly, however, they are both referred to simply as **donor insemination (DI)**. Although DI is fairly routine nowadays (about 30,000 U.S. babies per annum are born by means of DI),[9] it continues to raise some ethical concerns. By examining DI through the moral lenses of both those who disfavor it and those who favor it, we can better appreciate the moral complexity of even this relatively uncontroversial method of assisted reproduction.

1. Ethical Arguments Against Donor Insemination

DI critics are relatively few in numbers nowadays; however, they remain firm in their opposition to the technology. First, they argue that using DI to procreate may serve to jeopardize good marital and parental relationships. When a couple has a DI child, the mother is the child's beget-ter, bearer, and rearer but the father is only the child's rearer. Depending on how important genetic connections are to both parents, such a mother–father asymmetry may generate some difficulties. For example, one man, whose wife was pregnant with their DI child, confessed that he had hoped his wife would deliver a girl, because a son would highlight his loss.[10] "Junior" would not really be his junior. Such reactions may not be atypical. Indeed, studies indicate that a relatively high percentage of DI parents view the mother as the child's primary parent and the father as the child's secondary parent or even stepfather.[11]

Second, DI critics claim that children conceived by means of this proce-dure often suffer psychologically. Judging it best to hide their DI secret, some couples do not tell the child that the man rearing them is not their genetic fa-ther. However, secrets of this type rarely stay secrets, and when the truth is fi-nally disclosed, some DI children are reportedly traumatized. Comments Suzanne Rubin: "No one considers how the child feels when she finds that her natural father was a $25 cup of sperm. The fantasies revolve around what the donor was thinking while he was filling the cup. There is no passion, no human contact in such a union; just cold calculation and manipulation of an-other person's life."[12] Clearly distressed by the circumstances of her concep-tion, Rubin concludes that healthy family relationships cannot be built on a "foundation of deliberate lies,"[13] and that if anyone suffers in a DI family, it is typically the child who may never come to terms with the anonymous sperm donor in their background.

Third, DI critics speculate that many sperm donors live to regret their decision to donate or sell their gametes to others. They may find themselves pursued by a genetically related child who threatens to disrupt their own family life. Or they may start longing for connections to their genetic child, wondering whether the child is being reared by loving parents, or whether he or she has fared well in life.

Fourth, DI critics note that couples may want to use the procedure for unacceptable eugenic purposes—that is, not simply to avoid passing on a hereditary disease or disorder, but to gain access to superior donor genes.[14] Ironically, such a quest may prove misguided for several reasons including the fact that sperm-screening techniques are far from perfect. Although re-sponsible health care professionals screen sperm donors stringently for genetically- and sexually-transmitted diseases (so much so that they reject anywhere from 85%–95% of them), less responsible health care professionals screen sperm donors far more haphazardly. Much the same can be said about sperm banks. The reputable ones aim to provide only healthy sperm to cou-ples; but the less careful ones often negligently or even recklessly sell inade-quately screened sperm.[15]

Fifth, and finally, DI critics object that since the procedure is available to single women, lesbian couples, and unmarried heterosexual couples, it permits the creation of a variety of alternative family structures that fail to serve the best interests of children. To bolster their point of view, they refer to reports such as the one the Warnock Commission produced in Great Britain. That report concluded "the interests of the child dictate that it should be born into a home where there is a loving, stable, heterosexual relationship and that, therefore, the deliberate creation of a child for a woman who is not a partner in such a relationship is morally wrong."[16] Moreover, DI critics think it is particularly deleterious for children to be deliberately conceived and raised exclusively by women. In their estimation, children without a regular male presence in their lives may develop a distorted view of sexuality and procreation.[17]

2. Ethical Arguments For Donor Insemination

Advocates of DI tend to dismiss DI critics as alarmists who want to make mountains out of molehills. Unlike DI critics, they claim, first, that the kind of husband–wife tensions DI couples experience subsequent to the birth of their child are no worse than those that trouble other couples, and these can be resolved successfully if DI couples are honest with each other and with their children. In fact, if DI parents explain the insemination procedure to their children in a matter-of-fact way, their children are likely to view their DI origins positively rather than negatively. Comments one well-adjusted DI child:

> Knowing about my AID [DI] origin did nothing to alter my feelings for my family. Instead I felt grateful for the trouble they had taken to give me life. And they had given me such a strong set of roots, a rich and colorful heritage, a sense of being loved. With their adventure in biology, my parents had opened up the fairly rigid culture they had brought with them to this country. The secret knowledge of my "differentness" and my sister's may have helped our parents accept . . . the few deviations from their norms that we argued for.[18]

Second, DI advocates doubt the procedure is particularly harmful. Most sperm donors gladly sell their sperm in exchange for cash. Any harm done to them will probably stem from a breach of confidentiality, a relatively rare event nowadays because of society's commitment to protecting people's privacy. Moreover, a proper balance between DI children's interest in knowing their genetic heritage and sperm donors' interest in remaining anonymous can be struck. For instance, DI children can be given access either to only nonidentifying medical information about their genetic fathers, or to that identifying information their genetic fathers wish to disclose to them.

Third, DI advocates insist that, as things stand, most couples who use the procedure do not ordinarily request genetically superior donors. In fact, few of them express any interest in using sperm from sperm banks like the Hermann J. Muller Repository for Germinal Choice in California, which was

created to store the sperm of Nobel Prize winning men for the purpose of in-
seminating selected women.[19] Instead, most couples ask only that they be
matched with a person of the same race, ethnicity, body type, and intellect as
the husband. In the estimation of DI advocates, such requests are morally defensible. They simply permit the couple to procreate a child who resembles
the child they would have procreated had the man been fertile.

Fourth, DI advocates claim that one of the procedure's advantages is
precisely that it does permit the creation of alternative family structures.
They see the inclusion of single female parents and lesbian parents within the
meaning of family as a move toward greater equality in a society where single mothers and, particularly, lesbian couples still suffer from prejudice and
discrimination. They also see value in affirming the deliberate decision of
some women to be mothers but not wives or even sexual partners of men,
inasmuch as this decision helps correct the mistaken view that without a
man a woman cannot successfully raise a happy and socially adjusted child.

B. Legal Dimensions of Artificial Insemination

Like most types of assisted reproduction, DI is of legal as well as of ethical interest. In the early twentieth century, some U.S. courts still classified DI
children as illegitimate—"born out of wedlock," so to speak. Because the real
father of the child was arguably the genetic father (the sperm donor), the
child's mother was viewed as an adulteress, and her husband was viewed as
a betrayed spouse rearing another man's child. It did not matter whether the
child's rearing father regarded the child as his own. Not until the 1940s was
this conception of DI abandoned in *Strnad v. Strnad*,[20] a New York divorce
case. A woman sued to limit her ex-husband's right to visit their child who
had been conceived through DI with his consent. Although the court did not
explicitly rule that the child was legitimate, it held that the ex-husband,
though not the genetic father of the child, was "entitled to the same rights as
those acquired by a foster parent who has adopted a child, if not the same
rights as those to which a natural parent under the circumstances would be
entitled."[21] Later, in a 1968 California case, *People v. Sorenson*,[22] a woman sued
her ex-husband for child support. He refused to support the child on the
grounds that the child was not his, even though he had consented to his ex-
wife's use of DI. The Supreme Court of California ruled against the man. It
held that because he had consented to his wife's insemination by donor, the
child was his in the eyes of the law.

Although decades have passed since the Sorenson case, a comprehensive federal statute governing DI has yet to be written. Most states have,
however, enacted a variety of laws to regulate certain aspects of DI. Despite
the variations in these laws, most states agree that both partners must

consent to DI and that, if they both consent, the child born to them is legitimate. Some states go farther. They explicitly legislate that the sperm donor is not the legal father of the child. Other attempts to regulate the practice of DI include requirements for (1) documenting the informed consent of sperm recipients and/or their spouses or partners to DI; (2) keeping the personal identity of sperm donors confidential; (3) limiting the number of times any one man may serve as a sperm donor in a certain geographical area; (4) regulating the quality of sperm used in DI; and (5) confining the performance of DI to an authorized or licensed person, generally a physician.[23]

Of the requirements listed above, the fifth has been particularly controversial. In the past, a significant number of infertility clinics restricted DI access to married heterosexual couples, on the grounds that such couples are best suited to successfully rear children to adulthood. Frustrated by this policy, many single women and lesbian couples resorted to **self-insemination (SI)**. They asked male acquaintances for sperm which they then used to inseminate themselves. Or they got sperm from open sperm banks such as the Sperm Bank of Northern California which provides sperm to any woman, regardless of her marital status, sexual preference, or physical disability.[24]

Although SI has certain advantages—the woman not only decides who the donor will be, she also avoids the cost of physician-controlled DI (typically $400 to $600 per cycle)—[25] it also has definite disadvantages. Specifically, a woman who directly secures live sperm from a male acquaintance cannot be sure of their quality, as she would be were she to use frozen sperm from a reputable sperm bank which deals directly with only physicians. At present, physicians rarely use live, unscreened sperm for DI. Instead, the standard of practice is to use frozen sperm which have been carefully screened for genetic defects and diseases, sexually transmitted diseases, and the HIV virus.[26]

Another disadvantage of SI is using a known donor who may later demand access to his genetic child. For example, in a 1977 case, a man gave some of his sperm to a long-term woman friend who, after she was nearly 3 months pregnant, broke off contact with him. When the child was born, the sperm donor sued for visitation rights. A New Jersey court not only granted him visitation rights but also declared him the child's legal father.[27]

In another case over a decade later, a man from Oregon gave some of his sperm to a long-term lesbian friend who allegedly agreed to his playing an active role in the child's life. After the child was born, however, the woman, who no longer wanted the man in her life, blocked his access to the child. She claimed she had never regarded the man as anything more than a sperm donor. Subsequently, the man filed a parental-rights suit against the woman. Although a lower Oregon court dismissed his suit, an Oregon appeals court reversed the decision. It ruled that the man had parental rights to the child even though he had "fathered" his child by means of artificial insemination instead of natural sexual intercourse. The woman appealed the man's victory to the U.S. Supreme Court which upheld the Oregon appeals court's ruling and gave the man the right to try to prove in an Oregon court that the lesbian woman had originally agreed to let him help rear the child.[28] Although this decision does not affect married women who use DI, it does affect unmarried women who use the procedure. Caution would suggest, then, that it is prudent for single women to use the sperm of anonymous rather than known donors.

Interestingly, one of the most controversial legal issues that has recently emerged in the assisted-reproduction arena concerns not DI but AIH. An increasing number of widows want to use their deceased husband's or partner's sperm for procreative purposes. For example, in 1984 Corinne Parplaix, a French woman, sued a sperm bank to release her dead husband's sperm to her, even though he had left no specific instructions about their use. The state prosecutor argued that Mrs. Parplaix had no more right to her dead husband's sperm than to his feet or ears. Mrs. Parplaix's lawyer countered that Mr. Parplaix knew he was dying of cancer when he deposited his sperm. By so doing, he implied a contract with his wife, a contract to bear his child after his death. The court agreed with Mrs. Parplaix's lawyer. When apprised of the decision, Mrs. Parplaix said: "I'll call him Thomas . . . He'll be a pianist. That's what his father wanted."[29]

More recently, some women have requested physicians to retrieve sperm from their near-dead or dead husbands. Recently, the Northeast Organ Procurement Organization asked more than fifty other organ procurement organizations if they had ever been requested to recover sperm from organ donors. More than 80% of these organizations reported they had. In seven of the reported forty-six cases, **posthumous sperm retrieval** was attempted, but only three of these retrievals succeeded. None of the procurement organizations knew whether any of the three widows who requested the sperm actually used them to get pregnant and have a child.

Because requests for posthumous sperm retrieval may increase in significant numbers in future years, clear policies need to be developed for posthumous sperm retrieval. After all, a woman does not have an automatic right to claim her deceased husband's sperm if there is reason to think he did not want any offspring, including ones born posthumously. In this connection, Maggie Gallagher of the Center for Social Thought has commented: "It really does violate the principle of reproductive choice. A man can't tell his wife she can't have an abortion, and a woman can't tell her husband he can't have a vasectomy. I question making a man a father when he has never indicated he would want to be a father under these circumstances."[30] Yet, despite the strengths of Gallagher's line of reasoning, the counterpoint may be made that some men would welcome the opportunity to "father" a child posthumously. For example, Pam Maresca, widowed shortly after her marriage, argued cogently that her deceased husband, Manny, had very much wanted to have children. With the support of Manny's family, she convinced Manny's physicians to remove his sperm from his body for her future use. Although Pam has not ruled out marrying again, she insists that "it will have to be someone special enough to accept Manny's child."[31]

Closely related to a discussion of specific laws that govern DI/AIH is a related discussion of the formal and informal policies and attitudes behind this form of assisted reproduction. At present, the identities of sperm donors are kept anonymous, and most sperm donors are paid for their gametes in the range of $50 per ejaculation.[32] A policy of commercial, anonymous sperm donation supposedly serves sperm donors' best interests, including their interest in avoiding an unwanted financial or personal relationship with the child. In recent years, however, many sperm donors, psychologists, and counselors have questioned whether anonymous sperm donation really serves *all* sperm donors' best interests. They point out that an increasing number of sperm donors seem quite willing to share *identifying* as well as *nonidentifying* information about themselves with their genetic children. For example, in one study of sperm donors, psychologist Patricia P. Mahlstedt discovered that over 60% of them wanted to be contacted by their genetic offspring when they (the offspring) reached age 18.[33] Mahlstedt's research findings are bolstered by some media portrayals of sperm donors. For example, in a 1990s episode of the television show, "St. Elsewhere," a physician decides to donate his sperm to the hospital's infertility clinic. Through a complicated chain of events, he first discovers the identity of the woman who received his sperm and then follows her pregnancy obsessively. Eventually, he assigns himself to her case, at which point he begins to act like an expectant father. The pregnant woman's husband is bewildered by the physician's inappropriate behavior and asks the chief of residents to remove the physician from his wife's case. As a result, the physician nearly has a nervous breakdown, protesting that the woman is carrying his child and that he has a right to be involved in his child's life.

Empirical studies such as Mahlstedt's and media portrayals such as the *St. Elsewhere* episode suggest that a more open policy of sperm donation may well be in the best interests of at least some sperm donors. Moreover, such a policy may be in the best interests of DI children. At present, an asymmetry exists between children who have been adopted and children who have been produced through DI. In most jurisdictions, adopted children have the right to know nonidentifying medical information about both of their genetic parents at any time; and in an increasing number of jurisdictions, adopted children, who have reached legal adulthood, also have the right to identifying personal information about their genetic parents, provided that their genetic parents agree to reveal their identities. Assuming that the interests of adopted children are roughly equivalent to those of DI children, it would seem that DI children, like adopted children, should have the same rights, provided that the sperm donor is a "yes-donor"—that is, a man who identifies himself as willing to disclose identifying as well as nonidentifying information to his adult child.[34]

IV. ETHICAL AND LEGAL DIMENSIONS
OF *IN VITRO* FERTILIZATION

Donor insemination has become a relatively routine practice in infertility treatment clinics and does not attract much public attention. This state of affairs is in stark contrast to the explosive public reaction that occurred in 1978 in England, following the birth of the first "test-tube baby," Lesley Brown. At the time, it seemed as if everyone had an opinion about *in vitro* **fertilization**, particularly about creating human life in a petri dish. Advocates of IVF applauded this new form of assisted reproduction as yet another way for infertile couples to have a child genetically related to at least one of them. In their estimation, IVF was simply a technique that permitted infertile couples to do outside of the woman's body that which is ordinarily done within a woman's body. Critics of IVF disagreed. They presented IVF as the beginning of Huxley's *Brave New World*, a world in which human beings would be mass produced *ex utero*. In the end, IVF advocates won the day. As of yet no one has opened a human-being assembly plant, and IVF has become as accepted as DI.[35] But just because IVF has been relatively routinized does not mean that it is without ethical, legal, and social problems. On the contrary, IVF still poses many questions that need to be answered.

A. Ethical Dimensions of *In Vitro* Fertilization

1. *The Problems of Surplus Preembryos*

As we noted above, one of the main reasons that IVF has prompted far more ethical debate than artificial insemination is simply the fact that it facilitates the creation of life ex utero; that is, life outside the womb. Thus, it is not surprising that the IVF controversy has centered on the moral status of the so-called **preembryo**, a 2- to 3-day-old blastocyst consisting of approximately eight cells. Specifically, people have questioned whether it is permissible to discard surplus preembryos; that is, those preembryos that are not transferred into a woman's womb but instead are frozen or otherwise "put on hold." Are these preembryos mere tissue, full human persons, or something in-between?

In the early days of IVF, infertility specialists typically followed a more-the-merrier rule with respect to preembryos. In hope of achieving at least one full-term pregnancy and live birth, they routinely implanted in the woman's womb all the eggs that successfully fertilized in the petri dish. But as IVF techniques improved and more pregnancies were achieved, infertility specialists began to implant only the best-quality fertilized eggs in the woman's womb. They discarded the rest for fear of causing either a problematic multiple pregnancy (to be discussed below) or a pregnancy likely to result in a seriously defective newborn. When critics of IVF realized that clinicians were discarding surplus preembryos, they objected that clinicians were killing human persons.

One early response to the problem of discarding surplus embryos involved the development of a variation on IVF. Through **gamete intrafallopian transfer**, which we mentioned above, eggs and sperm were directly inserted into the woman's womb, after which nature was allowed to take its course. Thus, GIFT seemed to solve the problem of discarding surplus preembryos. But for several reasons, including the fact that GIFT requires surgery and general anesthesia, which put the woman's life and health at heightened risk, GIFT has not become the assisted-reproduction technique of choice.[36]

Another response to the problem of discarding surplus preembryos also involved a technological fix. Techniques for **cryopreservation** (the freezing of surplus preembryos) were developed in the 1990s. Not only did cryopreservation put on temporary hold the problem of what to do with surplus preembryos, it also had other advantages. It helped couples avoid problematic multiple pregnancies and it spared women, who did not get pregnant during the first cycle of IVF, from the physically taxing three or four cycles of IVF that otherwise might be necessary to achieve a pregnancy. For example, assume that a couple has produced six or seven preembryos. Most infertility specialists will transfer only two or three of them into the woman's womb, freezing the rest for possible use in the future. In the event the selected preembryos do not result in a live birth, the infertility specialists simply thaw some of the frozen preembryos for transfer into the woman's womb.

As we noted above, cyropreservation only postpones the surplus pre-embryo problem, it does not resolve it. As soon as, or even before, the woman in an IVF program gives birth to one or more children, she and her husband/partner may no longer want to use their surplus cryopreserved preembryos. Then the issue becomes whether to keep the surplus preembryos frozen indefinitely, to discard them, to put them up for adoption, or to use them for research.

Keeping surplus preembryos frozen indefinitely raises concerns about their condition. Do they deteriorate over time or not? Most infertility specialists believe both that preembryos can be safely stored indefinitely and that couples should have the option of keeping their preembryos stored for as long as they wish for a reasonable fee. Still, only so many surplus preembryos can be frozen and stored before an infertility clinic runs out of space. In the United Kingdom, a major controversy erupted in 1996 when 3,300 frozen preembryos were discarded subsequent to the passage of a law which made it possible for infertility clinics to discard any frozen preembryo that had been stored for over 5 years and whose storage bill had been unpaid. The same law also permitted the infertility clinic to discard 5-year-old preembryos whose genetic parents expressed no interest in determining their fate.[37]

Reflection on the U.K. controversy reminds us that couples who elect to discard their surplus preembryos may be viewed as abortionists by those who believe that human life, indeed, human personhood, begins the moment egg and sperm unite. Still, an elective abortion of a preembryo would be a very early abortion and one legally protected by *Roe v. Wade*,[38] the court ruling that permits first-trimester elective abortions. Interestingly, *if* discarding a preembryo is morally equivalent to aborting a fetus, then it would seem that men as well as women can make and be responsible for some abortion decisions. Because the surplus preembryo is outside of the woman's body, a persuasive case can be made that the woman's husband/partner has equal responsibility for a joint discard decision, or total responsibility for any unilateral discard decision he makes.

Rather than discarding their unwanted surplus preembryos, some couples elect to either put them up for adoption or give them to scientists for biomedical research, particularly stem-cell research. At present the decision to put one's preembryos up for adoption is easier to make than to operationalize. Very few infertility programs have embryo adoption programs, usually called "snowflake" programs. This situation may change in the near future, however, as the possibility of preembryo adoption is publicized more widely, and as adopting couples realize that this arrangement permits them to personally experience pregnancy.

More controversially, some couples choose to give their surplus preembryos to research scientists rather than to adopting couples. They do not want their preembryos to be born and to exist as persons who may try to enter their lives at some point of time. Instead, they want their preembryos to be destroyed and then used for research purposes. They reason that it is better that their preembryos be used meaningfully rather than merely discarded. But not everyone agrees with these couples' rationale. In particular, those who believe that life begins at the moment of conception view them as baby killers. Struggling to mediate between those who think that preembryos are persons and those who think they are more akin to biological material, the President's National Bioethics Advisory Commission (NBAC) has recommended that research on surplus preembryos "is permissible where there is good reason to believe that this destruction is necessary to develop cures for life-threatening or severely debilitating diseases and, when appropriate, protections and oversight are in place in order to prevent abuse":[39] better that a preembryo be used for humanity's well-being than that it simply be discarded.

2. IVF, Reasonable Risk Assumption, and Informed Consent

As many health care ethicists see it, another major moral issue to address in any discussion of IVF is its risk–benefit ratio. Although staunch IVF defenders insist that babies produced through IVF are at no greater risk for genetic damage than babies produced naturally, some recent studies suggest otherwise. According to a 2002 report in the *New England Journal of Medicine*, babies produced through IVF have an 8.6% risk of major birth defects—including heart and kidney problems, cleft palate, and undescended testicles—whereas babies produced naturally only have a 4.2% risk of these conditions. In addition, IVF babies are 2.6 times more likely than naturally conceived babies to be born with a very low birth weight, a significant risk factor for cardiac and cognitive problems. Yet, even if this study is accurate, 91% of IVF babies (as compared to 95% of naturally conceived babies) are still born healthy. Comments Dr. Zev Rosenwaks, director of New York Presbyterian Hospital's infertility program, "If you ask a couple if they would rather not have a child at all or try to have a child that over 95% of the time will be normal, I think they will choose to have the child."[40]

Probably higher than the risks posed to IVF babies, are the risks posed to the adults who use the procedure. Many people do not realize how emotionally taxing, physically demanding, and financially costly IVF can be. Not atypical is the IVF experience of Jennifer and Andrew Hale as told to a reporter for a popular women's magazine:

> The Hales knew shortly after they were married in 1991 that they were going to need IVF. Jennifer's tubes, tests had shown, were completely blocked. What they didn't know, though, was that Andrew also had a problem, something they learned three years later during their first IVF attempt, when only two out of a dozen eggs were successfully fertilized. Two more attempts (one with ICSI, one using frozen embryos) also failed. At that point, the Hales thought they might turn to adoption. But deciding to give IVF with ICSI one more shot, in 1997, they consulted the Pacific Fertility Medical Center in San Francisco. 'This time we had an angel on our side,' says Jennifer. Last July 4, Julia Elizabeth Hale was born.[41]

As happily as this story ended, omitted from it are the emotional ups and downs the Hales probably experienced, to say nothing of the likely disruption of their work schedules and marital relations as well as the bodily risks to which Jennifer was subjected. Women who are enrolled in IVF programs generally are exposed to the side effects of powerful, egg-stimulating hormones such as Clomid, anesthesia, possible surgery to retrieve eggs, and an increased risk of ectopic pregnancy.[42]

Perhaps the most disturbing fact about the kind of IVF miracles stories that appear in many popular women's magazines is that little, if any, mention is made of the IVF stories that do not have happy endings. In 2002, the Centers for Disease Control (CDC) reported that IVF clinics, of which there are approximately 390 in the United States, performed 115,392 IVF cycles in order to produce 45,000 live births for an average success rate of 35%.[43] Clearly, about two-thirds of IVF users are spending a lot of money only to be frustrated or disappointed, and because this is the case, the importance of informed consent to IVF cannot be overstressed.

3. The Problem of Multifetal Pregnancies

Almost or equally as bad as the prospect of having no baby is the possibility of having too many babies. In the United States, 55% of all assisted-reproduction births are **multifetal pregnancies**.[44] Barbara Seaman observes that "besides upping our infant death rates (five times higher for twins than for singletons and nine times higher for triplets),"[45] multiples are prone to serious health problems including cerebral palsy and certain types of blindness. Moreover, multiples are typically far more expensive than singletons. In a much publicized 1998 case, a woman in an IVF program gave birth to octuplets. Seven of the babies survived their premature birth, each of them with a 50% chance of a serious medical problem. During the first 2 months of their 4-month hospital stay, the octuplets' hospital bill amounted to more than two million dollars.[46]

Faced with the possibility of enormous medical costs as well as a radically altered lifestyle, couples who discover their pregnancy is multifetal are encouraged to carefully explore all their options. Sometimes health care professionals advise such couples to consider **selective reduction** and abort one or more of the fetuses for the benefit of the mother as well as of the surviving fetuses. But the selective reduction decision is not a decision that is easily made by couples in IVF programs. Precisely those couples who most want children are asked to abort one or more of their fetuses. For reasons such as these, the American College of Obstetricians and Gynecologists emphasizes the need for health care professionals to counsel couples in IVF programs about the likelihood and risks of a multifetal pregnancy. In some instances, it may be better for a couple to decide to remain childless rather than to risk having several, very needy children.

4. Egg Donors

Sometimes overlooked in discussions of IVF's risk–benefit ratio are the risks posed to **egg donors**. When infertile women in IVF programs fail to produce eggs, or produce few or unhealthy eggs, as is the case with many women over the age of 40, infertility specialists suggest using an egg donor, typically, a young woman with a generous supply of healthy eggs. Egg donors assume many of the same risks that IVF enrollees do, but without receiving the same benefit, namely, a much-wanted child. In contrast to sperm donation, which has traditionally used anonymous and commercial donors, egg donation initially involved known and altruistic donors. Infertility specialists thought that only female relatives or friends of women in IVF programs would be willing to serve as egg donors. But when it became evident to infertility specialists that some of their patients had pressured relatives or friends to serve as egg donors, they began to think that egg donation, like sperm donation, should be anonymous and commercial.[47]

Although using anonymous and commercial egg donors may be less emotionally entangling than using known and altruistic egg donors, choosing to do so is not without its own set of problems. Critics of IVF fear that many egg donors sell their gametes because they are financially strapped and in serious need of the thousands of dollars clinics pay for eggs.[48] They are particularly concerned about "super donors" who sell their eggs routinely, exposing themselves to very high levels of medical risk, and mercenary donors who use middlemen to advertise their high-priced "superior eggs." Reportedly, some infertile couples are willing to pay fees as high as $50,000 for the perfect egg.[49] In addition, critics of IVF worry that a significant percentage of egg donors may be unstable women burdened with heavy emotional baggage. In fact, a recent empirical study found that a statistically significant number of egg donors, perhaps as many as one-third, may be the survivors of a major reproductive loss (for example, abortion, miscarriage, or giving up a child for adoption).[50]

B. Legal Dimensions of IVF

1. General Legal Issues

Just as complex as the ethical issues that surround IVF are the legal issues. Philosopher Le Roy Walters notes that two sets of legal issues have surrounded IVF procedures: first-generation ones and second-generation ones. For the most part, first-generation IVF legal issues involved society's initial reactions to the thought of test-tube babies. People had concerns about playing God, and/or about creating lives that were somehow not fully human; however, as one healthy IVF baby after another was born, talk of imposing a ban on IVF ceased, as a new set of concerns about IVF began to emerge. According to Walters, these second generation IVF legal issues included the following six: (1) screening prospective rearing parents; (2) selling and buying human gametes; (3) medically unnecessary use of the new reproductive technologies; (4) anonymity versus identification in cases involving third parties; (5) quality control in programs offering the new reproduction technologies; and (6) insurance coverage for the new reproductive technologies.[51]

Walters claims that "liberty-oriented" people approach second-generation IVF legal issues very differently than do "welfare-oriented" people.[52] Liberty-oriented people claim that any individual who needs a reproduction-assisting technology should have access to it and that any individual who wishes to buy or sell gametes should be free to do so, provided that minimum safety standards and informed consent requirements are met. Moreover, liberty-oriented people maintain that any individual who wishes to use a reproduction-assisting technology should be free to do so, even if they are fertile and simply trying to produce a child with better gametes than their own, or trying to bypass the gestational process by using a surrogate mother to carry the embryo to term. With respect to third parties involved in IVF, liberty-oriented people claim that IVF rearing parents, egg donors, or sperm donors should be permitted either to know or not to know each another. In addition, they claim that upon reaching the age of majority IVF children should be permitted either to know or not to know their genetic parents, provided their genetic parents have agreed to disclose identifying information about themselves. Finally, liberty-oriented people claim that IVF clinics should be free to operate and advertise for clients, subject only to the standards that govern good businesses, and that people who wish to use reproduction-assisting technologies should be free to purchase them out-of-pocket or with any insurance plan that covers such expensive services.[53]

In contrast to liberty-oriented people, welfare-oriented people are very much in favor of screening prospective IVF parents. Many of them wish to exclude from IVF programs child abusers, poor people, single women, nontraditional couples (for example, homosexual couples), and unmarried heterosexual couples. The fact that the infertile people would not be subject to screening if they were fertile does not strike welfare-oriented people as discriminatory, since, as they see it, no one has a right to any and all medical services. Moreover, welfare-oriented people are opposed to the sale and purchase of human eggs and sperm. They favor a voluntary, nonprofit system for donating eggs and sperm. They claim that nonprofit systems symbolize social solidarity, whereas for-profit systems simply tempt people to sell gametes for as much as the market permits. Welfare-oriented people also are opposed to elective use of IVF and embryo transfer. In their opinion, IVF should be limited to infertile or genetically diseased couples in order (1) to conserve a relatively scarce medical resource for those who really need it; (2) to prevent the exploitation of poor women as egg donors; and (3) to discourage either a designer-baby approach or an animal-breeding approach to human reproduction. With respect to third parties involved in IVF, welfare-oriented people claim that the less gamete sellers and buyers know about one another the better, and the less IVF children know about their genetic parents the better. Finally, welfare-oriented people recommend that IVF programs be either certified by a professional organization (for example, the American Fertility Society) or licensed by a public body (for example, the Health and Human Services Department). They also insist that society has a moral obligation to provide infertile people with "infertility insurance" because "infertility seriously disrupts their life plans and diminishes their happiness."[54]

Interestingly, official groups, including health care societies, associations, and institutions, have tended to adopt a welfare attitude toward second-generation IVF legal issues. In contrast, the general public increasingly manifests a liberty attitude toward second-generation IVF issues. Certain groups of citizens, including several women's groups and minority groups, however, continue to have serious reservations about letting the market regulate the practice of IVF.

2. Special Legal Issues

Most of the specific legal issues surrounding IVF have involved inheritance and custody cases. In a case dating back to 1981, Mario and Elsa Rios entered an IVF program in Melbourne, Australia. Physicians there retrieved and fertilized with donor sperm several of Mrs. Rio's eggs. One of the fertilized eggs was placed in Mrs. Rios's womb. The two remaining fertilized eggs were frozen for possible future use. When Mrs. Rios miscarried, she told her physicians that she was not ready to have the frozen preembryos transferred into her womb. She and her husband then left for a vacation trip, which ended tragically in their death. Questions were immediately raised about the legal status of the orphaned frozen preembryos. Did they have a right to inherit a share of the couple's considerable estate? And who, after all, had the right to determine the frozen preembryos' future? Was it the couple's grown son, Michael, who had filed for guardianship? Or was it a right-to-life group willing to provide surrogate mothers for the frozen preembryos?[55] Ultimately, the state of Victoria assumed responsibility for this decision, ruling that the preembryos should not be discarded but, instead, should be anonymously donated to a woman unable to produce her own eggs.[56] Whether any woman actually bore a child from the frozen preembryos is not known, however.

Sometimes, as in the case of Mr. and Mrs. Rios, one or both of the genetic parents of the frozen preembryos die, but this is a rare event. It is much more likely that a frozen preembryo will become the object of a custody dispute than an inheritance dispute. In a widely discussed Tennessee divorce case, *Davis v. Davis* (1989), a couple had no prior agreement about the disposition of their seven frozen preembryos in the event of divorce. As it happened, the couple did divorce and the wife insisted that the frozen preembryos be available to her for thawing and placement in her womb or the womb of a surrogate mother. Meanwhile, her ex-husband vociferously objected to the idea of children from his failed marriage being born. The trial judge awarded custody of the frozen preembryos to the wife on the grounds that it was in their best interests, because she wanted them to live whereas her ex-husband wanted them to die. When the husband appealed the decision, the Tennessee Supreme Court ruled that the couple should have joint custody over the frozen preembryos. It also ruled that, absent a prior agreement about the fate of the frozen preembryos in the event of divorce, a person's right (in this case the husband's right) to "procreational autonomy" outweighed the state's "at best slight" interest in "the potential life embodied by these four- to eight-cell preembryos."[57] The court also stressed that if one member of a couple does *not* want to be a parent, his or her wishes outweigh the other person's interest in being a parent, unless the other person cannot become a parent in any other way. Subsequent to this decision, the wife carried her appeal to the U.S. Supreme Court, which affirmed the state court ruling and disappointed her. After further unpleasantness, the husband's wishes were honored. The frozen preembryos were destroyed in June 1993. In this instance, it seems correct to say that the husband chose to abort the preembryos.

Clearly, the law is struggling to determine if frozen preembryos have rights. So far, the trend is to regard frozen preembryos as the genetic parents' property, over which they have control. But it is not clear that frozen preembryos are mere property. To the degree their moral status is more akin to that of a person than, say, human tissue, it would seem desirable to develop **egg-freezing techniques**. At present, a limited number of infertility specialists remove the maximum number of available eggs from a woman, fertilize only a few of them to implant in her womb, and freeze the remaining unfertilized eggs for later use if the pregnancy fails or no child is born. Because eggs have the same neutral moral status as sperm, discarding unused eggs does not violate the moral sensibilities of those who believe that human persons come into existence with the union of sperm and egg.[58] Egg-freezing is not a well-developed technique, however. In fact, only 100 babies have been born from it, since it was first tried in 1990. Apparently, the process, which costs about $10,000, often results in damaged eggs, and most infertility specialists are reluctant to attempt it.[59]

V. The Ethical and Legal Dimensions of Surrogate Motherhood

Like artificial insemination and *in vitro* fertilization, **surrogate motherhood** has generated considerable ethical debate. Surrogate motherhood is a form of assisted reproduction that typically involves three persons: a married infertile couple (the intended parents) and a surrogate mother. There are two basic types of surrogacy: **traditional surrogacy** and **gestational surrogacy**. In traditional surrogacy, the surrogate mother is artificially inseminated with the sperm of the man who plans to rear the child with his wife or partner. Because the surrogate mother is the child's genetic as well as gestational mother, at some point after birth she must legally terminate her parental rights, and the intended mother must adopt the child. In gestational surrogacy, both the intended father and the intended mother have a genetic connection to the child. The surrogate mother simply gestates the couple's embryo after it has been produced through the process of *in vitro* fertilization. In a rare variation on gestational surrogacy, the intended parents would ask a surrogate mother to gestate an embryo they have adopted. In such a case, neither the intended parents nor the surrogate mother have a genetic connection to the child.[60]

An intended mother who gestates an embryo that she and her husband have adopted, or an embryo that is the product of her husband's sperm and a donor's egg, is not considered a surrogate mother. The fact that she became pregnant with the intention of keeping the baby distinguishes her from a surrogate mother, who became pregnant with the intention of relinquishing the baby to those who commissioned her reproductive services.

Unmarried couples (including lesbian and homosexual couples), married *fertile* couples who do not want to interrupt their lives with a pregnancy, and single men or women may also want to use a surrogate mother; however, because many centers for surrogate parenting limit their services to infertile, married, heterosexual couples, they may meet with resistance. Physicians are particularly reluctant to assist couples who have no *medical* reason for seeking the services of a surrogate mother; center and clinic administrators are disinclined to assist individuals other than heterosexual couples for fear of compounding the legal risks and ethical concerns that already surround surrogacy arrangements.

The fact that some surrogate mother arrangements are commercial while other are noncommercial further complicates surrogacy arrangements. **Commercial surrogacy** arrangements involve monetary payments to the surrogate mother and to the third parties who facilitate the pregnancy. In 2000, the average cost of such an arrangement was $60,000. The surrogate mother's fee, including expenses, is approximately $20,000 to $25,000, with the rest of the monies being paid out to physicians, lawyers, and the surrogacy brokers.[61] In contrast, **noncommercial surrogacy** arrangements, sometimes called gift or altruistic surrogacy, are privately negotiated, usually between an infertile married couple and one of their close female relatives or friends. No money passes hands for the surrogate mother's gestational services, although, typically, the couple covers the surrogate mother's medical expenses.

A. Ethical Perspectives on Surrogate Motherhood

Surrogate motherhood has many opponents as well as advocates. Although more controversies have erupted about commercial surrogacy arrangements than noncommercial surrogacy arrangements, gift or altruistic surrogacy has not gone unchallenged. In addition, both opponents and advocates of surrogate motherhood tend to have different moral intuitions about gestational surrogacy as opposed to traditional surrogacy.

1. *Ethical Arguments Against Surrogate Motherhood*

Most arguments against surrogate motherhood are based on the harms the practice is thought to produce. First, it is claimed that surrogate motherhood risks harms to the resulting children. Critics speculate that because the surrogate mother is not gestating the child for herself but for others, she may be less motivated to take care of herself and the fetus throughout the pregnancy and less emotionally committed to the fetus, should the pregnancy become too difficult for her to continue. For example, in one of the few peer-reviewed retrospective studies of surrogate motherhood in the medical literature to date, two-thirds of the forty-one surrogate mothers in the sample had at least one or more of the following perinatal risk factors: smoking, low income, unmarried, and/or prone to miscarriage.[62] Harm to the resulting child may also occur if the intended parents and/or the surrogate mother are not medically and psychologically screened for parental fitness as they would be in the course of traditional adoption proceedings. Finally, the resulting child may be harmed if he or she becomes the object of an acrimonious child-custody suit; is rejected by both the intended couple and the surrogate mother because he or she is in some way abnormal; or desires a stronger relationship with the surrogate mother than either the intended parents are willing to permit or the surrogate mother is willing to accept.

Second, it is claimed that the practice of surrogate motherhood risks harm to the intended parents and/or the surrogate mother and her family. Specifically, it is argued that introducing third parties into the process of human reproduction may weaken certain marital and familial relationships. If only one of the intended parents is genetically connected to the child, that parent may view himself/herself as having a greater claim to the child—a claim that may be recognized by the courts in the event of a divorce, for example. In rare instances, it is conceivable that an intended father may form an inappropriate psychological bond with the surrogate mother, viewing her—rather than his wife—as the "real" mother of his child. Other possible harms to the intended parents may occur if, for example, the surrogate mother deliberately exposes the fetus to harm, threatens to terminate the pregnancy unless she is paid more money, or refuses to relinquish the child at birth.

Possible harms to the surrogate mother include attempts by the intended parents to impose autonomy-restricting contracts on her that require her not only to agree to prenatal care but also to have amniocentesis, and depending on the results, to abort or not to abort the fetus. Although such contracts are legally nonbinding, a poorly informed surrogate mother may not realize the strength of her rights to refuse treatment or to have an abortion. In addition, the intended parents may refuse to pay the surrogate mother, or refuse to accept the child at birth either because the child is not to their liking or simply because they have lost interest in being parents. In cases of altruistic surrogacy, the intended parents may unduly pressure a friend or relative to prove her love for them by giving them the gift of a child.

Harm may also befall the family of the surrogate mother. If the surrogate mother is married, her husband may not approve of his wife serving as a surrogate mother, particularly if he views his wife as carrying another man's child, or if he regards the pregnancy as a risky undertaking for his wife. If the surrogate mother has children, they may start expressing concerns about why mommy isn't going to keep the baby and what mommy's decision portends for their security.

Over and beyond these possible harms to individuals, there are, in critics' estimation, the larger social harms that surrogate motherhood invites. As they see it, surrogacy arrangements may harm women in general. First, these arrangements may exploit women who need money. Although reputable surrogacy agencies and brokers refuse to accept markedly poor women into their programs, some less than morally stellar agencies and brokers actually prefer to use poor women. They reason that unemployed women or women on welfare, especially if they are single mothers, are highly unlikely to forsake their surrogacy fee in order to add to their family yet another mouth to feed.[63] Indeed, John Stehura, president of the Bionetics Foundation, Inc., an agency that contracts surrogate mothers, asserts that as far as he is concerned, a surrogate mother can never be poor enough. Because the going rate for surrogate mothers is high even by middle-class American standards, he thinks the surrogacy industry should move either to impoverished regions of the United States, where women might be willing to gestate fetuses for one-half the standard fee, or to developing nations where women are desperate for money.[64] In one of the few U.S. Office of Technology Assessments of surrogacy programs, it was reported that seven out of the thirteen programs surveyed were willing to accept as surrogate mothers women on welfare, and that the average income of all the surrogate mothers accepted by the thirteen programs was $18,000 in 1987.[65]

Second, altruistic surrogate mothers may also be exploited, though in a more subtle way. According to philosopher Uma Narayan, surrogate motherhood, in its altruistic form, involves "gender-role exploitation," whereby "the very aspects of 'femininity' used to glorify motherhood—views of women as loving, nurturing, and self-sacrificing" are deployed to motivate women to serve as surrogate mothers. Because only women can bring a human life into the world, surrogate motherhood often becomes a "compassion trap" for women.[66] Frequently, the call for surrogate mothers is accompanied by images of incredibly lonely, tragically unfulfilled infertile couples. Generous women are implored to step forward to give the gift of life, a baby, to these unfortunate couples; the fact that approximately one-third of all the women who answer this appeal have either had an abortion or given up a child for adoption strengthens some critics' suspicion that the desire to assuage past grief may sometimes inappropriately ground a woman's "choice" to be a surrogate mother.[67]

Over and beyond raising concerns about the exploitation of women, critics of surrogate motherhood raise concerns about the commodification of children. Rather than adopting a child or coming to terms with their childlessness, an infertile couple may protest that only a genetic child will do, offering to pay whatever they have to pay to get the kind of child they desire. Or, simply for reasons of convenience or vanity, a fertile woman may ask another woman to undergo the risks and discomforts of pregnancy for her. Under such conditions, observe the critics, parental love becomes quite conditional, and there is reason to challenge the intended parents' ability to make necessary sacrifices for their child. Babies, say the critics, ought not to be viewed as "products" to be manufactured in women's wombs for a price. They are not "Ken" and "Barbie" dolls to be ordered from a catalog.

2. Ethical Arguments For Surrogate Motherhood

Advocates of surrogate motherhood claim that the "concerns raised about surrogate motherhood are rashly speculative and bear no relation to the arrangements as they currently exist."[68] Specifically, those who favor surrogacy arrangements note that it is highly unlikely that the children resulting from them will in any way be harmed. For example, reproductive rights lawyer Lori Andrews claims that the surrogate mothers she has interviewed have uniformly described themselves as treating their surrogacy pregnancy with greater care than they would probably treat one of their own pregnancies *precisely* because they are carrying someone else's child.[69] Moreover, Andrews, like other advocates of collaborative reproduction, maintains that it is not fair to require collaborative reproducers to be medically and psychologically screened for parental fitness, because couples who are able to reproduce naturally are permitted to do so with no screening whatsoever. To be sure, proponents of surrogacy arrangements concede there have been some cases of children being rejected by both the intended parents and the surrogate mothers, as in the notorious Malahoff case. In this instance, a child born with microencephaly was initially rejected by all its parents.[70] Another famous surrogate custody dispute of Solomonic proportions was the sensationalized Baby M case,[71] which we will consider later in this chapter. But in most instances, all goes well and a very wanted child is brought home to the nursery that the intended parents have lovingly furnished.

Advocates of surrogacy arrangements also argue that there is little or no empirical evidence for claims that the intended parents, the surrogate mother, or the surrogate mother's family is harmed by surrogate motherhood. In their estimation, there is instead every reason to think that such parental arrangements are of considerable benefit to all the parties involved. The main beneficiaries are, of course, the intended parents who would otherwise not have the possibility of having a child genetically related to them. But the surrogate mother is also a major beneficiary of surrogacy arrangements. Advocates of surrogate motherhood claim that contrary to largely speculative reports, most surrogate mothers are financially secure, rigorously screened, and thoroughly informed women who wish to sell or give away their valuable reproductive services. Moreover, most surrogate mothers have little, if any, difficulty relinquishing the child to the intended parents. Rarely does a surrogate mother report experiencing anything like the psychological trauma that many birth mothers report experiencing when they decide to give up their child for adoption. Whereas 75% of birth mothers in the adoption setting decide to keep their child, available data indicate that fewer than 1% of surrogate mothers change their mind about giving the child to the intended parents.[72] Finally, it is simply not true that the surrogate mother's own children assume she has intentions of giving them away to the first bidder. On the contrary, the speculation is that children of surrogate mothers are proud of their mothers for giving a childless couple the opportunity to have a baby of their own.

Defenders of surrogacy arrangements also claim that far from creating divisions between women, there is evidence that such arrangements can actually bring women closer together or otherwise positively affect their lives. For example, in one study of over 2,000 couples and 2,000 surrogate mothers, psychologist Hilary Hanafin observed "the intended mothers, who have usually been working women, learn about child-rearing from the surrogate and deemphasize career once they have a family. The surrogate mothers, on the other hand, are motivated by the intended mothers to expand their horizons. Many pursue further education or make career advances after being surrogates."[73]

Finally, those who support surrogate motherhood insist that just because intended parents pay the surrogate mother and other third parties for their services, it does not mean that they view themselves as buying a "thing" or "toy" manufactured for their pleasure. Indeed, as Lori Andrews notes, "there is no evidence that the couple who pays $10,000 to a surrogate is any more likely to treat the child as a commodity than the couple who pays $10,000 to an *in vitro* fertilization doctor."[74]

B. Legal Remedies for Surrogate Motherhood

Because surrogate motherhood breaks the line between genetic, gestational, and social parenthood, it challenges the standard legal assumption that the woman who gives birth to a child is necessarily the genetic mother of that child. Among the legal remedies that have been proposed for surrogate motherhood are the following: (1) **criminalization** of commercial surrogate motherhood, but some form of legal recognition for altruistic surrogate motherhood;

(2) **nonenforcement** of both commercial and altruistic surrogate motherhood; (3) **enforcement** of both commercial and altruistic surrogate motherhood through **contract**; and (4) **regulation** of both commercial and altruistic surrogate motherhood as a form of **adoption**. Opponents of surrogate motherhood support either remedy (1) or remedy (2), whereas proponents of surrogate motherhood endorse either remedy (3) or remedy (4).

1. *Criminalization of (Commercial) Surrogate Motherhood*

Some opponents of surrogate motherhood maintain that commercial surrogate motherhood should be criminalized because it is a disguised form of baby-selling which more often than not involves the exploitation of financially needy women. In general, those who support criminal penalties for surrogate motherhood favor statutes such as the United Kingdom's Surrogacy Arrangements Act. Passed by the House of Lords in 1985, this statute imposes criminal sanctions not on those who provide or utilize surrogacy services but, rather, on those who serve as the middlemen in commercial surrogate motherhood negotiations. Accordingly, lawyers, physicians, and social workers are subject to fines and/or imprisonment if they "(a) initiate or take part in any negotiations with a view to the making of a surrogacy arrangement, (b) offer or agree to negotiate the making of surrogacy arrangement, or (c) compile any information with a view to its ease in making, or negotiating the making of, surrogacy arrangements."[75] In addition, publishers, directors, and mangers of newspapers, periodicals, and telecommunication systems are subject to fines and/or imprisonment if they put into print ads such as "wombs for hire" or "couple willing to pay royalty for host womb."[76]

The authors of the Surrogacy Arrangements Act justified it largely on the basis of the principle of legal moralism, according to which a person's liberty may be restricted to prevent immoral conduct on his or her part. They proclaimed, in the manner of Kant:

> [e]ven in compelling medical circumstances the danger of exploitation of one human being by another appears to the majority of us far to outweigh the potential benefits, in almost every case. That people would treat others as a means to their own ends, however desirable the consequences, must always be liable to moral objection. Such treatment of one person by another becomes positively exploitative when financial interests are involved.[77]

Although a few U.S. jurisdictions such as Michigan have made it a felony to serve as a surrogate broker—the penalty being a maximum $50,000 fine and 5-year imprisonment—[78] most U.S. jurisdictions have not rushed to impose bans on surrogate motherhood in either of its two forms for several reasons. First, it is objected that there is a difference between treating someone as a *means* and treating him or her as a *mere means*. Students treat their teachers as a means to their end of gaining knowledge, but no one is ready to criminalize the student–teacher relationship. Presumably, the student–teacher relationship is morally unobjectionable because teachers willingly contract to instruct students in exchange for pay. The student–teacher relationship would become morally objectionable if, for example, students forced their teachers to teach them for no pay. Thus, if coercion is the feature that transforms a morally permitted means–end relationship into a morally forbidden mere means–end relationship, then commercial surrogate motherhood is morally justifiable provided the parties to it freely agree to its terms.

Second, it is objected that if commercial surrogate motherhood merits criminalization, then *everyone* who participates in the practice should be treated as a criminal. Philosopher Uma Narayan views as extremely weak the standard arguments offered in defense of exempting commissioning couples and surrogate mothers from criminal penalties. She comments:

> It should not matter that . . . parents 'act in response to personal vulnerability, pain and desperation;' such factors are not usually grounds for refraining from punishing those culpable of premeditated criminal conduct. The argument that criminal penalties should not apply to parents because it is not in the best interests of the child is equally problematic, since the effects on the children of having parents incarcerated are not usually grounds for withholding criminal penalties on parents.[79]

Finally, it is objected that gift or altruistic surrogate motherhood often poses harms equal to those posed by commercial surrogate motherhood. Just because a surrogate mother receives money for her services, it does not mean that someone has not exploited her. Indeed, according to Narayan, families are not necessarily havens in an otherwise heartless world, and friends can be "false" as well as "true." She stresses that cases like that of Alejandra Muñoz confirm that family members can be even more exploitative than surrogate brokers. Muñoz's relatives told her that if she were successfully impregnated with the sperm of her cousin's husband, the embryo would be flushed into the womb of her infertile cousin. When the promised embryo transfer did not occur, Muñoz wanted to terminate the pregnancy, but her infertile cousin's family threatened to expose her as an undocumented immigrant and forcibly confined her to the family home until she gave birth.[80]

2. Nonenforcement of Commercial Surrogate Motherhood

One of the best ways to explain the concept of nonenforceability is by focusing on the Baby M case mentioned above. The Baby M or Stern–Whitehead case involved a 40-year-old biochemist, William Stern, and his wife Elizabeth, a 40-year-old pediatrician who suffered from the effects of multiple sclerosis. Because Elizabeth Stern thought she could not sustain a pregnancy, she and her husband contacted the Infertility Center in New York in order to hire a surrogate mother. The Center arranged for them to contact Mary Beth Whitehead, a young married woman with two children of her own, to be artificially inseminated by William Stern. As a result of the artificial insemination, Whitehead became pregnant and agreed to carry the fetus to term for $10,000 and give it up after birth to the Sterns.

After giving birth to the child, whom she named Sara, Mary Beth felt she could not go through with her agreement. The Sterns were unwilling to accept Whitehead's change of heart. They secured a court order to gain temporary custody of the baby whom they decided to name Melissa. Realizing that Melissa/Sara was going to be taken away from her, Whitehead fled the state with her family. Within days, however, the police tracked down the Whiteheads and recovered the baby.

Since the Sterns' legal custody of the baby was only temporary, they as well as the Whiteheads asked a New Jersey District Court to decide on a permanent home for Melissa/Sara. In granting custody to the Sterns, District Judge Harvey R. Sorkow ruled that surrogate motherhood arrangements were legally binding, despite the fact that no state specifically authorized such contracts. On further appeal of the case, however, the New Jersey State Supreme Court overruled Judge Sorkow's decision. It voided the contract between Mary Beth Whitehead and the Sterns as against public policy, holding that such transactions are tantamount to illegal baby-selling under New Jersey adoption laws as well as "perhaps criminal and potentially degrading to women."[81] Therefore, the state has no business enforcing contracts for commercial surrogate mothers.

For a court to rule that a surrogate motherhood contract is nonenforceable is for it to declare that if the contract is breached by either the surrogate mother or the commissioning couple, the state will leave the parties as it finds them. It will not help them resolve their dispute. So, for example, if the commissioning couple fails to pay the surrogate mother her fee, the state will not help her collect it. Or if the commissioning couple refuses to take the child from the surrogate mother, the state will not force them to do so. Instead, the state probably will require the surrogate mother either to maintain her parental relationship with the child or to put the child up for adoption. In the former case, the surrogate mother may be entitled to child support from the genetic father; in the latter case, she may be entitled to his financial assistance.[82] Alternatively, if the surrogate mother refuses to take care of her health during the pregnancy, or if she threatens to abort or actually does abort the fetus, the commissioning couple will not be able to sue her for damages. Moreover, if the surrogate mother refuses to give the child to the commissioning couple, they will not be able to secure custody of the child based on the contract they made with the surrogate mother; however, they may be able to secure full or joint custody based on their genetic relationship to the child.[83]

Although a custody approach supposedly is neutral between the contending parties, in point of fact, custody approaches generally favor individuals who are viewed as equipped to engage in successful child rearing. For example, in the Whitehead–Stern dispute over Baby M, Judge Sorkow observed that the day Whitehead signed her name on the dotted line, she proved her unfitness as a "real" mother.[84] He implied that no woman worthy of being a mother would consider contracting away her child to secure a monetary fee. Moreover, even if such "evidence" of unfitness was not permitted in a court of law, the surrogate mother would probably still fare worse in a custody dispute than the commissioning couple would. U.S. courts generally give custody to the parent(s) who can provide the child with a higher economic standard of living. Thus, the fact that surrogate mothers typically are poorer than the commissioning couples who contract for their services often provides courts with a reason to give the child to the commissioning couple rather than the surrogate mother. Finally, in cases where the surrogate mother is not related genetically to the child she gestated, U.S. courts are unlikely to view her gestational relationship to the child as a more significant basis for parental claims than the commissioning couple's genetic relationship to the child. Genes and blood lines still matter more than gestational connections in most U.S. courts.

For all these reasons, as well as the one cited by Narayan above— namely, that it may be in children's best interests to maintain relationships with all their parents (genetic, gestational, and social)[85]—some commentators have urged that if custody law is to be relied upon, it should be reformed so that all of a child's parents can be involved in his or her upbringing. But as ideal as this remedy to a custody dispute may seem, in practice it will work only if all of the child's parents are child-centered enough to overcome any desire to be the child's *chief* or *main* parent. To the extent that a child's parents prove unable to cooperate in the collaborative rearing of their child, it is probably best that a court designate only one or two of them to be the rearing parents of the child.

3. Enforcement of Surrogate Motherhood

Some proponents of surrogate motherhood believe that enforcing, rather than not enforcing, contracts for the arrangement are most likely to further the best interests of all concerned. Specifically, they stress that enforceable contracts are an excellent way "to illustrate that childbearing and childrearing are two quite distinct human functions and that childrearing need and should not be assigned exclusively to the woman who bears a child."[86] Proponents of a contract approach to surrogate motherhood are particularly adamant that it is not unfair or cruel to require a surrogate mother who has emotionally bonded to the child to relinquish the child to the commissioning couple. On the contrary, they insist that if anything is unfair it is depriving the commissioning couple of the child. In this connection, lawyer Marjorie Schultz has claimed that the biological relationship the surrogate mother has to the child is offset by the intentional relationship the commissioning couple has to the child:

> To ignore the significance of deliberation, purpose and expectation—the capacity to envision and shape the future through intentional choice—is to disregard one of the most distinctive traits that makes us human. It is to disregard crucial differences in moral meaning and responsibility. To disregard such intention with reference to so intimate and significant an activity as prevention and child-rearing is deeply shocking.[87]

Clearly, proponents of surrogate motherhood contracts believe that mind should rule over matter and mental intention over biological connection. They also maintain that their view is the one actually favored by the general public, including most women. For example, during the Baby M court proceedings, many commentators noted that, for the most part, women as well as men had no sympathy for Mary Beth Whitehead, the surrogate mother. "A deal's a deal!" they said. "She signed the contract, didn't she? She knew what she was doing."[88] Apparently, these people sided with the commissioning couple whose intentions seemed more compelling to them than the emotional turmoil of the surrogate mother.

Proponents of surrogate motherhood contracts further bolster their view with the argument that if a married infertile couple needs the gestational services of a surrogate mother in order to procreate a child that is genetically related to at least one of them, then forbidding the couple to pay a surrogate mother for her reproductive services may violate the equal protection clause the due process clause, and the right to privacy, all of which serve to protect people's fundamental procreative rights. As lawyer John Robertson has noted, paying surrogates is probably necessary if infertile couples are to obtain surrogacy services.[89] Proponents of commercial surrogate motherhood contracts also claim that banning pay for reproductive services is likely to "reactivate and reinforce the state's power to define what constitutes legitimate and illegitimate reproduction,"[90] whereas allowing payment is likely to "recognize a woman's legal authority to make decisions regarding the exercise of her reproductive capacity."[91]

Importantly, proponents of surrogate motherhood contracts emphasize that such agreements must be voluntary and respectful of the rights of everyone involved. They should, for example, guarantee the surrogate mother's freedom (1) to engage in self-chosen activities during pregnancy; (2) to refuse or accept proposed medical treatments during pregnancy and delivery; and (3) to continue or terminate the pregnancy. In addition, surrogate motherhood contracts should specify that the surrogate mother will not be liable for damages or subject to a lawsuit in the event that the fetus is spontaneously aborted, delivered stillborn, or born with defects. The contracts should also set a fairly high fee for the surrogate mother's reproductive services in order to adequately compensate her for the risks and discomforts that typically accompany pregnancy, labor, and delivery.[92] Finally, the contracts should be predicated upon securing the informed consent of all the parties to them. Physicians and psychologists should clearly outline to prospective surrogate mothers and commissioning couples all of the physical and psychological risks that may accompany collaborative reproduction. In addition, lawyers should clearly outline what will count as a breach of contract and how such breaches will be penalized.

4. Assimilation of Surrogate Motherhood Arrangements into Adoption Law

Another way to address surrogate motherhood arrangements is to assimilate them into an adoption paradigm. Proponents of an adoption approach to surrogate motherhood claim it is a mistake to dismiss the bonds that some surrogate mothers forge with the fetus during pregnancy as *merely* biological or hormonal. They cite with approval philosopher Iris Young's view of pregnancy. According to Young, pregnancy may appear to observers to be "a time of waiting and watching, when nothing happens,"[93] but for the pregnant woman "pregnancy has a temporality of movement, growth and change . . . . The pregnant woman experiences herself as a source and participant in a creative process. Though she does not plan and direct it, neither does it merely wash over her; rather, she is the process, this change."[94] Because of views of pregnancy such as Young's, proponents of an adoption approach to surrogate motherhood arrangements believe it is misguided to speak as if the relationship between a mother's body and her growing fetus is totally analogous to the "relationship" that might exist between an artificial womb and a fetus developing within it.[95] As they see it, for every surrogate mother who maintains that throughout her whole pregnancy she viewed herself merely as a fetal container, there is a surrogate mother more like the one described by writer Anne Taylor Fleming:

> She had meant to be unfazed, meant to make her parents and friends proud of her generosity, meant to make the couple she had the baby for like her so much that "afterwards" she would be part of their extended family and could watch her son grow up. But none of it, not one piece of that, had come out the right way. Her parents were not particularly proud. The couple did not want her around. And she was not unattached from her son and clearly never would be.[96]

Proponents of an adoption approach to surrogate motherhood concede that the rules and regulations governing adoption would have to be modified in order to accommodate the unique features of surrogate motherhood;

however, they claim these adjustments would be minimal. As in private adoptions, the surrogate mother would be paid only reasonable medical expenses and given only a limited amount of time after the birth of the child in which to decide whether or not to relinquish the child to the commissioning couple. Importantly, proponents of an adoption approach to surrogate motherhood believe a change-of-heart period should be granted to gestational as well as to traditional surrogate mothers. In their estimation, gestational connections trump genetic connections.[97]

Among the arguments that support the above view are those of philosopher Sara Ann Ketchum. She claims that as soon as scientists develop gene-splicing and chromosome-splicing techniques, it will be possible to procreate children with enormously complex genetic backgrounds. Who, then, will count as the genetic parents of each child? Only the donors who contributed the most genes to the child, or also those donors who contributed just a few genes to the child? Under this set of genetic circumstances, the uniqueness and intimacy of the gestational relationship will be revealed. Ketchum also notes that our intuitions suggest that at least in the case of rape, it is implausible to regard genetic connection as conferring parental rights. Finally, Ketchum emphasizes that to identify genetic connection as the essential criterion for parenthood is to suggest that the kind of relationship an anonymous sperm donor has with a child is just as close as the one between a woman and the child to whom she gives birth after a 9-month pregnancy. It is also to imply that adoptive parents are less real than genetic parents.[98]

Bolstering Ketchum's arguments in favor of privileging the gestational, and to some extent, the rearing connection, over the genetic connection, lawyer George Annas maintains that there are at least two moral reasons why the gestational mother rather than the commissioning couple should be legally presumed to have primary parental rights to rear that child. First, because it is the gestational mother and not the commissioning couple who assumes the major responsibility for bringing a new life into the world, she deserves to maintain her relationship with the child unless there is evidence of child abuse on her part.[99] Second, because the gestational mother "will of necessity be present at birth and immediately thereafter to care for the child," designating her the legal or "natural" mother of the child is more likely to protect the child's interests than any alternative arrangement.[100] What makes a person a parent, therefore, is the degree to which that person has shown through some sort of sweat labor that his or her commitment to a child is more than a matter of either mere genetic connection or mere intention.

Opponents of an adoption approach to surrogate motherhood agree with its proponents that it is wrong to trivialize the gestational connection, as California Judge Parslow did when he equated gestating an embryo with providing day care or "nanny" services for it.[101] Nonetheless, they insist it is equally wrong to dismiss as insignificant adults' genetic and/or intentional connections to a child, for at least three reasons. First, many women and men derive comfort from their genealogy—that is, from the fact they belong to a family who share a physical identity that stretches back into the past and forward into the future. Seeing one's physical characteristics reflected in one's children provides a sense of corporeal immortality—a sense that part of one's material as well as psychic identity will live on in a new and different form. Second, when a couple commissions the services of a surrogate mother their intentions to rear the child are more than mere intentions. The fact that they cannot show a "physical" commitment to their future child does not mean their commitment to the child is less serious than that of the surrogate mother. Some commissioning couples buy baby furniture and baby clothes in advance; others set up savings accounts for their future children; and still others routinely spend time musing about how life will be when their future child exist in the present tense. Third, and most significantly, the kind of care a gestational mother provides the child *in utero* can be readily supplemented and gradually replaced by other caring acts of parental commitment. Although commissioning couples cannot provide nutrients to their children *in utero*, they can bottle-feed, diaper, caress, and comfort them subsequent to birth. As soon as the child is born, the gestational mother's 9 months of labor can be matched minute for minute by the commissioning couple.

In addition to claiming it is misguided to automatically privilege gestational connections over genetic and intentional connections, opponents of an adoption approach to surrogate motherhood claim that it might not be in *women's* best interests to overemphasize the importance of the gestational connection. In the first place, if women want men to spend as much time caring for children as women generally do, then it is probably a mistake to repeatedly remind men that women have a connection to infants that is totally unavailable to men—indeed, a connection that makes men second-class parents until sometime after a child's birth. Second, stressing the importance of the gestational connection invites state authorities to seek more control than they already have over women's pregnancies. In recent years, national attention has focused on a wide range of issues arising from actions taken by women during pregnancy that may have harmful consequences for their children. These issues include: (1) medical interventions (such as refusal of a recommended cesarean section or insulin treatment for gestational diabetes); (2) innovative therapies (such as fetal surgery); (3) prenatal diagnosis; and (4) lifestyle concerns (such as alcohol, tobacco, or narcotic use during pregnancy). Since many people already believe that pregnant women have a moral responsibility to care for their fetuses *in utero*, they would be only too happy to join in the celebration of the gestational connection.

A final consideration raised by some opponents of an adoption approach to surrogate motherhood is that surrogate motherhood is not really like adoption after all. According to Phyllis Chesler, adoption should be regarded as a child-centered practice whereby adults, willing to give children the kind of love they need to thrive, take into their homes and hearts already-existing children. It should not, insists Chesler, be regarded as an adult-centered practice whereby children are deliberately conceived and brought into existence so that adults can have someone to love them.[102]

VI. CONCLUSION

Assisted-reproduction technologies, like all technologies, are neither entirely beneficial nor entirely harmful. When used properly and realistically, they can provide infertile couples with a child they could not otherwise have. The satisfaction and sense of human purpose and meaning that accompanies genetic parenthood should not be underestimated, even though it is certainly not the only form of parenthood available to people. Nevertheless, because of the ways in which some assisted-reproduction technologies have been priced and marketed, and because of numerous articles about women who would rather be dead than childless ("Give Me Children or I Shall Die!" reads the title of a 1996 *Hastings Center Report* article),[103] we should at least ask ourselves why more research dollars are not being used to address the underlying causes of infertility such as sexually transmitted diseases and environmental toxins. Corrections of these problems, as well as a measured assessment of the disadvantages as well as advantages of waiting until one is older to start a family, would probably spare many couples the heartache that all too often accompanies infertility.

Discussion Questions

1. Should women who are not infertile be allowed to use a surrogate mother to bear them a child?
2. If surrogate motherhood is legal, then why should we not consider the practice a potential occupation for women? Discuss the social ramifications of a job market for surrogate mothers.
3. Which of the following restrictions should be placed on using a surrogate mother: age; ethnicity; class; health (both psychological and physiological)?
4. Critics of surrogate motherhood argue that commercial surrogacy commodifies women and children. Would prohibiting any financial exchange address such problems? What problems might arise because financial exchange is prohibited?
5. Surrogate motherhood is typically defended as a contractual arrangement. How much control should the contracting couple have over the actions of the surrogate? Should family law or contract law dictate how surrogacy contracts are handled?
6. Discuss the advantages and disadvantages of surrogate motherhood arrangements for nontraditional relationships and marriages (gays, lesbians, single women, and single men).

7. Is parenthood a right? Should infertility be approached as a desire? Discuss the ethical implications for assisted reproduction in terms of these questions.

8. To what degree should assisted reproduction clinics furnish clients with complete information about success and failure rates?

9. Should any couple, fertile or infertile, have access to assisted reproduction technologies?

10. Who should have the right to decide the fate of embryos in disputed custody cases?

11. In your estimation, which of the following connections most makes someone the real parent of a child: genetic connections; gestational connections; rearing connections?

12. Can someone ever want a baby too much?

13. Would you ever donate or sell your gametes to someone? Why or why not? Would you in any way consider yourself the parent of the child, were one born?

14. In your estimation, do parents have a total right to discard their unwanted frozen embryos? Is discarding a frozen embryo any different than aborting a fetus? Why or why not?

15. Should women over 60 be permitted to use *in vitro* fertilization? Why or why not?

16. Should gamete donation be as anonymous as possible or as open as possible? Explain your choice.

Case Studies

1. Oakland, California is the site of the Oakland Feminist Women's Health Center—a sperm bank founded to make AID available in a manner consistent with feminist ideals. Women may secure sperm from the bank directly for purpose of self-insemination.

a. Is the Oakland Women's Health Center founded on a morally sound philosophy? Should single women and/or lesbians couples self-inseminate?

b. Should all assisted reproduction centers be legally required to provide their services to anyone who wants to use them, no questions asked?

2. Gayle is a 60-year-old retiree who has been married for 12 years to Tim. Both she and her husband retired comfortably and are in good health. They are looking forward to these years and have decided they would like to raise a child. After reading some articles about postmenopausal pregnancies, they have decided upon a course of action that employs egg donation, IVF with Tim's sperm, and embryo transfer into Gayle's womb. Although Gayle will not be genetically related to the child, Tim will. After explaining their plan to Dr. Wise, she expresses concerns about their proposal. Although Dr. Wise has successfully produced pregnancies in women in early menopause, she is uncomfortable with the idea of a postmenopausal pregnancy that will

require possibly harmful hormone treatments for Gayle and a pregnancy likely to be quite difficult.

a. Should the assisted reproduction clinic and Dr. Wise support Gayle and Tim in their attempt to have a child?

b. From a moral point of view, is Gayle and Tim's plan ethically justified? Justify your response.

c. Consider the age Gayle and Tim will be when their child enters college. Do you think they are in any way acting irresponsibly? Why or why not?

3. Quinn and her husband Joshua are in their mid-thirties and have not had success starting a family. After repeated cycles of IVF and repeated miscarried pregnancies, they have decided to invest their remaining hope for a child in their one remaining embryo, frozen in the embryo bank. They request that it be split into four cells so that each can begin the process of division and growth. Implantation will be attempted with two of the newly formed embryos. The other two will be frozen. If Quinn becomes pregnant and gives birth to a healthy child, they propose that in 3 years they be allowed to achieve pregnancy with the remaining two embryos. The plan could result in genetically identical children of different ages.

a. Is embryo splitting as an adjunct to IVF morally sound?

b. Is embryo splitting less morally problematic than cloning?

c. Should the clinic act in accordance with the couple's wishes? If not, why not?

d. Should Quinn and Joshua abandon this project and consider remaining childless, seeking their happiness in other ways than biological parenthood? Should they consider adoption?

4. Gina Kolata described the following case in *The New York Times* (August 5, 1991):

A South Dakota woman, Arlette Schweitzer, 42 years old, was the gestational surrogate mother of twins for her daughter, who was born without a uterus. The eggs came from her daughter and the sperm from her son-in-law. The embryos that resulted from IVF were then implanted in Schweitzer's womb. This was the first time in the United States that a woman gave birth to her own grandchildren. Schweitzer did not receive any payment for serving as a surrogate mother and said she bore the children out of love for her daughter.

a. Keeping this case in mind, discuss if there should be any restrictions on a family member being either a traditional surrogate mother or a gestational surrogate.

b. What social issues does this case raise regarding surrogate motherhood?

c. Is the family arrangement discussed in the best interests of the twins? Is the network of relationships into which they are born any more complex and challenging than the network of relationships that exist in so-called blended families? Explain why or why not.

5. Mr. and Mrs. Fiburnacci are in their late thirties. Because they both suffered from thalassemia, a debilitating type of hereditary anemia, and because Mrs. Fiburnacci was not able to sustain a pregnancy, they decided to adopt a child. Although it was only a matter of time before they would be accepted as adoptive parents by an adoption agency, they grew tired of waiting. They decided to secure the services of an off-shore surrogate mother agency. For the fee of U.S. $40,000, the agency provided them with sperm, eggs, and the services of a gestational surrogate who gave up any claim to parental rights. The problem is that during the third trimester of the gestational mother's pregnancy, the Fiburnaccis filed for divorce. Upon divorcing, neither Mr. nor Mrs. Fiburnacci wanted the child. To complicate matters, the gestational surrogate did not want the child either.

a. Who, if anyone, is the legal parent of the child?
b. What are the moral obligations of the Fiburnaccis to the child? What are those of the gestational mother to the child? What are those of the sperm and egg donors to the child?
c. Is the surrogate agency in anyway at fault in this type of situation? What about the health care professionals who assisted this particular reproduction? Are they in any way responsible?
d. Is the gestational mother, a non–U.S. citizen, legally entitled to have an abortion in the third trimester of the pregnancy? Is she morally justified?

Endnotes

1. Ronald Munson, *Intervention and Reflection: Basic Issues in Medical Ethics*, 6th ed. (Belmont, CA: Wadsworth/Thomson Learning, 2000), p. 662.
2. John Robertson, *Children of Choice: Freedom and the New Reproductive Technologies* (Princeton, NJ: Princeton University Press, 1994), p. 97.
3. Temma Ehrenfeld, "Infertility: a guy thing," *Newsweek* (March 25, 2002): 61–62.
4. John Robertson, *Children of Choice: Freedom and the New Reproductive Technologies* (Princeton, NJ: Princeton University Press, 1994), p. 97.
5. Allen A. Mitchell, "Infertility treatment: more risks and challenges," *New England Journal of Medicine*, 346 (2002): 769–770.
6. David A. Grainger and Bruce L. Tjaden, "Assisted reproductive technologies," in: Marlene B. Goldman, Marlene Goldman, and Maureen C. Hatch (eds.), *Women and Health* (San Diego: Academic Press, 2000), pp. 215–225.
7. Jusae Horsburgh, Sosan Schiradehette, Joanne Fowler, Macon Morehouse, and Jennifer Frey, "The next generation miracle babies," *People Magazine* (October 11, 2004): 218.
8. Ronald Munson, *Intervention and Reflection: Basic Issues in Medical Ethics*, 6th ed. (Belmont, CA: Wadsworth/Thomson Learning, 2000), p. 662.

9. Jennifer Wolff, "Sperm donor ruling could open door for offspring," *USA Today* (June 15, 2004): 13A.

10. Barbara Menning, "Donor insemination: the psychosocial issues," *American College of Gynecology and Obstetrics*, 18 (1981): 155–171.

11. Ibid.

12. Robin Rowland, "The social and psychological consequences of secrecy in artificial insemination by donor (AID) programmer," *Social Science Medicine*, 21, no. 4 (1985): 395.

13. Ibid.

14. George Annas, "Beyond the best interests of the sperm donor," *Child Welfare*, 13, no. 13 (March, 1981): 7.

15. L. T. Styron, "Artificial insemination: a new frontier for medical malpractice and medical products liability," *Loyola Law Review*, 32 (1986): 411–446.

16. Mary Warnock, *A Question of Life: The Warnock Report on Human Fertilization and Embryology* (Oxford: Basil Blackwell, 1985), p. 11.

17. Maureen McGuire and Nancy J. Alexander, "Artificial insemination of single women," *Fertility and Sterility*, 43, no. 2 (1985): 182–184.

18. Robin Rowland, "The social and psychological consequences of secrecy in artificial insemination by donor (AID) programmer," *Social Science Medicine*, 21, no. 4 (1985): 395.

19. Gena Corea, *The Mother Machine: Reproductive Technologies from Artificial Insemination to Artificial Wombs* (New York: Harper & Row, 1985), p. 25.

20. *Strnad v. Strnad*, 78. N.Y. Supplement, 2nd Ser. (1948) at 391–392.

21. Ibid.

22. *People v. Sorenson*, 68 Cal. 2nd 280, 66 Cal. Rpt. (1968) at 437.

23. B. J. Jensen, "Artificial insemination and the Law," *Brigham Young University Law Review* (1982): 955–956.

24. Robin Hemran, "When the 'Father' is a sperm donor," *Washington Post Health*, (February 11, 1992): 10.

25. Lawrence J. Kaplan and Carolyn M. Kaplan, "Natural reproduction and reproduction-aiding technologies," in: Kenneth D. Alpern (ed.), *The Ethics of Reproductive Technology* (New York: Oxford University Press, 1992), p. 24.

26. Robin Hemran, "When the 'Father' is a sperm donor," *Washington Post Health* (February 11, 1992): 14.

27. *C.M. v. C.C.*, 170 N.J. Superior Ct. 586, 407A. 2nd 849, 852 (Juv. and Dom. Rel. Ct. 1979).

28. Ruth Marcus, "Court lets sperm donor sue for parental rights," *New York Times* (April 24, 1990): A4.

29. Otto Frederick, "A legal, moral, social nightmare," *Time Magazine* (September 10, 1984): 55.

30. Laura Muha, "She lost her husband but saved their dream," *Redbook Magazine* (May 1995): 80.

31. Ibid., p. 83.

32. Nadine Brozan, "Babies from donated eggs: growing use stirs questions," *New York Times* (January 18, 1988): 9.

33. Patricia P. Mahlstedt, cited in Robin Hemran, "When the 'Father' is a sperm donor," *Washington Post Health* (February 11, 1992): 10.

34. Alison Kornet, "Should donors be anonymous?" *New Women* (November 1995): 144.

35. John A. Robertson, "Recommitment strategies for disposition of frozen embryos," *Emory Law Journal*, 50, no. 4 (Fall 2001): 991.

36. Michael C. Brannigan and Judith A. Boss, *Healthcare Ethics in a Diverse Society* (Mountain View, CA: Mayfield Publishing Company, 2002), p. 270.

37. Ronald Munson, *Intervention and Reflection: Basic Issues in Medical Ethics*, 6th ed. (Belmont, CA: Wadsworth/Thomson Learning, 2000), p. 663.

38. *Roe v. Wade*, 410 U.S. (1973).

39. National Bioethics Advisory Commission, "Ethical issues in human stem cell research," *Report and Recommendations of the National Bioethics Advisory Commission*, Vol. I (Rockville, MD: National Bioethics Advisory Commission, September 1999).

40. Michael D. Lemonick, Janice M. Horowitz, Alice Park, and Sora Song, "Risky business?" *Time* (March 18, 2002).

41. Toni Gerber Hope, "The ultimate fertility guide," *Redbook Magazine* (2002): 149.

42. Christine Overall, *Reproduction: Principles, Practices, Policies* (Toronto: Oxford University Press, 1993), p. 181.

43. "Assisted Reproductive Technology Reports," *Centers for Disease Control and Prevention* (February 17, 2005) *http://www.cdc.gov/reproductivehealth/art.htm* [accessed March 25, 2005].

44. Barbara Seaman, "Treating infertility," *The Women's Review of Books*, 22, no. 1 (October, 2004): 9.

45. Ibid.

46. Leigh Hopper, "Eleven-month-old chukwus honored," *Houston Chronicle* (November 7, 1999).

47. L. N. Schover, N. L. Collins, M. M. Quigley, J. Blanstein, and G. Kanoti, "Psychological follow-up of women evaluated as oocyte donors," *Human Reproduction*, 6, no. 10 (1991): 1491.

48. Michelle Blackely, "Eggs for sale: the latest controversy in reproductive technology," *USA Today Magazine* (July 2003): 56.

49. Claudia Kalb, "Baby boom: the $50,000 egg," *Newsweek* (March 15, 1999): 64.

50. L. N. Schover, N. L. Collins, M. M. Quigley, J. Blanstein, and G. Kanoti, "Psychological follow-up of women evaluated as oocyte donors," *Human Reproduction*, 6, no. 10 (1991): 1488.

51. LeRoy Walters, "Test-tube babies: ethical considerations," in: Richard T. Hull (ed.), *Ethical Issues in the New Reproductive Technologies* (Belmont, CA: Wadsworth Publishing, 1990), pp. 110–111.

52. Ibid., p. 114.

53. Ibid., p. 114–117.

54. Ibid.

55. Peter Singer and Deane Wells, *Making Babies: the New Science and Ethics of Conception* (New York: Charles Scribner's Sons, 1984), p. 86.

56. Ibid., p. 87.

57. *Davis v. Davis*, 842 S.W. 2d 588, 602-03 (Tenn. 1992).

58. Richard Jerome and Giovanna Brev, "In the bank," *People* (July 1, 2002): 48–50.

59. Jusae Horsburgh, Sosan Schiradehette, Joanne Fowler, Macon Morehouse, and Jennifer Frey, "The next generation miracle babies," *People Magazine* (October 11, 2004): 120.

60. John A. Robertson, "Surrogate mothers: not so novel after all," *The Hastings Center Report*, 13, no. 5 (October 1983): 28–34.

61. *Center for Surrogate Parenting, Inc* (November 9, 2004), *http://www.creatingfamilies.com/index.HTML* [accessed March 25, 2005].

62. Ethics Committee of the American Fertility Society, "Ethical considerations of assisted reproductive technologies," *Fertility and Sterility*, 62, 5 Suppl. 1 (1994): 15–125S.

63. R. H. Miller, "Surrogate parenting: an infant industry presents society with legal, ethical questions," *Ob-Gyn News*, no. 3 (February 1–14, 1983): 4.

64. Gena Corea, *The Mother Machine: Reproductive Technologies from Artificial Insemination to Artificial Wombs* (New York: Harper & Row, 1985), p. 214.

65. United States Congress, Office of Technology Assessment, *Infertility: Medical and Social Choices* (Washington, D.C.: U.S. Government Printing Office, OTA-BA-358, May 1988).

66. Gena Corea, *The Mother Machine: Reproductive Technologies from Artificial Insemination to Artificial Wombs* (New York: Harper & Row, 1985), p. 231.

67. Patricia A. Avery, "Surrogate mothers: center of a new storm," *U.S. News & World Report* (June 6, 1983): 76.

68. Lori B. Andrews, "Beyond doctrinal boundaries: a legal framework for surrogate motherhood," *Virginia Law Review*, 81 (November 1995): 8.

69. Ibid., p. 13.

70. Singer and Wells, *Making Babies: The New Science and Ethics of Conception.*

71. In re *Baby M* (1988) 537 A.2d 1227, N.J.

72. Lori B. Andrews, "Beyond doctrinal boundaries: a legal framework for surrogate motherhood," *Virginia Law Review*, 81 (November 1995): 10.

73. Andrews, *Between Strangers: Surrogate Mothers, Expectant Fathers, & Brave New World Babies* (New York: Harper and Row, 1989), pp. 71–72.

74. Lori B. Andrews, "Beyond doctrinal boundaries: a legal framework for surrogate motherhood," *Virginia Law Review*, 81 (November 1995): 20.

75. Surrogacy Arrangements Act 1985, United Kingdom, chapter 49, p. 2: section (1), (a), (b), and (c).

76. Ibid., p. 3: sections (1) through (5).

77. Ibid., p. 46.

78. Phyllis Chesler, *Sacred Bond: The Legacy of Baby M* (New York Times Books, 1988), p. 197.

79. Uma Narayan, "The 'gift' of a child: commercial surrogacy gift surrogacy, and motherhood," in: Patricia Boling (ed.), *Expecting Trouble: Surrogacy, Fetal Abuse & New Reproductive Technologies* (Boulder, CO: Westview Press, 1995), p. 189.

80. Ibid., p. 180.

81. Phyllis Chesler, *Sacred Bond: The Legacy of Baby M* (New York Times Books, 1988), pp. 197–203.

82. Lori B. Andrews, "The aftermath of baby M: proposed state laws on surrogate motherhood," *Hastings Center Report,* 17 (October–November 1987): 32.

83. Barbara Cohen, "Surrogate mothers: whose baby is it?" *American Journal of Law and Medicine,* 10, no. 3 (Fall 1984): 255.

84. Phyllis Chesler, *Sacred Bond: The Legacy of Baby M* (New York Times Books, 1988), p. 38.

85. Uma Narayan, "The 'gift' of a child: commercial surrogacy gift surrogacy, and motherhood," in: Patricia Boling (ed.), *Expecting Trouble: Surrogacy, Fetal Abuse & New Reproductive Technologies* (Boulder, CO: Westview Press, 1995), p. 194.

86. Mary Lyndon Shanley, "'Surrogate mothering' and women's freedom: a critique of contracts for human reproduction," in: Patricia Boling (ed.), *Expecting Trouble: Surrogacy, Fetal Abuse, & New Reproductive Technologies* (Boulder, CO: Westview Press), p. 157.

87. Majorie Maguire Schultz, "Reproductive technology and intention-based parenthood: an opportunity for gender neutrality," *Wisconsin Law Review,* 2 (1990): 377–378.

88. Phyllis Chesler, *Sacred Bond: The Legacy of Baby M* (New York Times Books, 1988), p. 164.

89. John Robertson, *Children of Choice: Freedom and the New Reproductive Technologies* (Princeton, NJ: Princeton University Press, 1994), p. 140.

90. Carmel Shavlev, *Birth Power* (New Haven, Conn.: Yale University Press, 1989), p. 94, 157.

91. Ibid.

92. Laura M. Purdy, "Another look at contract pregnancy," in: Laura M. Purdy (ed.), *Reproducing Persons: Issues in Feminist Bioethics* (Ithaca, NY: Cornell University Press, 1996), p. 211.

93. Iris M. Young, "Pregnant embodiment: subjectivity and alienation," in: Iris M. Young (ed.), *Throwing Like a Girl and Other Essays in Feminist Philosophy and Social Theory* (Bloomington: Indiana University Press, 1990), p. 167.

94. Ibid.

95. Mary Lyndon Shanley, "'Surrogate mothering and women's freedom: a critique of contracts for human reproduction," in: Patricia Boling (ed.), *Expecting Trouble: Surrogacy, Fetal Abuse, & New Reproductive Technologies* (Boulder, CO: Westview Press), p. 162.

96. Anne Taylor Fleming, "Our fascination with baby M," *New York Times Magazine* (March 20, 1987): 38.

97. Barbara Katz-Rothman, *Recreating Motherhood: Ideology and Technology in a Patriarchal Society* (New York: W.W. Norton, 1989), pp. 254–255.

98. Sara Ann Ketchum, "New reproductive technologies and the definition of parenthood: a feminist perspective," Paper presented at *Feminism and Legal Theory: Woman and Intimacy*, a conference sponsored by the Institute for Legal Studies at the University of Wisconsin, Madison (1987).

99. Sherman Elias and George J. Annas, "Noncoital reproduction," *Journal of American Medical Association*, 225 (January 3, 1986): 67.

100. George J. Annas, "Death without dignity for commercial surrogacy: the case of baby M," *Hastings Center Report*, 18, no. 2 (1988): 23–24.

101. Lawrence J. Nelson and Nancy Milliken, "Compelled medical treatment of pregnant women: life, liberty, and law in conflict," in: Richard T. Hull (ed.), *Ethical Issues in the New Reproductive Technologies* (Amherst, NY: Prometheus Books, 2005), pp. 224–240.

102. Phyllis Chesler, *Sacred Bond: The Legacy of Baby M* (New York Times Books, 1988), pp. 109–146.

103. Cynthia B. Cohen, "'Give me children or I shall die!': new reproductive technologies and harm to children," *Hastings Center Report*, 26, no. 2 (1996): 19–27.

chapter eight

Genetic Screening, Counseling, and Therapy

I. INTRODUCTION

In many ways, this is the Golden Age of medicine. Before the twentieth century, medicine consisted largely of painful amputations and cauterizations, massive doses of morphine, bloodlettings, and various water and rest cures that were probably less comforting and no more efficacious than Mom's chicken soup. The discovery of antibiotics and vaccines changed this dismal state of affairs, at least in those areas of the world with access to them.[1] Thanks to seemingly miraculous medications and vaccinations, whole classes of diseases were virtually eliminated and many epidemics were successfully controlled. Yet the truly amazing developments in medicine are only beginning. As a result of the completion of the **Human Genome Project** (HGP) and several spin-off projects in the emerging field of genomics, an increasing number of people throughout the world may be able to lead longer and healthier lives.[2]

The HGP, a 15-year, $3.1-billion effort to map the entire genome and to sequence all its genes, began in 1990 and was completed ahead of schedule in 2003.[3] Both the enormity and significance of this project are hard to exaggerate, given that the human body consists of about ten trillion cells. The nucleus of each of these cells contains twenty-three pairs of chromosomes. Each chromosome consists of two long and twisted strands of DNA, the chemical compound that passes on genetic information from one generation to the next. Human DNA is divided into clusters called genes, the total number of which is unknown but thought to be approximately 30,000. These genes are composed of four types of nucleotides called adenosine (A), thymine (T), guanine (G), and cytosine (C). About three billion nucleotides constitute the human genome, which is most easily understood as the blueprint for a human being. *Sequencing* consists of the break down of DNA into its nucleotides. *Mapping* entails the assignment of genes to their location on a chromosome.[4] Although the number changes daily, as of April 2000 more than 8,000 human genes had been located.[5]

Knowing where genes are located on the chromosomes is, of course, only part of the story. Genetic researchers do not value cartography for cartography's sake. On the contrary, their purpose in mapping the human genome is to gain knowledge about the nature and function of all the human genes, particularly those that are correlated with diseases, defects, and disorders. As they see it, the more they understand the mechanisms that determine human identity, behavior, and health status, the better they will be able to control them.

II. GENETIC TESTING AND SCREENING

Even as ordinary people struggle to understand not only the scientific but also the economic, political, social, and cultural consequences of the HGP, scientific experts are fast at work developing techniques for testing and/or screening human beings' genetic composition. Whereas **genetic testing** is conducted on *individuals* who are at a higher than average risk of carrying or having a genetic problem, **genetic screening** is conducted on an entire *population*, including individuals at low risk for the targeted genetic disease, defect, or disorder.[6] Significantly, fetuses, embryos, and even preembryos as well as children and adults can be genetically tested and/or screened for a variety of conditions.

A. Types of Genetic Testing and Screening

1. *Carrier Testing and Screening*

Through **carrier testing and screening**, health care professionals help people understand their risk for transmitting certain genetic diseases to their offspring. If one member of a couple is a carrier for a *dominant* disorder such as Huntington's disease, the couple has a 50% chance per pregnancy of procreating an affected child, and a 50% chance per pregnancy of procreating an unaffected child. In contrast, if one member of a couple is a carrier for a *recessive* disorder such as cystic fibrosis, Tay–Sachs disease, or sickle-cell anemia, the couple is not at any risk for procreating an affected child, though they are at 50% risk per pregnancy for procreating a carrier of the disorder; however, if both members of the couple are carriers for the disorder their odds worsen. They have a 25% chance per pregnancy of procreating an affected child as well as a 50% chance per pregnancy of procreating a carrier of the disorder.

Once a couple knows how great or small their risks of having an affected child are, they can choose in an informed way among several options. Among these options are: (1) not marrying or even divorcing; (2) marrying but deciding to remain childless; (3) marrying but deciding to adopt or to use either donor gametes; or (4) marrying and taking the risk of procreating with their own gametes.[7] The fourth one of these options is more likely to be taken by carriers of a recessive disorder than those of a dominant disorder.

2. Preimplantation Genetic Diagnosis

Couples with at least one carrier, who want to procreate with their own gametes and are enrolled in an IVF program, may request health care professionals to use **preimplantation genetic diagnosis (PIGD)** to test their preembryos. This method enables physicians to test the genetic condition of a twelve-cell preembryo before it is transferred from the petri dish to a woman's womb. At present it is possible to test preembryos for a limited range of serious, single-gene diseases such as cystic fibrosis, Duchenne muscular dystrophy, Tay–Sachs disease, hemophilia A and B, beta-thalassemia, sickle-cell disease, alpha-antitrypis deficiency, and Lesch–Nyhan syndrome.[8] It is also possible to test them for nonmedical conditions such as sex.

3. Prenatal Genetic Diagnosis

Much more developed than the technique for preimplantation genetic diagnosis are those for **prenatal genetic diagnosis (PGD)**. At present, most prenatal testing is done *in utero* (in the womb) using one of three approaches to identify a fetal genetic defect. The first approach involves visualization, which can be either noninvasive (ultrasonography) or invasive (embryoscopy, fetoscopy, and endoscopy). The second approach involves analysis of fetal tissues (amniocentesis, chorionic villus sampling [CVS], cordocentesis [fetal blood sampling], skin biopsy, liver biopsy, and muscle biopsy). The third approach involves laboratory studies (cytogenetics, biochemical analysis, and DNA analysis). All three of these approaches enable physicians to determine whether a fetus has a certain chromosomal abnormality such as Down's syndrome, an unbalanced translocation, a mosaic, a sex-chromosome disorder, a biochemical abnormality such as Huntington's disease (HD), sickle-cell anemia, Tay–Sachs disease, or a neural tube defect.[9]

Of the three approaches mentioned above, analysis of fetal tissues is the most common one. Increasingly, couples use **amniocentesis** and/or **chorionic villus sampling** to ascertain the health status of their future children. In amniocentesis, the membrane (amnion) surrounding the fetus is punctured with a needle. Some of the amniotic fluid is sucked out for DNA analysis. Typically, amniocentesis is performed sometime between the 14th and 16th week of pregnancy. The test is relatively risk-free to the woman and fetus. In fact, miscarriages occur only about one in every 200 times and infections are rare. Chorionic villus sampling involves retrieving hairlike villi cells from the developing placenta. The advantage of CVS is that it can be performed between the 6th and 10th week of pregnancy. It is somewhat less informative than amniocentesis, however, and there has been some debate about whether fetuses subjected to CVS are at higher risk for abnormalities than infants not subjected to CVS.[10]

Currently, most health care professionals do not routinely offer either amniocentesis or chorionic villus sampling to all pregnant women. They claim that (1) the risks of these tests, though small, should not be imposed on people very unlikely to have an impaired child, and (2) the costs of these tests (for example, $1000 to $2500 for amniocentesis) should not be imposed on people for services that are probably medically unnecessary. For the two reasons just stated, most health care professionals advise prenatal genetic testing only when at least one of the following conditions enters into the procreative calculus: (1) advanced maternal age (age 35 and upwards); (2) a family history of genetic abnormalities; (3) membership in an at-risk ethnic group (for example, Tay–Sachs in Askenazi Jews and sickle-cell anemia in African-Americans); (4) a family history of infants with birth defects; and/or (5) multiple miscarriages.[11]

The present policy of restricting access to prenatal genetic testing may change in the future, however. Researchers claim they are on the verge of developing a highly accurate, risk-free maternal blood test to separate fetal cells from maternal cells. Should this blood test become available to clinicians, obstetricians will be able to test very young embryos for a great variety of genetic problems without risking harm to them or subjecting their mothers to major bodily intrusions.[12]

4. Neonatal Testing and Screening

Another form of genetic testing/screening targets newborns. The neonatal conditions screened for are relatively serious. For instance, all fifty U.S. states routinely screen infants for phenylketonuria (PKU), a disorder that, if undetected and untreated by a special diet low in phenylalanine, can lead to severe mental retardation. Other disorders routinely screened for in the United States are galactosemia, a disorder affecting the body's ability to process lactose in dairy products; congenital hypothyroidism, an endocrine disorder; and sickle-cell anemia, a blood disorder that can be fatal even before 1 year of age.[13] Significantly, all of these disorders can be effectively treated or at least ameliorated if detected as early as possible. Equally important is the fact that as soon as prenatal diagnosis becomes safer, more effective, and even easier than it is now, it will probably replace **neonatal testing/screening** entirely.

5. Presymptomatic Testing and Screening

Yet another type of genetic testing/screening aims to uncover genetic diseases before symptoms appear. Testing of individuals is particularly appropriate in families plagued by a particular genetic disease, the symptoms of which can be ameliorated or even averted if proper preventive measures are taken. For example, at present it is possible to test for familial polyposis of the colon, a condition that can be managed by frequent colonscopies and removal of the colon, if necessary. Similarly, it is possible to test for familial hypercholesterolemia (extremely high cholesterol) and hemochromatosis (too much iron in the blood). Both of these potentially life-threatening conditions can be managed successfully by diet, drugs, and/or relatively simple therapies.[14] It is also possible to test for some of the genes known to be associated with familial breast cancer, specifically BRCA1, which may be responsible for about 50% of hereditary breast cancers, and BRCA2, which may be responsible for about 30%–40% of hereditary breast cancers. Although persons with BRCA1 and/or BRCA2 do not necessarily develop breast cancer, their chances of not doing so can be improved by altering their environment. Changes in diet, alcohol consumption and exercise, frequency of mammograms, and, more controversially, undergoing a prophylactic double mastectomy can help.[15]

Even more questionable than some of the above examples of **presymptomatic testing/screening** are those that involve diseases, the ravages of which cannot be successfully treated. Huntington's disease is probably the best known example of a testable disease for which there is no preventive measure, no efficacious treatment, and certainly no cure. HD usually manifests itself in a person sometime between the age of 35 and 45 years, after which a 10- to 20-year course of deterioration begins. People with HD gradually lose control of their motor functions and cognitive capacities. In addition, they tend to suffer from depression, apathy, or obsessive-compulsive disorders. Most disturbing, over 25% of the people who suffer from HD attempt suicide and 10% actually succeed.[16]

In the future, it will be possible to test/screen presymptomatically not only for more single-gene disorders such as HD but also for many diseases controlled by multiple genes and/or a complex combination of hereditary and environmental factors. Indeed, genetic testing may become available for virtually every gene that the HGP has identified. Thus, it is not surprising that Dr. Norman Fost, a professor of pediatrics at the University of Wisconsin, predicts, "Soon you'll have blood drawn and you'll get a CD-ROM back that reads, 'You have 275 mutant genes. Here's how to find out more about these diseases.'"[17]

B. Clinical, Ethical, Legal, and Social Issues Surrounding Genetic Testing and Screening

Although health care professionals and ethicists favor genetic testing and screening for serious medical conditions, they stress that it needs to be done responsibly.[18] They favor limiting the availability of certain genetic tests and screens until their accuracy is verified and their cost is assessed. In addition, the consensus of these experts is that no test or screen should be offered unless it can be administered in a manner that respects patients' autonomy, safeguards patients' confidentiality, and values patients' quality-of-life judgments.

1. Scientific Accuracy and Economic Cost Issues in Genetic Testing and Screening

Oftentimes, people ask for a genetic test or screen without realizing that interpreting its results is more like an art than a science. A patient may leave a geneticist's office thinking she is dying when, in point of fact, nothing could be farther from the truth; or, alternatively, a patient may leave a geneticist's office thinking he is in tip-top shape, only to be struck down by the ravages of a genetic disease a few months later. The consequences of either a **false positive** (saying a condition is present when it is actually absent) or a **false negative** (saying a condition is absent when it is actually present) can be quite harmful. For example, an infant who is incorrectly identified as having PKU may be put on a very restrictive diet which is not only not very appetizing but also lacking in a variety of nutrients necessary for optimal health; a woman who is incorrectly identified as having either the BRCA1 gene or the BRCA2 gene may rush into an unnecessary prophylactic double mastectomy; or a man who is incorrectly identified as not having the HD gene may proceed to marry and genetically father several children whom he would not have procreated had he known his actual health status.

Not only are the results of some genetic tests and screens misleading, they are often quite costly, especially if they are offered to one and all. For example, a *broad-based* prenatal screening program for cystic fibrosis (CF) *alone* would probably cost from $250,000 to $1,250,000 per identified CF fetus *averted*.[19] Therefore, most health care ethicists recommend genetic tests and screens not be offered to individuals unless they are at relative risk for a serious genetic disease.[20] Individuals should not be genetically screened and tested simply because they are curious about each and every detail of their genetic endowment.

2. Autonomy Issues in Genetic Testing and Screening

In addition to worrying about the accuracy and cost of certain genetic tests and screens, many health care professionals and ethicists express concerns about whether these tests and screens are simply being *offered* to people, or whether they are instead being *imposed* on people against their wills. Among other experts, health care lawyer and ethicist George J. Annas insists that "autonomy requires that all screening [testing] programs be voluntary, and that consent to them is sought only after full information concerning the implications of a positive finding is both disclosed and understood."[21] He claims that forcing unwanted genetic information on unwilling individuals may result in one or more of the following harms: (1) an erosion of such democratic values as liberty and individual choice; (2) feelings of hopelessness, because there are few treatments or cures for most detected diseases; (3) discrimination toward persons identified as victims of, or carriers for, genetic diseases; and (4) the unnecessary anxiety or unjustified relief of individuals who are incorrectly screened.[22]

a. Mandatory versus Voluntary Genetic Testing and Screening Programs

Annas's concerns about genetic testing and screening are important ones. No one wants to recreate the kind of **mandatory genetic testing and screening programs** that appeared in the 1970s. When an inexpensive test was developed to identify carriers of the gene for sickle-cell trait, many African-Americans initially urged state and federal authorities to provide them with government-subsidized sickle-cell anemia screening programs. Sickle-cell anemia is, after all, a disease that is prevalent among African-Americans in particular. It is an autosomal recessive blood disorder that results in a painful form of anemia that weakens the immune system and contributes to premature strokes and heart attacks. Some of its sufferers can live well enough with it, but others are totally debilitated by it.

Between 1971 and 1972, twelve U.S. states enacted mandatory sickle-cell anemia screening laws and secured federal funds to set up major screening programs, typically at marriage license bureaus. Unfortunately, the results of these tests were not always reserved for the screened individuals' eyes only. On the contrary, information about carrier status often was sent to insurers and employers without securing the carriers' consent. Because some health care insurers did not want to cover individuals with a high probability of procreating children affected with sickle-cell anemia, they started to reject carriers' application for health care insurance. In addition, some employers began to practice their own version of "cherry-picking." Not understanding that carriers for a recessive genetic disease do not themselves have the disease, some employers refused to hire sickle-cell anemia carriers because they thought these individuals were too sick to keep up with a demanding workload.

Serious misunderstandings and overreactions such as the ones described above led many African-Americans to think that the real aim of mandatory sickle-cell screening programs was not to help them manage a health problem specific to their community but rather to discriminate against them. Largely in response to the African-American community's concerns about possibly racially motivated sickle-cell anemia screening policies, the National Sickle-Cell Anemia Control Act was passed in 1972. States swiftly dropped their mandatory screening programs. In some instances, they initiated voluntary programs in their stead.[23]

At present, most health care professionals and ethicists recommend that *all* genetic tests and screens should be voluntary. The strongest proponents of voluntary screening even reject mandatory newborn screening programs for conditions such as PKU that if left untreated will cause severe harm. As they see it, the state is not really needed in the nursery. They reason that because virtually all parents want their newborns to be screened for treatable devastating genetic diseases, there is no need to involve state authorities in their decision-making process. Only if all, or most, parents started to adamantly turn down offers of newborn screening for conditions such as PKU would it be necessary to resort to state coercion.[24]

In addition to challenging well-established mandatory newborn screening programs, the most committed defenders of an exclusively voluntary system of genetic testing and screening claim that just because a genetic test and screen is described as voluntary does not necessarily mean it *is* voluntary. For example, they point to the private-sector Tay–Sachs carrier-screening program known as **Dor Yeshorim** or "Generation of the Righteous."

Presented by its supporters as a model voluntary screening program for carriers of genetic diseases, *Dor Yeshorim* claims that it seeks to maintain confidentiality; to avoid discrimination; and to respect the ethnic, religious, and cultural values of the Ashkenazi Jews, a tightly bound community that favors matchmade marriages. The program coordinators visit predominantly Jewish high schools and encourage students to be screened for Tay–Sachs, a painful genetic disease that progressively destroys nerve cells in the brain and spinal cord and results in death usually before the age of two. Blood samples taken from the students are coded by a number that is given to the screened individual; no name is associated with the sample and no genetic counseling is provided. When a young man and woman begin to date, or when parents enter into matchmaking negotiations, someone (usually the matchmaker) calls up the numbers of the two individuals and the system indicates whether they are a suitable match. Continued dating or marriage between the individuals is discouraged if they are identified as being at risk for procreating a child afflicted with Tay–Sachs. Over the last two decades, the *Dor Yeshorim* program has reportedly reduced the number of children born with Tay–Sachs to Ashkenazi Jews by between 65% and 85%.[25]

Despite the beneficial results of *Dor Yeshorim*, some health care ethicists and professionals nonetheless object to it on the grounds that it is coercive. Specifically, they claim that the brochures for *Dor Yeshorim* present carrier screening as a religious duty, implying that marital and procreative decisions are not so much a matter of individual choice as of social responsibility. Thus, to the extent that Ashkenazi Jews are exhorted to do the *righteous* thing, they may feel they have no choice other than being screened.

b. The Right Not to Know Personal Genetic Information versus the Right to Know Personal Genetic Information

Closely related to the subject of voluntary versus mandatory screening is the matter of the **right not to know** versus the **right to know** personal genetic information. Whereas some people experience genetic knowledge as power, other people experience it as horror. Therefore, we need to develop good policies for not communicating as well as communicating personal genetic information.

1. The Right Not to Know   People have many reasons for not wanting to know the details of their genetic destiny. Some fear their genetic information may be passed on to family members who might view them as potential liabilities or to employers or insurers who might discriminate against them. Others worry about their psychic well being. They claim that knowing too many details about their genetic condition would throw an enormous wet towel over their lives, especially if what they had to look forward to was a debilitating, untreatable disease such as Huntington's disease, amyelotrophic lateral sclerosis (ALS), or Alzheimer's.

Although the desire to make one's marriage, procreation, and career plans in a carefree manner is understandable, it is not necessarily morally justifiable. For example, as we have previously noted, HD is a debilitating neurological disorder that includes loss of motor coordination and diminishing of intellectual capacities over a decade or more and ends with an exceptionally harsh death. Still, only 15% of the people who suspect they are at risk for HD choose to be genetically tested for the condition,[26] and only a fraction of them let third parties know their health status. But if people fear they are at risk for HD, is it not their responsibility to be tested for HD and to disclose the results to certain third parties? Might not a man's fiancée want to know her future husband's HD status in order to make a fully informed decision about entering a marriage arrangement with him or having children with him? Similarly, might not the director of personnel of a major airline want to know the HD status of the pilots who routinely fly the company's large jets?

In the course of answering such questions, philosopher Rosamond Rhodes concludes that individuals who refuse to be genetically tested for fear of getting bad news about themselves are morally irresponsible. As she sees it, individuals who suspect they are at high risk for a genetic disease should be tested for the condition and communicate the results to at least their intimate associates. Rhodes claims that individuals' duty to inform their present or future family members about their genetic condition stems from kinship bonds and the duties of nonmaleficence and fidelity. She also argues that far from enhancing autonomy, a right not to know, particularly in cases that involve devastating diseases like HD, is incompatible with the value of autonomy. She draws an analogy between a person who drives blindfolded and a person who goes untested for HD even though he suspects he has the disease. In Rhodes' opinion, autonomy does not give either of these people the right to remain ignorant of states of affairs that put others as well as themselves at significant risk. Unless individuals have correct information about their circumstances, they are not in a position to act autonomously.[27]

Although Rhodes' points are with merit, it is one thing to claim that individuals have a *moral* duty to know and share their genetic destiny and quite another to impose upon individuals a *legal* duty to know and share their genetic destiny. One can imagine wives suing husbands for having tricked them into a marriage full of hardships, or children suing parents for having burdened them with a serious genetic disease for which there is no treatment.

2. The Right to Know   For every person who does not want to know about their genetic status, there is at least one person who does. For the latter individuals, the crucial issue is access to genetic testing and screening. They want to be tested and screened, even if the information they get is less than accurate, very costly, or medically unnecessary. These are the kind of people who believe that bad news as well as good news is empowering, and that the more they know about their health status, the more they can prevent or at least prepare for a disease. These are also the kind of people who, if they are denied information from health care professionals, will try to get it from someone else. Indeed, there is already considerable concern among geneticists and genetic counselors that pharmaceutical companies will try to market genetic tests and screens directly to the public. After all, everything from pregnancy tests to cocaine tests is already being marketed to the general public.

Recently, the right to know has been invoked by parents who claim they should have access not only to their own genetic information but also to their children's. The current view held by most health care professionals is that diagnostic tests on children for presymptomatic diseases for which no treatment is available should be discouraged.[28] Usually parents are given access to information about their children's medical condition so they can decide which treatments are in their children's best interests. But when no treatment is available for a presymptomatic disease such as HD, for example, there exists no persuasive *medical* reason to provide parents with information about their child—information their child may prefer not to know. If adults have the right not to know their genetic condition, should not this same right be extended to children? Perhaps parents will treat their child as an invalid if they discover he or she has the HD gene, even though their child is otherwise healthy and wants to be treated like a *normal* kid. Alternatively, the child may not be able to handle the HD diagnosis. He or she may fall into a depression, or decide it makes no sense for him or her to try to do well in school or to pursue close friendships, particularly those that could lead to sexual relations.

Yet, even though parents may harm their children if they secure presymptomatic genetic information about them, parents may, just as likely, benefit them. One reason to test a child for a presymptomatic genetic condition for which there is currently no treatment is to permit financial planning by the parents. Another reason to test such a child is that experimental treatments for genetic conditions are developing rapidly, and that "if parents know their child has a genetic condition, they will be on the alert for experimental treatment programs in which to enroll their child."[29] Two final reasons to ascertain a child's genetic health status, perhaps the most compelling ones, are that parents who know their child's genetic destiny "can help their child cope with the problem;"[30] and that some mature minors are eager to know their own genetic health status sooner, rather than later, so they can make good decisions about the course of their own lives as soon as possible. When such considerations are added to the fact that genetic tests may soon be available to screen everyone, young or old, not only for serious genetic diseases but also for relatively minor genetic diseases, susceptibilities to genetic disease, and even nondisease genetic characteristics, it appears that we will have to rethink our ideas about whom should be told what about their own or someone else's genetic status.

3. Confidentiality Issues in Genetic Testing and Screening

As we noted in Chapter 2, confidentiality is central to the patient–health care professional relationship. If patients cannot trust their health care professionals to safeguard their secrets (for example, sexual preference, bathroom habits, and drug prescriptions), they are not likely to be candid during office check-ups and hospital visits. As a result of patients telling health care professionals only some of the truth some of the time, health care professionals may treat them with less than efficacious or even harmful remedies. Patients' health will suffer and health care professionals may be sued for medical malpractice. To avoid this state of affairs, health care professionals need to reassure patients that their secrets, particularly their genetic secrets, will be held in strict confidence.

a. Confidentiality and Family Members

Patients sometimes tell their health care providers that they do not want their family members to know their genetic status for fear of alarming or alienating them. But problems may arise when patients hide their genetic status from family members. Oftentimes, family members cannot make informed decisions about matters important to them without the information that is being withheld from them.

Among the guidelines to which health care professionals appeal when they need to balance the value of maintaining patient confidentiality on the one hand against the value of not risking harm to related third parties on the other are the ones that were formulated by the President's Commission for the Study of Ethical Problems in Medicine in the early 1980s. According to this commission, patient confidentiality may be breached only if the following criteria are met:

(1) Reasonable efforts to elicit voluntary consent for disclosure have failed; (2) there is a high probability both that harm will occur if the information is withheld and that the disclosed information will actually be used to avert harm; (3) the harm that identifiable individuals would suffer would be serious; and (4) appropriate precautions are taken to insure that only the genetic information needed for diagnosis and/or treatment of the disease in question is disclosed.[31]

To be sure, it is easier to understand these criteria than it is to apply them in practice. If health care professionals are not sure which of the two values they are weighing against each other is heavier, they should consult with colleagues and representatives of their professional organizations. Collective wisdom usually produces better results than an individual's educated guess.

b. Confidentiality and Health Care Insurers

Patients' concerns about sharing their genetic information with family members pale when compared to their concerns about divulging their genetic status to unrelated third parties. In particular, they worry about sharing their genetic secrets with health care insurers. They fear their candor will be rewarded with either an increased health care insurance premium or no health care insurance premium.

Although it is difficult to determine how frequently health care insurers actually discriminate against individuals, some cases have been documented. In defense of these discriminatory actions, the health care insurance industry has noted that, with the exception of certain state mandates, it has no obligation to cover individuals who have high-cost diseases, be they genetic or environmental in origin. Thus, it is not surprising that the U.S.

private health care insurance industry gradually has shifted from a **community-rating system** (which averages a particular community's losses and determines a fair rate for a geographical area) to a **risk-based system** (which charges different prices to different individuals depending on their health status, or even refuses to insure individuals who need or will need expensive health care).

Many health care ethicists and professionals regret the shift to a risk-based system of private health care insurance because of the moral assumptions presumably underlying it. Under the older, community-based model, the "moral assumption was that a community shared the risks of its members . . ."[32] Healthy people subsidized unhealthy people's care on the grounds that, one day, they might need help when disease struck them low. In contrast to this "we're-all-in-the-same-boat" view of private health care insurance, the risk-based model of health care insurance is based on a "why-should-I-have-to-pay-for-you?" view of health care insurance. According to this latter view of health care insurance, healthy people should not have to pay high premiums to subsidize unhealthy people.

Today's health care insurers insist that, in order to survive in the marketplace, they must have complete access to prospective subscribers' health status information, including their genetic information. They stress that unless prospective subscribers are required to reveal this information to them, prospective subscribers will likely engage in **adverse selection**. Variously defined, adverse selection is best understood as "the tendency of people who know they are at higher risk to over purchase [insurance] relative to the rest of the population and the tendency of people at lower risk to under purchase [insurance] . . ."[33] As health care insurers see it, if a significant proportion of their prospective subscribers engage in adverse selection, they will have to charge very high premiums to all their subscribers, no matter how healthy or unhealthy they may be. In order to avoid this state of affairs, which many subscribers view as unjust, health care insurers argue that they must have access to their subscribers' genetic information.

In the estimation of most people outside the insurance industry, however, there is a major flaw in health care insurers' reasoning about adverse selection; namely, virtually everyone is programmed with a large number of unhealthy genes, just waiting to express themselves at an inopportune time. Thus, it is not surprising that Americans have united in their efforts to get legislation passed such as HIPAA, which we discussed in Chapter 3. An increasing number of rules and regulations prevent not only health care insurers but also employers and other interested third parties from having automatic or easy access to Americans' genetic information in particular. Importantly, but not always stressed enough, these rules and regulations do not prevent health care insurers from denying coverage to individuals who refuse to voluntarily submit their personal health information to them.[34]

Clearly, we need a better way to provide unhealthy as well as healthy people with adequate, affordable health care insurance without destroying the private health care insurance industry in the process. Some commentators, among them bioethicist and lawyer John A. Robertson, think that the "genetic dust" will gradually settle, and Americans will grow accustomed to voluntarily providing their genetic information to health care insurers and other interested third parties.[35] Other commentators disagree. They think that the confidentiality problems created by genetic testing are so great that the private health care insurance industry's best chances for survival rests in its returning to a community-rating system. As they see it, precisely because we know that most people are genetic "time bombs," the rationale for spreading risks across large populations is even more compelling today than it was years ago when risk-based rating systems first appeared. A final group of commentators think that the only sensible course of action is to replace private health care insurance with public health care insurance, a view that the private health care insurer industry rejects, but that people fearful of being left without health care insurance generally applaud.

c. Confidentiality and Employers

Like health care insurers, employers have interests in obtaining medical information, including genetic information about their employees. Some of these interests harmonize with employees' interests, but others do not. Some employers may want to know their employees' genetic health status to prevent occupational injuries and illnesses or to prevent harm to coworkers or customers if the condition is one that, like Huntington's disease, can impair an employee's judgment and coordination. Other employers may use genetic tests because of concerns about worker productivity or employee retention. Still other employers may want genetic information about their employees simply to disenroll them from their company's health care insurance program. Comments Mark A. Rothstein:

> Employers often pay at least $2,500 per year per employee for health insurance. In some industries and in some companies, where the benefits are more generous the cost may be much higher. In any given year, five percent of health care claimants consume fifty percent of health care resources, and ten percent of claimants consume seventy percent of resources. It quickly becomes clear to health benefits managers that if they can eliminate a class of very high cost users, they are going to save the company a lot of money. And those high-cost users do not even have to be employees, they can be the dependents of employees.[36]

Because of this last consideration in particular, health care ethicists and professionals have serious reservations about giving employers access to their employees' medical information, including their genetic information. The issue is extraordinarily complex, says Morton Hunt. As he sees it, we can expect many moral dilemmas to arise in the workplace including the following five:

> (1) equal opportunity versus health protection dilemma; (2) equal opportunity versus free enterprise dilemma; (3) fairness to the handicapped versus the greatest happiness of the greatest number; (4) individual freedom versus social control; and (5) knowledge versus privacy/paternalism versus autonomy.[37]

Each one of the moral dilemmas Hunt lists is substantial enough to merit separate consideration.

The equal opportunity versus health protection dilemma arises, in Hunt's estimation, because we believe both that job discrimination on the basis of race, color, religion, sex, age, and national origin is wrong, and that employers and the government should protect workers from health risks in the workplace. Because members of certain ethnic minorities may be genetically "hypersusceptible" to some of the hazardous chemicals used at industrial plants, it would seem that employers should not hire them for work that threatens their health and perhaps even their life. But if employers fail to hire these individuals, a situation of *de facto* discrimination may result. The rejected individuals may even go without work. Does this possible state of affairs mean, then, that in the name of equality of opportunity, employers are obligated to hire people very likely to meet with harm in their workplace? If the employee becomes ill, whose fault is it? Is it the fault of the employer who decided to hire him or her despite their genetic hypersusceptibility? Or is it instead the fault of the employee who took the job knowing fully well about their genetic hypersusceptibility?[38]

The equal opportunity versus free enterprise dilemma arises in part from efforts to resolve the equal opportunity versus health protection dilemma we just noted. Hunt urges employers to offer hypersusceptible employees jobs that will not expose them to health risks but will provide them with pay and benefits comparable to those given for risky jobs. Although this recommendation may serve hypersusceptible employees' interests well, it is unlikely to serve employers' interests equally well. Are employers obligated to reserve all their industry's well-paying, safe jobs for hypersusceptible individuals? Are they obligated to create such jobs if they do not already have them?

The fairness to the handicapped versus "the greatest happiness of the greatest number" may be an even more difficult dilemma to resolve than the two we have already mentioned. According to Hunt, the **American Disabilities Act (ADA)** requires employers to make "reasonable accommodations" (for example, ramps, special computers, modified work schedules, work-from-home opportunities) for employees with disabilities. What happens, then, if genetic hypersusceptibilities or even genetic predispositions are classified as disabilities? How far will employers have to go to accommodate what could be a large number of people with very diverse needs? To be sure, going out of business would constitute an unreasonable price to pay for accommodating employees with genetic disabilities. But what about a 5% or even 10% less profitable bottom line? Would paying such a price be reasonable or unreasonable? Can employers in a slumping economy, for example, really afford to reasonably accommodate the needs of *all* hypersusceptible individuals?[39]

The fourth dilemma, **individual freedom versus social control**, is also a thorny one in Hunt's estimation. Americans value their right to take risks. If this were not the case, society would not permit people to be race car drivers, to work exceedingly long hours, or to serve as firefighters, rescue workers, or police officers. Does this mean, then, that a woman who knows she is at exceptionally high risk for lung cancer has a right to work in an industry that uses chemicals she knows will imperil her health? Is it fair to her coworkers that their paychecks will be smaller because of the employer's efforts to maintain a plant clean enough for her lungs? What about her coworkers' rights and interests? Is there a time to tell hypersusceptible individuals that what is owed to them is equal, not exceptional, consideration and respect? After all, hypersusceptible individuals are not more worthy than individuals with ordinary susceptibilities; they are simply *as worthy*.[40]

The final dilemma, **knowledge versus privacy/paternalism versus autonomy**, brings back the complex issue of the right to know one's genetic status versus the right not to know it. Individuals may wish not to be genetically screened not only for fear that their employers and/or coworkers may discriminate against them, but also for fear that they may hear some very bad news about themselves—news they would prefer not to know. The question then becomes whether, in the event that harm befalls them, hypersusceptible individuals who refuse to be genetically screened retain their right to sue employers. Fairness in this instance, as in the case of any of the other dilemmas we discussed above, would seem to demand much in the way of "compromise and barter," says Hunt.[41]

4. Eugenics Issues in Genetic Testing and Screening

Perhaps the greatest concern people have about genetic testing and screening is whether it will lead to a program of eugenics aimed to eliminate the unfit and to reproduce the fit. Many health care ethicists and professionals fear that the new **genomics** will replicate the mistakes the old **eugenics** made worldwide during the first half of the twentieth century. The eugenics programs that flourished in the United States from about 1890 to 1940, for example, grew in response to several misguided assumptions; namely, that (1) permitting an increasing number of people with genetic defects to live long enough to reproduce would weaken the human race; (2) not only mental and physical diseases but also social woes such as poverty, criminality, alcoholism, and prostitution were inheritable genetic traits; and (3) genetically inferior people were reproducing faster than genetically superior people and would eventually displace them.[42] These assumptions, which were eventually repudiated by most scientists, fueled early- and mid-twentieth century thinking and social programs. Specifically, they resulted in restrictive immigration laws. Northern Europeans were viewed as good stock, whereas Southern Europeans and Asians were viewed as bad stock, not fit to populate the United States. In addition, these same false beliefs led to judicial approval of rights-violating compulsory sterilization laws.

Because of the ways in which society misunderstood and misapplied genetics information in the past, we have worries about the new genomics. Is it less riddled with problems than the old eugenics was? We seek to reassure ourselves that our worries may be unnecessary, however, for at least two reasons. First, compared to the kind of *pseudo-science* that produced eugenics, the kind of science that guides the HGP in general and genomics in particular is *bona fide science*. Today's geneticists seem dedicated to improving humankind's health status, irrespective of individuals' race, gender, ethnicity, or wealth. Second, the language of the new genomics is the *rhetoric of choice*, whereas the language of the old genomics was the *rhetoric of coercion*. The old eugenics was about forced sterilizations, getting rid of undesirable people, and sacrificing the individual for the group's supposed good. The new eugenics is about controlling one's genetic destiny, choosing the kind of children one wants, and being as healthy and happy as possible. Yet, paradoxically, it may be the positive features of the new genomics—its scientific stature and its emphasis on autonomy—that should concern us most. Perhaps the new genomics is a wolf in sheep's clothing—a disguised version of the old eugenics, more powerful than its ancestor precisely because it is able to secure the general support of most of the populace, including even those persons whose reproductive powers it hopes to control.

Genomics enthusiasts often stress that the aim of reproductive genetic testing and screening is simply to inform prospective parents about the genetic health status of their future child and not to prompt prospective parents to eliminate defective fetuses. In point of fact, however, a high percentage of parents do choose to abort their fetus if it tests positive for a serious genetic disease.[43] There is also increasing evidence that a significant percentage of prospective parents would consider aborting their fetus if it had only a slight genetic disease, a susceptibility to a genetic disease, or a characteristic that did not mesh with one of their preferences (say, a preference for a male as opposed to a female child). In one study, researchers surveyed a sample of prospective parents about what type of genetic risks would lead them to terminate a pregnancy. They discovered that 1% of the surveyed couples would terminate a pregnancy if the fetus was not the sex they wanted;

6% would abort a fetus susceptible to Alzheimer's disease; and 11% would abort a fetus susceptible to obesity.[44] In another study, researchers discovered that 12% of potential parents in the United States would abort a fetus with a genetic predisposition to be fat.[45]

Studies, such as the two mentioned above, have triggered heated debates about the desirability of procreating less-than-normal children. Proponents of procreating only normal children stress that it can be emotionally and economically draining for individuals to bring less-than-normal children into the world, especially if they have a serious genetic disease or disorder. They also claim that it is not fair to ask a child with a serious genetic disease or disorder to be born simply because its parents want it to be born. In this connection, philosopher Laura Purdy has written:

> When I look into my heart to see what it says about this matter I see, I admit, emotions I would rather not feel—reluctance to face the burdens society must bear, unease in the presence of some disabled persons. But most of all, what I see there are the demands of love: to love someone is to care desperately about their welfare and to want for them *only* good things. The thought that I might bring to life a child with serious physical or mental problems when I could, by doing something different, bring forth one without them, is utterly incomprehensible to me.[46]

As reasonable as Purdy's line or argument may seem to many people, critics of the argument note that it serves to reinforce the views of those who long to live in a society where only perfect or nearly perfect people are welcome. They point out, as does lawyer Lori B. Andrews, that the concept of **normality** is a moving target. She claims that as genetic testing "is increasingly offered for less and less serious disorders,"[47] our understanding of what is normal and what counts as a life worth living will be continually "upgraded." She also seconds the speculations of Michael S. Lagan, a vice president of the National Organization for Rare Disorders, who has commented that, "Eventually there will be discrimination against those who look 'different' because their genes were not altered. The absence of ethical restraints means crooked noses and teeth, acne or baldness, will become the mark of Cain a century from now."[48]

Like others who wish to slow the march towards what they term "genetic perfectionism," Andrews and Lagan are particularly concerned that, increasingly, pregnant women feel they have not simply a *right* to test their fetus for genetic disorders and diseases, mild as well as serious, but a *duty* to do so, and to seriously consider aborting their fetus, should it prove to be less than completely normal. That this worry is not irrational is stressed by Andrews in particular. She points out the way the public reacted to the pregnancy of California TV anchorwoman **Bree Walker**. When Walker, who is affected with ectrodactyly, a mild genetic condition that typically fuses the bones in a person's hands and that can be effectively treated with surgery, decided to continue her pregnancy of a fetus with the same condition, she was condemned "as irresponsible and immoral, by a high percentage of her viewers."[49]

In view of Bree Walker's case and other similar cases, disability rights advocate Adrienne Asch advises pregnant women to withstand perfectionists' pressure tactics and to decide for themselves whether they want to abort a fetus that perfectionists, but not they, find lacking. Asch claims that if it is wrong to abort a fetus solely because it is female, for example, then it is also wrong to abort a fetus solely because it has the gene for Down's syndrome, *spina bifida*, cystic fibrosis, or muscular dystrophy (four genetic diseases that do not usually prevent those who have them from leading reasonably meaningful lives). Ableism is no less wrong than sexism, in Asch's estimation.[50]

Although most geneticists and genetic counselors believe it is indeed wrong to pressure prospective parents to abort their genetically defective fetuses, they also think it is equally wrong to pressure parents not to do so. Part of the explanation for this view is fear of civil suit for **wrongful life** or **wrongful birth**. In a wrongful life suit, the child asserts it would have been better never to have been born. In a wrongful birth suit, parents claim they were wronged when health care professionals did not provide accurate, timely information to enable them to avoid the conception or birth of a damaged child.

So far courts in twenty-two states have sustained wrongful birth suits; but only a few states have sustained wrongful life suits. For example, the parents of **Shauna Curlender**, who was born with Tay–Sachs disease, sued the physician and the genetics lab that told them they were *not* carriers of the Tay–Sachs gene. They claimed they would not have procreated with their own gametes had they known they were carriers for Tay–Sachs disease. In addition, Shauna sued the same physician and genetics lab, arguing that she would rather not have been born than to be born with the painful, fatal disease of Tay–Sachs.

Although a California lower court awarded the parents damages for Shauna's wrongful birth, it did not award Shauna damages for wrongful life. The court agreed that the physician and genetics lab breached their duty by failing to provide the Curlenders with the information they needed to make an informed choice to procreate or not to procreate; however, it did not agree with Shauna that some societal consensus exists which supports the view that nonexistence is preferable to existence with Tay–Sachs disease. When Shauna's lawyers appealed the lower court's decision to the California Supreme Court, it surprisingly overruled the lower court's decision. The court reasoned that because "doctors had gained the knowledge to avoid 'genetic disasters' and decrease the health care system's burden of caring for children with genetic disease,"[51] Shauna did, after all, have a legitimate wrongful life claim against the physician and the genetics lab. In addition, the California Supreme Court speculated that children with a serious genetic disease like Tay–Sachs may be able to sue their parents for wrongful life if their parents knew they were carriers of the disease.

Of course, it is not only judicial rulings that motivate many health care professionals to willingly disclose to prospective parents their fetus's entire genome. It is also their belief that prospective parents have a right to procreate the child of their dreams. Many geneticists and genetic counselors emphasize that couples' views differ about the seriousness of genetic diseases. They also reason that if a woman wants to exercise her right to have an abortion in the first trimester of her pregnancy, it matters not to the law whether she does so because her healthy fetus is female, or because she and her husband do not have the means to rear a child, or because her fetus has tested positive for Tay–Sachs disease. Finally, they reason that if health care professionals prevent prospective parents from learning everything they want to know about the genetic status of their child, prospective parents will simply turn to non–health professionals for this information. Better, they say, for prospective parents to be properly counseled and advised by trained geneticists and genetic counselors who can help them make wise reproductive decisions than to leave them to the vagaries of individuals eager to make money by satisfying every curiosity of prospective parents about their fetus's genetic status.

Because many health care professionals are increasingly inclined to spill all the genetic beans about a fetus to its procreators,[52] critics fear that health care professionals will soon become employees of the "Designer Child" industry. In order to prevent this state of affairs from occurring, health care ethicist Carson Strong recommends a policy according to which "physicians should honor requests for prenatal tests for disease, including relatively minor diseases and susceptibilities to diseases, but not requests pertaining to nondisease characteristics."[53] Strong defends his view on the grounds that the purpose of genetic diagnosis and also genetic counseling (see next section) is to help patients and their families with respect to *health* and *disease* issues. Therefore, health care professionals may justifiably refuse to perform tests for nonmedical characteristics such as sex, unless special conditions exist. In this connection, it is interesting to note that "special" conditions may not be that hard to find. Departing from the position of the **American College of Obstetricians and Gynecologists**, which as of 2002 still voiced firm opposition to meeting requests for preimplantation (as well as prenatal) sex selection for personal and family reasons,[54] the **American Society for Reproductive Medicine (ASRT)** recently decided to accept preimplantation sex selection for "family balancing" purposes in nations such as the United States where there is not a marked preference for one sex of child over another.[55] Apparently, the ASRT supports the view that when "special conditions" such as an all-girl or all-boy family exist, it is permissible to help a couple choose the sex of their next child.

III. GENETIC COUNSELING

Our discussion of issues related to genetic testing and screening brings us to the subject of **genetic counseling,** a relatively new field and one that is rapidly evolving. Whereas genetic counseling was provided mainly by obstetricians and gynecologists in the past, today it is most often provided by trained genetic counselors. Genetic counseling is best defined "as the interaction between a health care provider and patient or family member on concerns about the birth of a child with medical problems, reproductive testing options, a family history of ill health, or the diagnosis of an inherited condition."[56] This interaction has three components (1) a diagnostic component during which clinical geneticists gather genetic information from patients' family histories, medical records, and clinical examinations or test results; (2) an educational component during which genetic counselors discuss with patients a range of issues related to the genetic condition of their fetuses, embryos, preembryos, or yet unconceived descendants; and (3) a psychosocial component during which genetic counselors explore patients' emotional responses to information they have just received.[57]

Although genetic counselors are sometimes particularly disturbed by the reproductive decisions prospective parents make after they receive information about the genetic status of their embryo, they have traditionally espoused a "no-comment" policy. This policy, forged at the zenith of the patients' rights movement, may no longer be as desirable as it seemed in the past, however. As people become increasingly focused on having the child of their dreams, genetic counselors are likely to encounter prospective parents who want to use the new genomics in arguably harmful ways. Eventually, genetic counselors may be forced to ask themselves whether nondirective genetic counseling is truly a morally responsible way for them to advise patients. Comments health care ethicist Arthur Caplan:

> If families come seeking testing and counseling so that they can indulge their taste for a child of a particular sex, or if, for some personal reasons, they want a child with a particular disease or handicap, or because they hope to create a tissue donor, the counselor bound by strict value neutrality can say nothing. As the range of traits and conditions correlated with genetic states begins to grow, the requests of parents are likely to grow as well. At some point parents are likely to begin making requests for testing and counseling that clearly fall in the realm of genetic improvement and enhancement rather than in the domain of dysfunction and disease. An ethic of value neutrality provides no foundation for counselors to try and dissuade parents from making choices that are frivolous, silly, or malicious.[58]

Largely on the basis of his reflections above, Caplan recommends that genetic counseling move toward a more deliberative style of counseling in which, for example, counselors and patients candidly exchange their personal views on genetic diseases, defects, and disorders before the patient makes a final decision about whether or not to terminate a pregnancy.[59] Autonomous decision-making does not need to be solitary. In fact, there is reason to believe that decisions made in isolation from the input and reactions of others are not fully autonomous, but merely lonely.

IV. GENE THERAPY

Since the beginning of the 1990s, gene therapy, like genetic counseling, has been a matter of considerable controversy and debate. In the future, we may not have to accept our own, our children's, or even our remote descendants' genetic status. Instead, we may be able to use gene therapy to alter ourselves and/or our descendants. But how far should we go in our attempts to redesign ourselves? Should we use gene therapy only to alter disease-causing genes of particular, presently alive individuals? Or should we also use it to repair and/or enhance the genetic material within our reproductive cells, thereby passing on our genetic changes to our descendants? Clearly, these are difficult questions to answer. They require us to understand the differences between somatic cell gene therapy and germ cell gene therapy. In addition, they require us to ask ourselves if there are significant differences between using gene therapy for purposes of treating disease on the one hand and using it for purposes of enhancement or self-improvement on the other.

A. Gene Therapy for Treatment Purposes: Somatic Cell and Germ Line Therapies

1. *Somatic Cell Gene Therapy for Treatment Purposes*

To date, only one kind of gene therapy has been attempted in the United States; namely, **somatic cell gene therapy**. This type of gene therapy treats already differentiated defective cells (for example, defective blood cells) with normal-functioning genes. It can be accomplished *ex vivo*, *in situ*, or *in vivo*. In the *ex vivo* method, the most widely used method of gene therapy, researchers remove defective cells from the patient and add normal-functioning genes to them. The corrected cells are then put back into the patient's body. In the *in situ* method, researchers directly insert normal-functioning genes into the patient's body at the disease site. Because it is extremely difficult to locate disease sites, this technique has been attempted only rarely. Finally, in the *in vivo* method, which remains a *hypothetical* procedure at present, researchers inject viral vectors with normal-functioning genes into the patient's bloodstream.

The bloodstream then carries the vectors and genes directly to the disease site in the patient's body.

After many years of genetic testing on animals, somatic cell gene therapy first was performed in the United States in 1990 on two girls, aged four and nine, who were unable to produce adenosine deaminase (ADAM), an enzyme that eliminates harmful metabolic products from the bloodstream. Because it permits toxic substances to accumulate and destroy immune-system T cells, the absence of ADAM typically causes Severe-Combined Immuno-deficiency (SCID). The girls' SCID had been kept under control through very costly, weekly injections of PEG-ADAM, a synthetic enzyme. Yet, despite this treatment, neither of the girls was in good health because PEG-ADAM can do only so much to compensate for ADAM deficiency. A team of researchers tried to help the girls by extracting immune system T cells from them. They then inserted normal ADAM genes into the T cells before injecting them back into the girls. The treated T cells began producing natural ADAM, enabling the girls' immune systems to function more effectively; however, the researchers feared they had not permanently cured the girls. Because the life span of treated T cells is only several months, they instructed the girls' parents to keep their daughters on a reduced-dosage regimen of PEG-ADAM injections as "back-up" treatment just in case the gene therapy experiment ultimately failed.[60]

Despite the fact that the first U.S. attempt at gene therapy was not entirely successful, it was successful enough to inspire the submission of approximately 600 clinical protocols throughout the world. Of these protocols, 10% have focused on single gene disorders, most of them very rare with the exception of cystic fibrosis.[61] The other 90% have focused on diseases such as malignant cancers, which are caused by several genes interacting with a range of environmental conditions. Progress has been slow, and successes such as the development of a promising treatment for hemophilia B, a rare type of bleeding disorder,[62] have been offset by tragedies such as the death of a young man in a University of Pennsylvania study. He suffered from a metabolic disorder and died from a reaction to a vector used to deliver genetically altered cells to him.[63]

The fact that gene therapy can and has resulted in serious harm and even death has signaled conscientious researchers that somatic cell gene therapy should be guided by the same considerations, constraints, and ethical principles that govern experimental treatment in general. According to LeRoy Walters and Julie Gage Palmers, seven questions need to be addressed before giving the green light to a proposal for somatic cell gene therapy:

1. What is the disease to be treated?
2. What alternative interventions are available for the treatment of the disease?
3. What is the anticipated or potential harm of the experimental gene therapy procedure?

4. What is the anticipated or potential benefit of the experimental gene therapy procedure?
5. What procedure will be followed to ensure fairness in the selection of patient subjects?
6. What steps will be taken to ensure that patients, or their parents or guardians, give informed and voluntary consent to participating in the research?
7. How will the privacy of patients and the confidentiality of their medical information be protected?[64]

Precisely because somatic cell gene therapy is experimental, health care professionals and ethicists agree it is appropriate only for sufficiently serious or life-threatening diseases. Thus, myopia is not a good candidate for gene therapy, whereas Fanconi's anemia is. Fanconi's anemia is a serious genetic disease which causes bone marrow failure, and typically results in death from leukemia before the age of six. At present, the best treatment for Fanconi's anemia is to replace the patient's faulty immune system with a healthy one through a bone marrow transplant. For the transplant to work, however, the donor's human leukocyte antigen (HLA) must closely match the recipient's HLA. Thus, it is not surprising that the survival odds of a nonrelated transplant are 30%, whereas the survival odds of a sibling transplant are 85%. So large is the differential between these two sets of survival odds that some parents of children with Fanconi's anemia have deliberately tried to conceive a child through IVF in order to use PIGD to screen their preembryos for the presence of the right kind of HLA. If a preembryo has the wrong HLA type, it is discarded, and only those preembryos with the right HLA type are implanted in the woman's womb. Regrettably, the pregnancy does not always succeed, and the entire, very lengthy, and taxing IVF process has to be repeated. Effective somatic cell gene therapy would obviate the need for otherwise unnecessary IVF treatments and also dissuade distressed parents from trying to have one child in order to save another.[65]

To be sure, using somatic cell gene therapy to treat Fanconi's anemia would be risky depending on the technique used. Incorrectly inserted genes might not function at all, or might lead to serious malfunctions. Yet were the therapy to work completely successfully, the odds of effecting a cure for Fanconi's anemia would increase from 85% to 100%, and many procedures quite painful to young patients could be avoided.[66] Moreover, selecting Fanconi's anemia patients for somatic cell germ therapy in a fair manner would be feasible. One woman, Arleen Auerbach, keeps a registry of all of the people (about 800) in the United States with Fanconi's anemia. She helps patients, physicians, and researchers get in touch with each other. She also helps patients' families understand the risks and benefits of specific experimental treatments for Fanconi's anemia, an informational process that is continued by the researchers and clinicians most directly involved in the experimental treatment of this disease. Although researchers and clinicians make it a point to be zealous protectors of their young patients' privacy, frequently the families of these children are not averse to sharing their story with others. They gain strength from the realization that they and their children are playing a key role in finding a way to treat, and perhaps even cure, a genetic disease that snuffs out a life well before it has been fully lived. In the estimation of most health care ethicists, if we overlook the high-dollar cost of somatic cell gene therapy for Fanconi's anemia, the disease is an ideal candidate for somatic cell gene therapy.

2. Germ Line Gene Therapy for Treatment Purposes

Because researchers have had difficulties perfecting somatic cell gene therapy, there is some pressure to move in the direction of **germ line gene therapy**, which may be easier to control than somatic cell gene therapy. Germ line gene therapy is the attempt to modify the DNA in reproductive cells (sperm and eggs), or in the cells of very early embryos—typically IVF preembryos developing in a petri dish. If a preembryo tested positive for Fanconi's anemia, for example, researchers would aim to correct the preembryo's genes *before* inserting the blastocyst into the womb of the woman who will gestate it. Should the experiment work, not only would the baby be born without Fanconi's anemia, all of its descendants would be born without the defect. In other words, the main difference between somatic cell gene therapy and germ line gene therapy is that the former constitutes treatment for the individual only, whereas the latter constitutes treatment for the individual's descendants as well. They too will be born without the condition that plagues the individual. Significantly, it is this particular difference between somatic cell gene therapy and germ line gene therapy that triggers at least six ethical concerns about germ line gene therapy.

Opponents of germ line gene therapy claim, first, that the technique poses too many unpredictable, ineliminable, and serious long-term risks to the altered individuals and their offspring to be justifiable.[67] In their estimation, the risk–benefit ratio is such that apart from last-chance or only-chance circumstances, there is no justification for using germ line gene therapy to eliminate conditions such as cystic fibrosis, for example. Like many genetic diseases, cystic fibrosis does not necessarily require germ line gene therapy. It can be addressed through the far less risky means of carrier screening, prenatal diagnosis followed by abortion, or somatic cell gene therapy (subsequent to the birth of the afflicted individual).

Second, opponents of germ line gene therapy insist that the technique places multiple human generations in the role of nonconsenting research subjects. As they see it, the present generation of human beings is not capable of determining the best interests of individuals who will be born 100 or even 500 years later. Future generations may find the traits this generation values decidedly disadvantageous or undesirable.[68]

Third, opponents of germ line gene therapy claim the technique violates individuals' right to a unique genetic identity. In other words, as they see it, germ line gene therapy substitutes for the individual who would have been born another individual. At the very least, it substitutes for the individual who would have been born a very different version of his or her original self.[69] For example, imagine a boy with Down's syndrome who wakes up one morning without Down's syndrome. Would he be the same boy he is now with cystic fibrosis?

Fourth, opponents of germ line gene therapy maintain that so long as the technique is performed on early *ex utero* embryos or, more problematically, on early *in utero* embryos, women will be exposed to serious health risks. Women as well as their embryos will be used as subjects for risky research experiments. Comments Dr. David Perlman:

> Fetus and mother are connected via the umbilical cord and exchange blood, nutrients, waste products and antibodies, among other substances. If a retrovirus containing spliced genes is used as the vehicle for delivering genetic changes to early concepti, sperm or ova, as has been proposed and recently attempted, then women may face the danger of having their own genetic material altered by these retroviruses. Since no one currently knows the mechanism of human genetic recombination and whether proto-oncogenes or other activating factors in adult women might interact with fetal retroversion and cause genetic recombination of normal adult and fetal genes, there is a chance of genetic endangerment.[70]

Finally, opponents of germ line gene therapy raise a fifth and sixth objection to it, both of which apply equally well to somatic cell gene therapy, namely, that germ line gene therapy will never be cost effective enough to warrant widescale use,[71] and that germ line gene therapy for treatment purposes will set the stage for scientists to use it for enhancement purposes that are likely to serve the interests of only some people. Merely because their parents could afford expensive germ line gene therapy for them, enhanced individuals would have social and economic advantages that nonenhanced individuals would lack. Over time, the gap between privileged and unprivileged individuals would grow and our world would become even more unfair than it is now.[72]

Although the case against germ line gene therapy has persuaded many health care professionals and government officials to seek moratoriums on it, germ line gene therapy does have its advocates. Advocates of germ line gene therapy claim, first, that the risks of the technique do not outweigh its probable benefits. Specifically, they argue that germ line gene therapy may be morally preferable to somatic cell gene therapy because it will obviate the need to perform equally costly, risky somatic cell gene therapy on multiple generations.[73]

There is, they insist, no reason to think that a dreaded disease such as HD will somehow become a blessing to the human community a hundred years hence. Thus, it makes sense to eliminate the gene for HD at the preembryo stage, so that when individuals reach adulthood, they can procreate descendants without the gene for HD.

Second, advocates of germ line gene therapy note that if we are willing to trust individuals to safeguard the well being of their *present* children, we should also be willing to trust individuals to act in the best interests of their *future* children, grandchildren, great grandchildren, and so on.[74] We will be on safe moral ground provided we make only those genetic modifications that are ethically acceptable to us now and highly unlikely to lead "to predictably bad consequences for future persons."[75]

Third, advocates of germ line gene therapy maintain that the technique does not result in the birth of a person other than the person who would have been born had germ line gene therapy not been performed. As they see it, preembryos in petri dishes are not individual persons, but merely clusters of undifferentiated cells. To alter them is not, therefore, to alter a person. The only person that will ever exist is the one that will result ultimately from changes made on some cells in a petri dish.

Fourth, advocates of germ line gene therapy stress that just because a woman knows that germ line gene therapy *might* ameliorate or cure her future child's genetic disease does not mean that she will necessarily risk her life or health to serve this end. To be sure, a woman may feel pressured to go the proverbial extra mile for her future child's well-being and consent to germ line gene therapy, but this pressure is not likely to be as high, for example, as the pressure to consent to a Caesarian section for the good of her fetus. Just because some women may agree to gene therapy for their future child's sake for fear of being labeled "selfish" does not mean that all women will so agree.

Fifth, advocates of germ line gene therapy maintain that "it is too early to know what the relative cost of germ line intervention will be when the technique is fully developed."[76] For all we know, germ line gene therapy may be quite a bargain when compared to the emotional and financial costs of caring for people with serious genetic diseases, and/or doing somatic cell gene therapy on one generation after another.

Sixth, and finally, advocates of germ line gene therapy maintain either that we can and should draw boundary lines between using germ line gene therapy for therapeutic purposes on one hand and using it for enhancement purposes on the other, or that we should feel free to use germ line gene therapy for whatever purposes we wish provided it is safe, effective, and no more inequitable than any other practice ordinarily permitted in a free and democratic society—for example, sending one's children to the best schools.[77] Because the last of these views on germ line gene therapy is quite controversial, it merits our full attention.

B. Gene Therapy for Enhancement Purposes: Somatic Cell and Germ Line Gene Therapy

1. *Somatic Cell Gene Therapy for Enhancement Purposes*

Increasingly, health care ethicists maintain that the line that separates therapeutic interventions from enhancement interventions is more signifi-cant ethically than the line that separates somatic cell gene therapy from germ line gene therapy. For them the crucial question to ask is whether gene therapy, be it somatic cell or germ line gene therapy, should be used only for *health-related reasons* (the modification or elimination of abnormal genes) or also for *non–health-related reasons* (the improvement or enhancement of nor-mal genes).

Examples of health-related genetic treatments are the *physical* one of eliminating the genes associated with diseases such as Tay–Sachs and cystic fibrosis; the *intellectual* one of eliminating the genes associated with senile dementia and mental retardation; and the *moral* one of eliminating the genes associated with sociopathetic tendencies. In contrast, examples of non–health-related genetic enhancements are the *physical* one of helping people sleep less than a normal amount of time; the *intellectual* one of increasing the efficiency of long-term memory; and the *moral* one of stimulating capacities for "friend-liness."[78] Although most health care ethicists believe that health care profes-sionals should be in the treatment business only, some disagree with what they view as an unnecessarily cautious position. As these more permissive health care ethicists see it, there is nothing obviously wrong about using ge-netic means to improve oneself or one's children since people routinely use environmental means for enhancement purposes. For example, people try to sharpen their minds through education; their physical appearance through cosmetics and cosmetic surgery; their character through self-help programs and spiritual counseling; and their bodies through diet and exercise. Some-times they use sheer will power to do this, but increasingly they rely on drugs. Moreover, people do these kinds of things not only to improve them-selves but also to improve their children. Parents send their children to the best schools possible, monitor their diet, take them to dermatologists and or-thodontists, and enroll them in a variety of enrichment programs. Thus, as-suming that genetic enhancement techniques become safe, effective, and beneficial, there would seem to be no reason to discourage their use. On the contrary, as lawyer John Robertson claims, there would be powerful reasons to encourage the use of genetic enhancement techniques, especially in the case of one's children or prospective children.[79] Rather than subjecting an existing child to cosmetic surgery to straighten her supposedly ugly nose, why not make sure instead that the child is born with an appropriately shaped nosed so that she never has to feel badly about her ugly nose?

Or why not use gene therapy to make sure a child is born friendly rather than counseling the child repeatedly about the value of being an outgoing person, or providing the child with Prozac to help him be more affable and good-natured?

Robertson's questions are challenging, but his critics think they have some good answers to them. For example, Dena Davis suggests that because genetic modifications of children typically are more permanent than environmental modifications of children, they are more problematic. She comments:

> Deliberately creating a child who will be forced irreversibly into the parents' notion of 'the good life' violates the Kantian principle of treating each person as an end in herself and never as a means only. All parenthood exists as a balance between fulfillment of parental hopes and values and the individual flowering of the actual child in his or her own direction. . . Parental practices which close exits virtually forever are insufficiently attentive to the child as an end in herself. By closing off the child's right to an open future, they deprive the child as an entity who exists to fulfill parental hopes and dreams, not his own.[80]

Other critics of Robertson employ a different line of reasoning than Davis's. They claim that Robertson's mistake is not to challenge sufficiently parents' purported right to shape the lives of their children. Specifically, they stress that whether parents impose modifications in their children *prenatally* through gene therapy or *postnatally* through some sort of treatment, therapy, or training is not the key moral issue. Rather, the crucial concern is the *imposition* of the modification *per se*. With what motive is it imposed and after how much reflection? Is it imposed to give parents more control over their child's life or, instead, is it imposed to give the child more control over his/her life?

Among the health care ethicists who claim that both pre- and postbirth enhancements/diminishments should be scrutinized with the same moral lens is philosopher Glenn McGee. He makes the case:

> . . . that reproductive genetic enhancement can best be understood within a wider range of other, more mundane parental decisions. The basic choices parents make about schools and nutrition and our ambitions for our offspring are inevitable and appropriate enhancement decisions. The question is not whether but how to enhance the lives and character of our children. All parental enhancements are subject to some dangers common to our cultural experiences of parenting.[81]

McGee claims that parents bent on enhancing their children are often prone to sins such as "calculativeness," "being overbearing," "shortsightedness," and "hasty judgment."[82] Such parents may hastily elect to enhance currently desirable traits in their children which society subsequently relabels as undesirable, or they may get so systematic and rational about improving their children that they deprive themselves and their children of a fully *human* parent–child relationship; they may put too much faith in the power of genetics, forgetting that the environment also plays a strong role in human development; or they might find themselves with a child who, despite all their interventions, still falls short of their expectations. Although such sins are "not-so-deadly," says McGee, they should nonetheless be avoided as much as possible by slow-paced, cautious, let's-see-how-well-it-works approach to genetic enhancement.

Some of McGee's points are reinforced by philosopher Maggie Little. She worries that parents might be tempted to use genetic interventions as well as environmental interventions to shape their offspring to fit societal standards of perfection which reflect racist, sexist, homophobic, and/or ableist attitudes. For example, in a worst case scenario, African-American parents might request lighter skin for their children, or plump mothers with mousy-brown hair might request thin bodies and blond hair for their daughters. Little views such requests as morally disturbing because "the norms of appearance at issue are grounded in or get life from a broader system of attitudes and actions that are in fact unjust."[83] In other words, for African-Americans to want their children to look White rather than Black is probably not "some aesthetic whimsical preference."[84] More likely, it is a function of a racist history in which being Black is devalued and being White is valorized. Similarly, for mothers to want their daughters to look like fashion models or movie stars probably is not some aesthetic whimsical preference either, but more likely, a function of a sexist history in which being an obese or even moderately plump woman is penalized economically and emotionally, and being a thin woman is rewarded. Rather than welcoming and encouraging diversity and change, enhancement interventions would, in Little's estimation, generally aim instead for homogeneity and the further ossification of the status quo, and an unjust one at that.

Concerns about justice also occupy Maxwell Mehlman and Jeffrey Botkin in their analysis of both somatic cell and germ line gene therapy. As they see it, gene therapy will be accessible only to those individuals who have adequate insurance coverage or who can afford to pay for them out of pocket. Mehlman and Botkin speculate that as a result of this state of affairs society gradually would separate into two classes: a "genetic aristocracy" and a "genetic underclass." They comment that the former group:

> . . . would be virtually free of inherited disorders, would receive powerful genetic therapies for acquired diseases, and would be engineered with superior physical and mental abilities; [and that the latter group] would continue to suffer from genetic illnesses and would have to content itself with less effective, conventional medical treatments. Its members would be able to improve their mental and physical traits only through comparatively laborious traditional methods of self-improvement.[85]

As bad as the consequences of this divide would be for the individuals in the genetic underclass, Mehlman and Botkin think its worst consequence would be the destruction of democratic society as a whole. As they see it, a genetically stratified society would undermine the American concept of social equality in a threefold way. First, it would increase actual inequality by enabling the genetic aristocracy to secure greater genetic health and talent than the genetic underclass. Second, a genetically stratified society would erode the belief in equality of opportunity by enabling the genetic aristocracy to make themselves the "best and the brightest" and then to pass on their genetic advantages to succeeding generations. Finally, it would destroy the hope for social mobility in the genetic underclass by making them increasingly resentful about their lot in life.[86]

Mehlman and Botkin consider the possibility of banning genetic therapies, particularly enhancement interventions, but come to the conclusion that legal bans and even health care professionals' refusal to provide certain treatments/enhancements will not work in the long run. Convinced that most people will want to use as much safe, effective, and supposedly beneficial gene therapy as they can afford, Mehlman and Botkin predict that legislators and judges will succumb to citizen pressure, and that health care professionals will respond gradually to their patients' demands. As the use of gene therapy increases, particularly for enhancement purposes, there will only be two possible ways to save democracy: some system of preferential treatment for the genetically nonenhanced, or a genetic lottery, open to one and all, the prize being a complete package of genetic services.[87] Because Mehlman and Botkin conclude that preferential treatment policies are feasible only when the people preferentially treated are qualified to do the job for which they are chosen, a state of affairs that may not obtain when one selects a genetically nonenhanced person over a genetically enhanced person, they endorse the genetic lottery approach to gene inequity. But one has to worry about a society that depends on games of chance to maintain the mere illusion of equality among its citizens.

V. CONCLUSION

Genetic screening, testing, counseling, and therapy promise to transform medicine in this century in the same dramatic way that antibiotics transformed medicine in the previous century. The knowledge gleaned from the Human Genome Project will help alleviate or even eliminate some of the diseases and conditions human beings most dread. But it also will challenge many of our ethical and legal norms, economic arrangements, political structures, and personal relationships. The new genomics will increase our range of choices. It will enable us to know much that we want to know about our own futures, and it will permit us to shape our descendants' fates in many ways; however, this knowledge carries a price tag. It imposes considerable new responsibilities on our shoulders. We have to make sure that we do not create a social and economic divide between the "genetic haves" and "genetic have-nots" when it becomes apparent that only the well-to-do have the financial means to eat anything they want on the menu of genetic products. In addition, we have to make sure that we do not tinker so much with our human nature that we shape beings that are not only entirely alien from us but also possibly worse than we are. To be sure, the current human species is very different from the human species when it first evolved from its primate origins. There is no reason to think that the human species as it is now incarnated is somehow the "best and the brightest" it can be. But if we decide to use the new genomics to alter ourselves, we cannot afford to be cavalier about the genetic modifications we choose to make. In choosing for ourselves, we will, as usual, be choosing for others. The ability to modify our genes as well as our environment brings this simple point into stark relief: like Prometheus, we are playing with fire. The benefits are probably worth the risks, but proceeding judiciously is still in order.

Discussion Questions

1. Should genetic counselors provide information about a child's sex to parents if there is no medical reason to provide them this information? What are the moral arguments in favor of telling the parents? What are those of not telling the parents?

2. When a married couple asks geneticists to screen their fetus for genetic disease and the chromosome studies indicate that someone other than the husband is the genetic father of the fetus, who, if anyone, has a moral obligation to tell the wife? Is it the husband? Consider all possibilities.

3. An HMO's policy for genetic testing is to cover the cost of the procedure and counseling only if the patient agrees to abort any pregnancy involving a fetus affected by a serious genetic disease. Is the HMO's policy legal? Is it moral? What is your position on this matter?

4. Do employers have a right to know their employees' genetic status? For example, does an airline company have the right to know that one of its pilots just tested positive for Huntington's disease? Do patients have a right to know that their surgeon just tested positive for Huntington's disease?

5. Do life insurers and/or health care insurers have a right to know their subscribers' genetic status? When, if ever, may life or health care insurance be denied a patient? Is it fair to charge people with certain genetic diseases more for their insurance than people without these diseases?

6. What if a man refuses to share genetic information with his brother when failure to do so may cause irreparable harm to his sibling? Can you think of any ethically sound reasons for one sibling to deny another sibling this kind of information?

7. Should gene therapy be used only for treatment purposes?

8. Construct arguments for and against "perfect babies." Do you hope to have a perfect baby? Why or why not?

Case Studies

1. Gaucher's Disease is a recessive metabolic disorder. Mr. and Mrs. F know they are both carriers for this disease, but they have not notified their children out of shame. Fortunately, neither of their children has developed this condition, which can be fatal, but their grandchildren are at risk.

    a. What should the genetic counselors and physicians do?

    b. Should anyone besides Mr. and Mrs. F know the diagnosis and what it means for the family?

    c. Should there be a public health mandate requiring physicians to notify persons at risk for genetic diseases?

2. Currently, women can be tested to determine if they have one or the other of two "breast cancer genes," BRCA1 and BRCA2. Having one of these two genes does not mean that a woman will not get another sort of breast cancer. Moreover, even if a woman has the BRCA1 or BRCA2 gene, this fact alone does not necessarily mean she will actually get breast cancer. Still, a noticeable number of women with one of the two "breast cancer genes" elect to have a double mastectomy simply because they know they are at substantial risk for breast cancer of a particular type. Present the strongest case you can for a young woman getting a double mastectomy when she finds out she has a "breast cancer gene." Then set out the strongest case against such a mastectomy.

    a. If you were a genetic counselor, how would you advise a woman who had just found out she has one of the "breast cancer genes"? How directive or nondirective would you be?

    b. Should physicians agree to perform double mastectomies on women just because they have a "breast cancer gene"? Are they following the Hippocratic principle, "Do no harm," if they remove a woman's breasts because of her excessive fear about getting breast cancer?

    c. Do you think U.S. citizens are knowledgeable enough about genes and their interaction with the environment to make wise health care decisions? Why or why not?

    d. What if a woman gets a double mastectomy only to discover that her lab results were incorrect? She does not have a "breast cancer gene," after all. Who, if anyone, should be liable for her tragedy? Is it the lab, the genetic counselors, the physicians, or only the woman?

3. The Human Genome Diversity Project (HGDP), which involves collecting DNA samples from hundreds of population groups, has been a controversial project in the eyes of many indigenous groups. Securing this information has the potential to provide insight into human evolution and act as a springboard for medical research. Concerns have arisen about how these research findings may be used against participants, however. For example, a public health report notes that health insurance might be denied to members of a group that are found to be predisposed genetically to a disease. Moreover, gene sequences might be patented for profit without any proceeds going to the group or individual donors from whom the genetic material was taken. The report recommends that the U.S. government limit its initial funding of HGDP to projects that originate in the United States, where experienced investigators, well-equipped laboratories, and ethics committees exist (*Public Health Reports*, volume 113, no. 1, January–February 1998).

a. If you were a member of a small minority population or tribe that suffers from a serious genetic disease, would you want your group to be studied by HGDP researchers? Why or why not?

b. What issues arise when scientists seek to patent gene sequences for profit without compensating individual donors? Do individuals own their genetic information? Are genes to be classified as property, a commodity, a natural resource, or a gift to share?

c. Who should have access to the information obtained by HGDP researchers?

4. On November 28, 1999, *The New York Times* reported a case involving the death of 18-year-old Jesse Gelsinger, who underwent somatic gene therapy for the treatment of ornithine thranscarbamylase deficiency (OTC) at the University of Pennsylvania. This is a genetic disorder in which the enzyme necessary for the metabolism of the amino acid ornithine is lacking. The result of this condition is that the liver cannot remove the toxic breakdown product, ammonia, which accumulates as proteins (composed of amino acids including ornithine) are metabolized. Jesse suffered from a mild form of the disease, which could be controlled through diet and drugs. A gene-altered virus meant to correct the enzyme deficiency triggered an adverse immune response in him that spiraled out of control. Neither Jesse nor his father was informed of the risks of the intervention. Nor were they told that despite 600 clinical trials, somatic cell gene therapy had never cured anyone of any disorder.[88]

a. When, if ever, is it ethically sound to describe somatic cell gene alteration as a *bona fide* treatment rather than just an experiment? When does an experiment become a treatment?

b. Does the fact that Jesse's condition could have been controlled through diet and drugs in any way influence your moral assessment of his participating in the experiment? Why or why not?

5. As a teenager, Dennis Bellamy witnessed both his parents die slowly from Huntington's disease. Dennis, who is 32 years of age, remembers how his mother lost her job due to symptoms associated with the then undiagnosed disease. After both parents were diagnosed, both were denied medical insurance by their employers. Dennis knows that he eventually will manifest symptoms of Huntington's Disease and wants to have a family (as does his wife). The problem is that Dennis's wife does not want to use a sperm donor any more than Dennis does. They volunteer to be subjects in a germ line gene therapy experiment using a retrovirus to replace Dennis's unhealthy gene with a healthy one. The experiment is a success. In a little more than 2 years they give birth to a son, who does not carry the gene for Huntington's disease.

   a. Was germ line gene therapy morally justified in this case? What if their son had been born seriously disfigured or worse?

   b. Should insurance companies be allowed to refuse coverage for people with genetic diseases such as Huntington's disease? Who should bear the burden of these costs? Do employers have the right to refuse to hire or provide health care coverage on the basis of genetic disorders?

   c. The Bellamys have seen some of their gay relatives suffer grievously due to social ostracism. In fact, one of their gay relatives committed suicide. The Bellamys have just heard there is a "gay gene." If their embryo has this gene, they want health care professionals to use germ line gene therapy to transform the "gay gene" into a "heterosexual gene" (assuming, of course, that either of these two kinds of genes exists). Would you have any objection to honoring the Bellamys' request? Why or why not?

Endnotes

1. Laurie Garrett, *The Coming Plague* (New York: Penguin Books, 1994), pp. 30–52.

2. Eric T. Juengst, "The Human Genome Project and bioethics," *Kennedy Institute of Ethics Journal*, 1, no. 1 (March 1991): 71.

3. Ivan Noble, "Human genome finally complete," *BBC News World Edition* (April 14, 2003), *http://news.bbc.co.uk/2/hi/science/nature/2940601/stm* [accessed March 28, 2005].

4. Eric T. Juengst, "Human Genome Project and bioethics," *Kennedy Institute of Ethics Journal*, 1, no. 1 (March 1991): 1.

5. Sharon Begley, "Decoding the human body," *Newsweek Magazine* (April 10, 2000): 54–57.

6. Dawn Vargo, "Genetic testing and screening," *Focus on Social Issues: Bioethics/Sanctity of Human Life* (May 18, 2004), *http://www.family.org/cforum/fosi/bioethics/facts/a0032058.cfm* [accessed November 9, 2004].

7. John A. Robertson, "Procreative liberty and human genetics," *Emory Law Journal*, 39 (1990): 698.

8. Alan H. Handyside, "Genetic testing and screening: pre-implantation diagnosis," in: Warren T. Reich (ed.), *Encyclopedia of Bioethics* (New York: Simon and Schuster/Macmillan, 1995), p. 985.

9. Alan H. Handyside, "Preimplantation diagnosis of genetic defects," in: James O. Drife and Alexander A. Templeton (eds.), *Infertility: Proceedings of the Twenty-Fifth Study Group of the Royal College of Obstetricians and Gynecologists* (London: Springer, 1992), pp. 331–344.

10. Kathleen Curry, "Peering into the womb," *Charlotte Observer* (March 21, 1994): E2.

11. Mark Lappé, "The predictive power of the new genetics," *Hastings Center Report*, 14 (October 1984): 19.

12. Sherman Elias et al., "First trimester prenatal diagnosis of Trisomy 21 in fetal cells from maternal blood," *Lancet*, 340 (1992): 1033.

13. Margaretta Seashore, "Newborn screening," in: Warren T. Reich (ed.), *Encyclopedia of Bioethics* (New York: Simon and Schuster/Macmillan, 1995), p. 991.

14. Kathleen Jo Guitierrez and Phyllis Gayden Patterson, *Pathophysiology* (Philadelphia, PA: W.B. Saunders, 2002), p. 487.

15. Deborah Schrag, Karen M. Kuntz, Judy E. Garber, and Jane C. Weeks, "Decision analysis—effects of prophylatic mastectomy and oophorectomy on life expectancy among women with BRCA1 and BRCA2 mutations," *New England Journal of Medicine*, 36, no. 3 (1997): 1465–1471.

16. D. Craufurd and R. Harris, "Ethics of predictive testing for Huntington's Disease: the need for more information," *British Medical Journal*, 293 (July 26, 1986): 249–251.

17. Quoted in Denise Gray, "The new way to predict your future health," *Redbook Magazine* (July 1994): 38.

18. George J. Annas, "Mapping the human genome and the meaning of monster mythology," *Emory Law Journal*, 39, no. 3 (Summer 1990): 641.

19. NIH Consensus Statement, *Genetic Testing for Cystic Fibrosis*, 15, no. 4 (April 14–16, 1997): 15.

20. John C. Fletcher and Dorothy C. Wertz, "Ethics, law, and medical genetics: after the human genome is mapped," *Emory Law Journal*, 39, no. 3 (Summer 1990): 787.

21. George J. Annas, "Mapping the human genome and the meaning of monster mythology," *Emory Law Journal*, 39, no. 3 (Summer 1990): 641.

22. Ronald Yezzi, *Medical Ethics: Thinking About Unavoidable Questions* (New York: Holt, Rinehart and Winston, 1980), p. 93.

23. Ronald Munson, *Intervention and Reflection: Basic Issues in Medical Ethics*, 6th ed. (Belmont, CA: Wadsworth/Thomson Learning, 2000), p. 579.

24. Neil A. Holtzman, "Genetic screening: criteria and evaluation—a message for the future," *Genetic Disease: Screening and Management* (New York: Alan R. Liss, Inc., 1986), pp. 3–18.

25. Michael Kaback, "The control of genetic disease by carrier screening and antenatal diagnosis: social, ethical, medicological issues," *Birth Defects: Original Article Series*, 18 (1983): 243–254.

26. Theresa M. Marteau and Robert T. Croyle, "Psychological responses to genetic testing," *British Medical Journal*, 316 (February 1998): 694.

27. Rosamond Rhodes, "Genetic links, family ties and social bonds: rights and responsibilities in the face of genetic knowledge," *The Journal of Medicine and Philosophy*, 23, no. 1 (1998): 10–30.

28. Dennis S. Karjala, "A legal research agenda for the human genome initiative," *Jurimetrics Journal*, 32, no. 2 (Winter 1992): 166.

29. Ibid., p. 167.

30. Ibid., p. 169.

31. President's Commission for the Study of Ethical Problems in Medicine and Biomedical and Behavioral Research, *Screening and Counseling for Genetic Conditions* (1983): 44.

32. Glenn McGee, *The Perfect Baby: A Pragmatic Approach to Genetics* (Lanham, MD: Rowman and Littlefield Publishers, Inc., 1997), p. 94.

33. Dennis S. Karjala, "A legal research agenda for the human genome initiative," *Jurimetrics Journal*, 32, no. 2 (Winter 1992): 172.

34. John A. Robertson, "Legal issues in genetic testing," *The Genome, Ethics and the Law: Issues in Genetic Testing, A Report of a Conference on the Ethical and Legal Implications of Genetic Testing, Coolfront Conference Center, Berkeley Springs, West Virginia, June 14–16, 1992* (Washington, DC: AAAS, 1992), p. 101.

35. Ibid., p. 96.

36. Mark A. Rothstein, "Genetic privacy and confidentiality: why they are so hard to protect," *The Journal of Law, Medicine and Ethics*, 26, no. 3 (Fall 1998): 199.

37. Morton Hunt, "The total gene screen," *The New York Times Magazine* (January 19, 1986): 56–60.

38. Ibid., p. 56.

39. Ibid., p. 59.

40. Ibid.

41. Ibid., p. 60.

42. Martin S. Pernick, *The Black Stork: Eugenics and the Death of 'Defective Babies' in American Medicine and Motion Pictures Since 1945* (New York: Oxford University Press, 1996), pp. 41–80.

43. Mary B. Mahowald, *Genes, Women, Equality* (New York: Oxford University Press, 2000), p. 144.

44. Carson Strong, *Ethics in Reproductive and Perinatal Medicine* (New Haven: Yale University Press, 1997), p. 138.

45. Lori B. Andrews, *The Clone Age: Adventures in the New World of Reproductive Technology* (New York: Henry Holt and Co., 1999), p. 154.

46. Laura M. Purdy, "Loving future people," in: Laura M. Purdy (ed.), *Reproducing Persons: Issues in Feminist Bioethics* (Ithaca, NY: Cornell University Press, 1996), p. 58.

47. Lori B. Andrews, *The Clone Age: Adventures in the New World of Reproductive Technology* (New York: Henry Holt and Co., 1999), p. 162.

48. Ibid., p. 147.

49. Ibid., p. 134.

50. Adrienne Asch, "Can aborting 'imperfect' children be immoral?" in: John D. Arras and Bonnie Steinbock (eds.), *Ethical Issues in Modern Medicine* (Mountain View, CA: Mayfield Publishing Company, 1995), pp. 386–387.

51. Lori B. Andrews, *The Clone Age: Adventures in the New World of Reproductive Technology* (New York: Henry Holt and Co., 1999), p. 151.

52. Ibid., p. 143.

53. Carson Strong, *Ethics in Reproductive and Perinatal Medicine* (New Haven: Yale University Press, 1997), p. 144.

54. ACOG Committee on Ethics (2003–2004), "Sex selection," *American College of Obstetricians and Gynecologists* (revised January 2004), *http://www.acog.org/from_home/publications/ethics/ethics037.pdf* [accessed March 28, 2005].

55. Ethics Committee of the American Society of Reproductive Medicine, "Sex selection and preimplantation genetic diagnosis," *Fertility and Sterility*, 72, no. 4 (October 1999): 595–598.

56. Barbara Bowles Biesecker, "Practice of genetic counseling," in: Warren T. Reich (ed.), *Encyclopedia of Bioethics* (New York: Simon and Schuster/Macmillan, 1995), p. 923.

57. Diane M. Bartels, Bonnie S. LeRoy, and Arthur L. Caplan (eds.), *Prescribing Our Future: Ethical Challenges in Genetic Counseling* (New York: Aldine deGruyer, 1993).

58. Arthur L. Caplan, "Neutrality is not morality: the ethics of genetic counseling," in: Diane M. Bartels, Bonnie S. LeRoy, and Arthur L. Caplan (eds.), *Prescribing Our Future: Ethical Challenges in Genetic Counseling* (New York: Aldine deGruyer, 1993), p. 163.

59. Ezekiel J. Emanuel and Linda L. Emanuel, "Four models of the physician–patient relationship," in: John D. Arras and Bonnie Steinbock (eds.), *Ethical Issues in Modern Medicine* (Mountain View, CA: Mayfield Publishing Company, 1995), pp. 67–77.

60. Jeff Lyon and Peter Gormer, *Altered Fates* (New York: W.W. Norton and Company, 1996), pp. 176–201.

61. Michael Boylan and Kevin E. Brown, *Genetic Engineering: Science and Ethics in the New Frontier* (Upper Saddle River, NJ: Prentice-Hall Inc., 2001), p. 110.

62. Marina Cavazzana-Calvo et al., "Gene therapy of human severe combined immuno-deficiency (SCID)-IX disease," *Science*, 228 (2000): 669–75.

63. Susan Sternberg, "Gene-therapy trial resumes at Stanford," *USA Today* (February 4, 2002): 8D.

64. LeRoy Walters and Julie Gage Palmer, *The Ethics of Human Gene Therapy* (New York: Oxford University Press, 1997), p. 37.

65. Lisa Belkin, "The Made-to-Order Savior," *The New York Times Magazine* (July 1, 2001): 40.

66. Ibid., p. 39.

67. Edward M. Berger and Bernard M. Gert, "Genetic disorders and the ethical status of germ-line gene therapy," *Journal of Medicine and Philosophy*, 16 (1991): 677–681.

68. Ray Moseley, "Commentary: maintaining the somatic/germ-line distinction: some ethical drawbacks," *Journal of Medicine and Philosophy*, 16 (1991): 642.

69. Kathleen Nolan, "Commentary: how do we think about the ethics of human germ-line genetic therapy?" *Journal of Medicine and Philosophy*, 16 (1991): 617–618.

70. David Perlman, "The ethics of germ-line gene therapy: challenges to mainstream approaches by a feminist critique," *Trends in Health Care, Law and Ethics*, 8 (Fall 1993): 43.

71. Bruce K. Zimmerman, "Human germ-line therapy: the case for its development and use," *Journal of Medicine and Philosophy*, 16 (1991): 596–598.

72. Edward M. Berger and Bernard M. Gert, "Genetic disorders and the ethical status of germ-line gene therapy," *Journal of Medicine and Philosophy*, 16 (1991): 679–681.

73. LeRoy Walters and Julie Gage Palmer, *The Ethics of Human Gene Therapy* (New York: Oxford University Press, 1997), p. 105.

74. Ray Moseley, "Commentary: maintaining the somatic/germ-line distinction: some ethical drawbacks," *Journal of Medicine and Philosophy*, 16 (1991): 643.

75. Ibid.

76. LeRoy Walters and Julie Gage Palmer, *The Ethics of Human Gene Therapy* (New York: Oxford University Press, 1997).

77. John A. Robertson, *Children of Choice: Freedom and the New Reproductive Technologies* (Princeton, NJ: Princeton University Press, 1994).

78. LeRoy Walters and Julie Gage Palmer, *The Ethics of Human Gene Therapy* (New York: Oxford University Press, 1997).

79. John A. Robertson, *Children of Choice: Freedom and the New Reproductive Technologies* (Princeton, NJ: Princeton University Press, 1994), p. 167.

80. Dena S. Davis, "Genetic dilemmas and the child's right to an open future," *Rutgers Law Journal*, 28, no. 3 (Spring 1997): 549–552.

81. Glenn McGee, *The Perfect Baby: A Pragmatic Approach to Genetics* (Lanham, MD: Rowman and Littlefield Publishers, Inc. 1997), p. 117.

82. Ibid., pp. 123–133.

83. Margaret Olivia Little, "Cosmetic surgery, suspect norms, and the ethics of complicity," in: Erik Parens (ed.), *Enhancing Human Traits: Ethical and Social Implication* (Washington, DC: Georgetown University Press, 1999), p. 166.

84. Ibid.

85. Maxwell J. Mehlman and Jeffrey R. Botkin, *Access to the Genome: The Challenge to Equality* (Washington, DC: Georgetown University Press, 1998), p. 99.

86. Ibid., p. 102.

87. Ibid., pp. 124–128.

88. Sheryl Gay Stolberg, "The biotech death of Jesse Gelsinger," *The New York Times Magazine* (November 28, 1999), *http://www.nytimes.com/library/magazine/home/19991128mag-stolberg.html* [accessed June 7, 2005].

chapter nine

Therapeutic Cloning, Reproductive Cloning, and Ectogenesis

I. INTRODUCTION

Depending on their moral and political values, social and economic conditions, and level of scientific development, citizens of different nations develop particular concerns about issues surrounding life. In the United States, we put an extraordinary emphasis on the value of each individual's life. We tirelessly debate the necessary and sufficient conditions for personhood and struggle to construct unique selves. We diligently write treatises on the question of personal identity and systematically develop technologies that promise to extend the human lifespan. Many of us fully believe that our own lives are so precious that the community should make enormous sacrifices to preserve them. Thus, it is not surprising that during the *Roe v. Wade* abortion debate (see Chapter 6), many Americans identified with the aborted fetus, imagining what it would be for them not to exist. Leaving aside the fact that had they not been born, "they" would not know "they" were nonexistent, it seems that a significant number of Americans believe that bringing a new life into the world is so important that women's right not to procreate may be severely limited to achieve this goal. Yet, by no means are all Americans convinced that preembryonic, embryonic, and fetal human lives are of the same moral order as human life outside the womb is. Indeed, in 2004, nearly one million people gathered in Washington, D.C. to protest President George W. Bush's abortion policies and to speak up for the reproductive rights of women in general. Still, most of these protesters would be reluctant to claim that human life in its early stages has *no* moral meaning or value; it is just that they do not think that human life in its earliest stages is as meaning-filled and rights-protected as human life is in its later, more developed stages. In other words, for them, the life of an adult pregnant woman has greater moral weight than, say, the life of a 3-day-old blastocyst.

Americans' preoccupation with life and its value is of interest to us because it helps explain why matters such as research on fetuses, using fetal tissue from aborted fetuses to treat living persons' diseases, stem-cell research,

216

cloning, and ectogenesis have taken center stage in many health care ethics debates. A discussion of these thorny issues is particularly important because they force us to confront the possibility that some kinds of valuable human life may need to be sacrificed in order to preserve other kinds of valuable human life.

II. Research on Fetuses

A. *In Utero* Research on Fetuses

1. In Utero *Research on Fetuses Intended for Birth*

Research on a fetus implanted in a woman's womb involves not only the fetus's body but also the body of the pregnant woman in which it exists. For this reason, *in utero* **fetal research/treatment** may not be conducted without the informed consent of the pregnant woman. Although some pregnant women willingly consent to *in utero* research/treatment on their fetuses, others do not. For example, many pregnant women refuse *experimental* treatments, surgeries, or drugs to correct a defect in the fetus, or to prevent it from succumbing to a life- or health-threatening disease. In addition, some pregnant women refuse more than this. They say no to *established* treatments, surgeries, or drugs for their *in utero* fetuses, even when prior research indicates that such interventions would spare their future infant the ravages associated with HIV-AIDS, for example.

Many people think pregnant women have both a legal and a moral obligation to consent to promising experimental as well as established medical interventions for the fetus. Yet, the fact of the matter is that although parents have clear moral and legal obligations to accept established and, more rarely, promising experimental medical interventions for their already-born children, pregnant women's obligations to their unborn fetuses are most likely less binding. Comments lawyer George Annas:

> . . . The [already born] child must be treated because parents have an obligation to act in the best interests of their children (as defined by child neglect laws), and treatment in no way compromises the bodily integrity of the parents. Fetuses, however, are not independent persons and cannot be treated without invading the mother's body. Treating the fetus against the will of the mother requires us to degrade and dehumanize the mother and treat her as an inert container.[1]

In other words, unlike parents of born children, pregnant women cannot keep their bodily best interests separate from those of the human life within their wombs. Thus, it is not fair to impose more in the way of bodily self-sacrifice on pregnant woman than on parents of born children.

2. In Utero *Research on Fetuses Intended for Abortion*

Although it is difficult to decide whether research on fetuses intended for birth is morally permissible, it is just as difficult to decide whether research on fetuses intended for abortion is morally permissible. Those who support non-therapeutic research on fetuses intended for abortion stress that such research is less harmful to fetuses than the fate that awaits them: namely, death. In contrast, those who oppose nontherapeutic research on fetuses intended for abortion point out that it is not necessarily true that these fetuses, in fact, will be aborted successfully or aborted at all. Occasionally, fetuses intended for death are born alive. Moreover, some pregnant women decide not to go ahead with their original plans to terminate their pregnancy. Therefore, the possibility exists that, due to nontherapeutic research conducted on it, a fetus may be born with severe defects. Thus, it would seem that researchers should treat fetuses intended for abortion with the same care they treat fetuses intended for birth.[2] This latter view is, by the way, the prevailing legal and moral view in the United States.

B. *Ex Utero* Research on Living, though Nonviable, Fetuses

In the same way that they are divided about the moral correctness of doing research on living, *in utero* fetuses, health care ethicists are divided about whether it is permissible to do *ex utero* **fetal research** on living, though nonviable, aborted or miscarried fetuses. Some claim that such research may be justified depending on the purposes of the research. For instance, it may be morally permissible to do research on a nonviable aborted fetus if the knowledge gained could be used to help save the lives of premature infants in the future. Others disagree with this view, however. They object to research on a nonviable aborted fetus on the grounds that it may feel pain, or that, in the case of elective abortion, the mother may permit research on the fetus because she lacks concern for its interests. But just because a woman plans to terminate her pregnancy, it does not mean she is incapable of acting in her fetus's best interests should it be born alive. Confronted with the fact that her fetus, though nonviable, is nonetheless alive, a woman may not want researchers to cause it pain or to treat it as a mere clump of tissue.[3]

C. Using Fetal Tissue from Dead, Aborted Fetuses to Treat Living Persons

Using fetal tissue from dead, aborted fetuses to treat living infants, children, and adults for diseases ranging from diabetes to Parkinson's disease is another research practice that is morally controversial. Some worry that pregnant women, who would not otherwise have an abortion, may decide to have one to help a relative or friend. In the past, for example, a woman had an abortion so that the tissue from the aborted fetus could be used to treat her father for Parkinson's Disease.[4] Others express the view that a woman may get pregnant in order to abort her fetus so that researchers can use its tissue to treat some disease from which she suffers. Allegedly, a woman did this in order to secure liver tissue to treat her severe aplastic anemia.[5] In order to prevent researchers and the larger society from viewing dead, aborted fetuses merely as unwanted clumps of cells that might prove medically useful, many health care ethicists recommend that researchers not use fetal tissue from an elective abortion unless the woman would have had the abortion even if her fetus's tissue was medically useless. They also recommend that no one approach a pregnant woman about using her dead fetus's tissue until after the abortion decision is made or, even better, until after the abortion procedure is completed. Then, and only then, is it proper for some persons other than the researchers to seek permission to use the dead fetus's tissue.

III. RESEARCH ON PREEMBRYOS

According to bioethicist LeRoy Walters, there are two contexts for research on preembryos (that is, embryos that have not been implanted in a woman's womb): namely (1) research followed by preembryo transfer into either the womb of a woman or, conceivably, some sort of artificial womb and (2) research not followed by preembryo transfer.[6] Although some of the ethical questions that arise in research not followed by preembryo transfer are quite different from those that characterize research followed by preembryo transfer, both types of research necessitate an analysis of the moral status of preembryonic life.

In general, there are three views about preimplantation embryonic human life. The first view is that from the moment of fertilization onwards, a preembryo has the same right to life and bodily integrity that any (adult) human being has. Therefore, no research should be performed on a preembryo that would not be performed on an adult human being. At the opposite end of the spectrum is the second view, that the preembryo is merely a cluster of cells. Regarded as mere biological matter, the preembryo has no interests of its own and it is perfectly justifiable to perform nontherapeutic as well as therapeutic research on it. Between these two extreme views of the preembryo is the view proposed by the U.S. National Institutes of Health Human Embryo Research Panel in 1994, which permitted some therapeutic but not nontherapeutic research on preembryos. The panel stated that although the preembryo is not a person, it is a form of human life that merits a considerable measure of respect because of the interests it may one day manifest.

Moreover, if there is any chance that the preembryo is sentient, researchers should not do research on it. Thus, like expert panels in several other nations, the Human Embryo Research Panel decided that researchers may conduct therapeutic studies on preembryos only for 14 days. At that 2-week juncture, the so-called primitive streak of consciousness occurs in the embryo, and it may be argued that the preembryo has developed one of the minimum necessary conditions for human personhood.[7]

A. Research on Preembryos Destined for Implantation

As we know from Chapter 7, preembryos are produced for reproductive purposes during the course of IVF. For the most part, health care ethicists no longer view the IVF process as experimental research but as an overall beneficial treatment which makes it possible for persons to be born who otherwise would not be born. But, if researchers announced plans to implant preembryos in an artificial womb, or to engage in gene therapy on IVF preembryos before their implantation in a natural womb, chances are that most health care ethicists would regard such interventions as extremely risky and as research of questionable value to the preembryo and to society. The same rules that govern research on embryos and fetuses *in utero* probably would be imposed on any preembryo selected for implantation in the woman's womb. Only therapeutic research on preembryos would be permitted, and this only if the promised benefits of the research clearly outweighed the possible harms to them.

B. Research on Preembryos Not Destined for Implantation: Stem-Cell Research, Including Therapeutic Cloning

Not all preembryos are produced and used for reproductive purposes, however. Some of them, including ones that were initially produced for reproductive purposes, are used for research purposes. For example, in November 1998, one research group, headed by Dr. James Thomson at the University of Wisconsin, announced success in culturing human embryonic stem cells which had been derived from unused IVF preembryos. Another research group, headed by Dr. John Gearhart at Johns Hopkins University achieved the same result using the tissue of aborted fetuses.[8] Neither of these two research groups was funded by the U.S. federal government. Instead, both of them were funded by the Geron Corporation, a California biotechnological firm eager to get an exclusive license for commercial use of Gearhart's and Thomson's study results. Geron's generosity to Gearhart and Thomas has not gone unrewarded. The scientists' preliminary results have been successful enough for Geron to reveal its plans to become the first U.S.

company to test treatments using human embryonic stem cells in people.[9] Specifically, it plans to file for FDA approval in 2005 to begin embryonic stem-cell studies on humans with new spinal cord injuries.[10]

Embryonic stem cells are pluripotent and, in some instances, totipotent primordial cells. They have the potential to develop either into *many* (pluri) or even *all* (toti) different types of human cells. Their cell lines are immortal in the sense that they can be cultured indefinitely, producing an arguably limitless supply of cells. According to many scientists, stem cells will prove useful in treating damaged human cells and tissues (including major organs), testing pharmaceuticals for safety, studying embryo development, and discovering new techniques for gene therapy. Indeed, according to the Stem Cell Research Foundation (SCRF), stem-cell research promises to create new treatments to help millions of Americans: 58 million with heart disease, 43 million with arthritis, 10 million with osteoporosis, 8.2 million with cancer, 4 million with Alzheimer's disease, 1 million with juvenile diabetes, and 0.25 million with spinal cord injuries.[11]

Although a limited number of stem cells are found in adults and in newborns' umbilical cord blood, most scientists think the best source of them is either in the inner mass of a blastocyst (a stage in the development of a preembryo that occurs approximately 4 days after fertilization) or in the gonadal tissue of aborted fetuses. Thus, it is not surprising that embryonic stem-cell research is morally controversial. It requires the prior destruction of preembryos or embryos that, as we noted above, have significant moral status in the view of many people.

There are three ways for researchers to secure preembryos for stem-cell research. The first way is to use the so-called spare or excess embryos from the IVF process. As we noted in Chapter 7, when a couple produces more preembryos than is prudent to transfer into the woman's womb, clinicians generally advise the couple to freeze some of their preembryos for possible future use. If the couple takes the clinicians' advice, they will be asked to sign a contract that specifies their wishes for the frozen surplus preembryos, should they decide not to use them after all. Their options include discarding their preembryos, putting them up for adoption, keeping them frozen for a fee, or letting others use them for research purposes. If a couple opts to have their preembryos used for research, then the question arises whether such research is morally permissible. In other words, just because a couple views a preembryo as their genetic product to do with as they please, it does not mean that everyone views preembryos as rightless commodities or property—that is, as "fair game" for research that would not be permitted on adult human persons.

The second source of preembryos for stem-cell research is outside of the IVF clinic. Researchers advertise for egg donors and sperm donors, and ask to use their genetic material for stem-cell research. Some health care ethicists maintain it is morally preferable to use preembryos deliberately created for reproduction. They reason that the consenting egg and sperm donors will be totally emotionally distanced from the preembryos created from their genetic material. Unlike some couples in IVF programs, they will be spared second thoughts about the fate to which they have regulated their frozen surplus preembryos; namely, death, as opposed to the possibility of life through the means of embryo adoption, for example. Other health care ethicists disagree. As they see it, it is more wrong to use deliberately created preembryos for research purposes than to use frozen surplus IVF preembryos that otherwise would be discarded. They reason that deliberately creating preembryos for research purposes may lead to a "cheapening" and "demeaning" of procreation and parenting, as well as the commodification of all embryonic life.[12] In contrast, using surplus frozen IVF preembryos otherwise destined for discard has the advantage of bringing some good out of an otherwise arguably evil act.

The third source of preembryos for research purposes is also outside the IVF clinic. Researchers claim that preembryos deliberately created by somatic cell transfer (SCNT) instead of standard IVF have the greatest therapeutic potential because they can be used to grow cells thoroughly compatible with the patient's cells. However, the technique of SCNT is a form of cloning. To create a research preembryo through SCNT, researchers must fuse the nucleus of one of the patient's somatic cells with an enucleated donor egg cell—that is, an egg cell whose own nucleus has been removed and then stimulated to fertilize. Although researchers involved in stem-cell research maintain they have no intention of using cloned preembryos for reproductive purposes, some U.S. bioethicists and policy makers distrust their promissory notes. As these critics see it, it is wise to prohibit **therapeutic cloning** for some length of time so that it does not facilitate the development of **reproductive cloning**,[13] which is generally condemned worldwide as well as in the United States.

In 2001, President George W. Bush attempted to steer a mid-course between those who have no objections to embryonic stem-cell research and those who oppose it in all instances. Specifically, he announced that federal funds may be used for adult stem-cell research, umbilical cord blood stem-cell research, and embryonic stem-cell research on sixty-four (later expanded to seventy-eight) existing stem-cell colonies.[14] A staunch antiabortion advocate, President Bush reasoned that because there was no way to bring back from the dead the preembryos that had been destroyed to create existing stem-cell colonies, some good (treatments for certain devastating diseases) might as well come from their evil origin. Finally, President Bush stated emphatically that no federal money would be available either to create additional stem-cell colonies from surplus IVF preembryos or to deliberately create embryos for research purposes.

Although overall public reaction was favorable to President Bush's ruling, his decision disappointed several groups as the months went on. On one side, some research lobbyists, particularly those hoping to find cures for devastating diseases such as Parkinson's, Amyotrophic Lateral Sclerosis (ALS), and Alzheimer's protested that Bush's decision constituted an unwarranted restriction on potentially life-saving research. They stressed that there were, in fact, not 78 stem-cell colonies to use, but only 23.[15] Of these, 7 were duplicates, 31 were in overseas laboratories that either were unwilling or unable to transfer them to the NIH for safekeeping and distribution, 16 died after being thawed, and 1 was withdrawn because the preembryo donor withheld consent.[16] They also pointed out that these 23 stem-cell colonies were neither genetically diverse nor entirely safe. They had, after all, been grown in mouse culture or "feeders," making them at risk for viral contamination.[17]

On the other side of the stem-cell debate, some staunch abortion foes argued that Bush's policy was flawed and not appropriate because it used research funding on the original 78 stem-cell colonies. Wendy Wright, the communications director of Concerned Women for America, stated:

> The President's position contradicts the Nuremberg Code . . . We should be horrified at the prospect of participating in research on embryos who are deliberately killed for the same reason that we are horrified that gold fillings were taken from the teeth of Holocaust victims.[18]

Some people who agree with Wright claim that they would not knowingly use treatments or medications developed from these stem-cell colonies even if failing to do so cost them their lives.

It is important to emphasize that President Bush's ruling forbade only *federal* funding for research on stem-cell lines derived after August 9, 2001; it did not forbid *private* institutions or states to fund such research. At present, a great deal of private money is supporting stem-cell research. In 2004, money from the Juvenile Diabetes Research Foundation and the Howard Hughes Medical Institute enabled Harvard scientist Doug Melton to create seventeen new stem-cell colonies, almost as many as the twenty-three at the NIH.[19] In addition, Geron and the University of California gave $800,000 to Dr. Susan Fisher at the University of California, San Francisco to create uncontaminated stem-cell colonies.[20]

Also actively supporting stem-cell research are several U.S. states. In February 2004, the Governor of New Jersey released a budget proposal that earmarked $6.5 million for stem-cell research.[21] New Jersey's efforts pale beside those of California, however. In November 2004, Californians passed Proposition 71, which provides up to three billion dollars in state taxpayer money over a 10-year period for stem-cell research.[22] The fact that producers Doug Wick and Jerry Zocker, eBay founder Pierre Omidyar, and Bill Gates were among Proposition 71's biggest supporters has not gone unnoticed.[23]

Alarmed by developments in the private sector and the states, some adamant opponents of stem-cell research in the U.S. House of Representatives and Senate have sought to go much farther than President Bush. They have sponsored bills banning therapeutic cloning (SCNT) which, as we noted above, is precisely the kind of stem-cell research scientists most want to do. As early as 2003, bills were proposed in both the House of Representatives and the Senate to ban therapeutic cloning as well as reproductive cloning. The House passed its version of the bill (HR 2505) on February 27, 2003. Often referred to as the Weldon–Stupak Bill, HR 2505 imposes fines of at least one million dollars and prison terms of up to 10 years on anyone who performs SCNT.[24] Significantly, in face of the U.S. public's increasingly favorable attitude toward stem-cell research, the Senate did not pass its version of HR2505. But even though the majority of the Senate does not favor a ban on therapeutic cloning, it does seem to favor a ban on reproductive cloning as is clear in S303, the February 5, 2003 bipartisan-supported "Human Cloning Ban and Stem Cell Research Protection Act."[25]

Brutal economic and political realities, rather than refined moral arguments, may ultimately decide the outcome of the U.S. stem-cell debate. The greatest strides in stem-cell research, particularly therapeutic cloning, are being made outside the United States. Specifically, South Korea is the current world leader. Researchers at Seoul National University demonstrated in 2005 that it is possible to create stem cells tailored to individual patients. They believe that in future, patient-specific stem cells could be used to grow replacements for failing organs and to develop treatments for a range of diseases. Because these medical products would be entirely compatible with the targeted patient's immune system, the patient would not reject them and could almost certainly benefit from them.[26]

The thought of South Korean scientists and scientists at laboratories in a variety of nations whose governments encourage rather than discourage embryonic stem-cell research has many U.S. federal and state public authorities rethinking their views on stem cells. It also has more than a few U.S. scientists considering relocation to a nation more receptive to their work. In fact, several top American scientists have already left for the United Kingdom, Sweden, and most recently, for Singapore. They point out that in the United States they are forced to spend too much of their time trying to get funds for their research—time that could be spent instead on actually doing their research.

Yet another reality that may end the embryonic stem-cell research debate is a scientific breakthrough. Dr. Robert Lanza has reported success removing just one cell from mice preembryos without destroying the preembryos in the process. Were it possible to perform this technique on human preembryos, embryonic stem-cell research would no longer necessitate the destruction of human life.[27]

IV. Reproductive Cloning

As we noted above, holding the line between permissible therapeutic cloning on the one hand and impermissible reproductive cloning on the other seems to be the general position of U.S. society. Most U.S. researchers as well as an increasing number of U.S. public officials seem comfortable with this compromise. They appear to believe that the line they have drawn in the sands of research will continue to hold. But the likelihood is that this line, like other boundary lines, may not hold forever. The siren call of scientific progress combined with the demand of the U.S. citizenry for reproducing in whatever way they want, may, sooner or later, tempt researchers to engage in reproductive cloning. In contrast to the purpose of therapeutic cloning, the purpose of reproductive cloning is not to get a petri dish full of brain cells, blood cells, or liver cells. Rather, it is to produce a "special" preembryo and implant it in a woman's womb. In other words, the ultimate aim of reproductive cloning is to secure a particular kind of child—namely, the identical twin of the person whose genetic material was used in the cloning process.

For many people, the idea of deliberately engineered twins (as opposed to naturally produced twins) is of great ethical concern. As critics of reproductive cloning see it, this technique is intrinsically wrong because it substitutes the process of human replication for human procreation. For centuries, two separate individuals, a male with sperm and a female with eggs, have physically united to co-create a unique person whose chromosomes are a distinctive blend of their two separate sets of chromosomes.[28] In reproductive cloning, however, two no longer have to become one for procreation to take place. A person can procreate in a solitary manner, as in the hypothetical case of a woman who asks that one of her eggs be enucleated, filled with the DNA from one of her somatic cells, and then inserted into her uterus at the blastocyst stage.

The thought of individuals replicating themselves in such a solitary manner troubles most people. They fear that an individual who desires to procreate his or her own twin alone may be rejecting all the good things human beings have traditionally offered each other in the way of community, companionship, and intimacy. Yet there are some people who disagree with this negative view of reproductive cloning. As they see it, it is not intrinsically wrong to replicate as opposed to procreate the human race. Lawyer and healthcare ethicist John Robertson, for example, notes that, like all children, cloned children do, after all, have two genetic parents; namely, the two genetic parents of the person who is cloned.[29] Specifically, if I am cloned for reproductive purposes and decide to get pregnant with "myself," the child to whom I give birth will be my identical twin and the genetic offspring of my genetic mother and genetic father.

Less debatable than the view that reproductive cloning is intrinsically wrong is the view that at present it is both very unsafe and highly ineffectual to clone a human being. In fact, cloning any mammal remains a relatively unsuccessful process. In order to produce Dolly, the world famous ewe, Dr. Ian Wilmut and his colleagues used 277 enucleated eggs. Only 29 of these enucleated eggs developed to the blastocyst stage, and only one of these blastocysts (Dolly) was brought to term successfully.[30] Moreover, reports indicate that because an adult somatic cell was used to clone Dolly, her body prematurely aged before she died in 2003. Unless efforts to clone sheep, cows, and monkeys, for example, become much more safe and efficacious, there is a significant reason not to attempt human reproductive cloning. According to experts, producing a single viable human clone would require scores of women to donate eggs and carry embryos, most of which would either not come to term or be born with major deformities.

Although both supporters and opponents of reproductive cloning agree that much more animal research is necessary before it is safe to attempt human reproductive cloning, opponents of the technique admit that safety issues are simply *one* of their concerns. Indeed, according to Robertson, among the other concerns that have been raised is the fear that the clone's **sense of individuality** will be threatened, so much so that the clone will not regard himself/herself as a separate and unique person, or that others will fail to view the clone as a distinct individual. But, as proponents of human reproductive cloning point out, there is no reason to think that a clone's sense of individuality will be any more threatened than an identical twin's sense of individuality. Presently, most identical twins do not regard themselves as one and the same person just because their genotype is identical; and others, particularly parents and family members, typically strive to differentiate one twin from the other. To be sure, there are exceptions to this rule. Some identical twins do try to fuse their separate identities, making a fetish out of dressing alike, for example. Moreover, some parents of identical twins do try to provide their twins with precisely the same experiences in a concerted effort to make their twins' phenotype as well as genotype identical. To the degree that such attempts and similar attempts to rear clones in the image and likeness of their genetic source are psychologically harmful to children, however, good counseling may be of assistance, says Robertson.[31] In his estimation, clones' identity issues will probably be no worse than those of ordinary people.

Related to the lack-of-individuality objection to human reproductive cloning is the **lack-of-autonomy** objection. There are, says Robertson, many variations on the lack-of-autonomy objection to reproductive cloning, but most of them have to do with rearers seeking to get the clone to think, act, and look the same way its genetic source thinks/thought, acts/acted, and looks/looked. Rather than letting the clone follow his or her own "preferences and paths in life,"[32] the rearers of the clone may be tempted to do everything in their power to get it to follow in the footsteps of the clone's genetic source. They may permit the clone to open only those doors that lead to having the same experiences the clone's genetic source had. As Robertson sees it, however, this objection to human reproductive cloning is overstated. He points out that at present many parents lock doors their children may wish to enter, shoving them through doors of their own selection instead. Once again, the solution to this type of problem, whether it arises in the family of a clone or in the family of a naturally procreated child, is, in Robertson's estimation, good counseling.

Another objection to human reproductive cloning is that it may lead to the **objectification** or **instrumentalization** of children in general. Some people assert that unless they can be guaranteed a child whose genotype is precisely the genotype they wish, they do not want a child after all. Only a child with what they view as the ideal genotype is of interest to them. Any other child would be a great disappointment. Clearly, people with this type of attitude toward children seem to view children as some sort of consumer item. Fortunately, most parents presently settle for the child that is in fact born to them. If it turns out that the rearing parents of a clone are far more likely than the rearing parents of a naturally produced child to view the child as a mere means to their own goals, then there may be good reason to challenge human reproductive cloning. For example, if parents routinely wanted to clone an existing child only to use it as a source of spare parts for an already existing child, then society would be well advised to think about a ban on human reproductive cloning.

An even more powerful objection to human reproductive cloning is the way in which it may undermine kinship, lineage, and family relations. Robertson analyzes the degree to which cloning an existing (or deceased) child, cloning an unrelated third party, rearing a clone of one's self, and cloning and rearing one's parents might threaten the (genetic) family as we know it. As he sees it, kinship issues do not loom at all when genetic parents clone an existing (or deceased) child because they are just as much the (genetic) parents of the clone as of the other child. Kinship issues do emerge, though not dramatically in Robertson's estimation, when the DNA of an unrelated third party is used in the cloning process. However, it is his view that if society is prepared to endorse embryo adoption, it should also be prepared to endorse cloning a third party. After all, if a couple is permitted to adopt embryo X rather than embryo Y simply because they prefer the genetic characteristics of embryo X, why should not a couple be permitted to gestate and rear the clone of a third party whose genetic characteristics they prefer? Still, despite his willingness to endorse many types of human reproductive cloning, Robertson does not necessarily accept *all* forms of human cloning. Specifically, he suggests that cloning oneself or one's parents may be perceived as too "deviant" from ordinary reproductive arrangements to fall within the protected sphere of procreative liberty.[33]

V. Ectogenesis

When the topics at hand are stem-cell research, including therapeutic cloning and reproductive cloning, preembryos that are 14 days old and younger are the proposed objects of biomedical research. But research on preembryos older than 14 days, including the ones that have been implanted successfully in women's wombs, has also been contemplated, though not pursued for technical as well as ethical reasons. Interest in **ectogenesis**—that is, gestating human beings *ex utero* in an artificial placenta—is spurred from both the end-side and the beginning-side of the gestational process. In 1984, Peter Singer, a philosopher, and Deane Wells, a member of the Australian Parliament, wrote a book, entitled *Making Babies: The New Science and Ethics of Conception*, in which they argued that ectogenesis was on the "fast track" for development for two main reasons.[34] First, fetal viability is shifting to ever earlier times due to developments in the Neonatal Intensive Care Unit (NICU). By the late 1980s it was possible to save babies born as early as 6 or even 5.5 months, and weighing less than 100 grams.[35] Singer and Wells reasoned that before long someone would develop an incubator able to sustain a 5-month or even a 4.5-month old human fetus. They pointed to the fact that some Japanese researchers had already incubated a partially developed goat kid from 120 days (the equivalent of the 20th to 24th gestational week of a human fetus) until it was ready to be born, 17 days later. Despite serious developmental problems with the resulting kid (it was unable to stand or breathe by itself), the researchers pronounced their experiment a near success.[36]

Singer and Wells's second source of optimism about the development of ectogenesis drew inspiration from the opposite end of pregnancy—that is, from the moment of conception rather than of birth. They pointed to the then relatively new procedure of IVF. As we noted in Chapter 7, in IVF a number of eggs are removed from a woman's ovaries and fertilized with sperm outside her body. When the fertilized eggs are developed to about the eight-cell stage, they are transferred back into either her uterus or the uterus of another woman. Although no human embryo transfer attempted more than 3 days after fertilization (the 32-cell stage) has implanted successfully in a woman's womb, some scientists have reportedly kept human embryos alive *in vitro* for up to 9 days.[37] Moreover, the fact that the United Kingdom, for example, currently forbids experimentation on human fetuses *in vitro* after 14 days suggests that some researchers have tried, perhaps successfully, to keep preembryos alive for at least 2 weeks and maybe longer.[38]

In an attempt to decide whether the overall benefits of ectogenesis exceed its overall harms, Singer and Wells weighed five proectogenesis arguments against five antiectogenesis arguments. They claimed there are two particularly strong arguments in favor of ectogenesis. The first of these arguments is that ectogenesis offers an alternative to surrogate motherhood. Rather than contracting for the services of a surrogate mother, a woman who has eggs but is unable to gestate them could instead use an artificial womb to bring the embryo to term. Supposedly, it would be advisable for her to exercise this option in order to avoid tug-of-war situations such as the one that arose in the Whitehead–Stern controversy over Baby M[39] (see Chapter 7). In Singer and Wells's estimation, had an artificial womb been available, both the Sterns and the Whiteheads could have been spared much grief. Mrs. Stern's eggs could have been fertilized with her husband's sperm *in vitro*.

The resulting embryos could then have been transferred into an artificial womb. There would have been no need to use Mary Beth Whitehead at all.

The second strong argument in favor of ectogenesis is that it has the potential to resolve the abortion controversy. Presently, there is no way to remove a first-trimester or early second-trimester fetus from a woman's body without killing the fetus. But subsequent to the development of an artificial womb, a fetus could be extracted from a woman's body for transfer and further development in the artificial womb. Singer and Wells think such transfers should be recommended on the grounds that although women have a right to be "rid of the fetus," they do not, therefore, also have a right to kill it.[40]

Having presented the two strongest arguments in favor of ectogenesis, Singer and Wells quickly dispatched three more debatable arguments in favor of it: (1) biological pregnancy is not in women's best interests because it confines women to the domestic sphere; (2) biological pregnancy is not in children's best interests because it causes parents (particularly mothers) to cling to their children as if they were possessions; and (3) adults may use *ex utero* fetuses for much needed replacement organs and tissues. Singer and Wells rejected arguments (1) and (2) on the grounds that presently there is no way to calculate the effects of ectogenesis on women's and children's best interests. For all we know, ectogenesis may be worse for both women and children than biological pregnancy. In addition, they dismissed argument (3) on the grounds that the majority of the public would find the idea of a fetal organ farm too repulsive to endorse.[41]

Among the antiectogenesis arguments Singer and Wells considered were the following ones: (1) at present ectogenesis is fraught with too many risks; (2) ectogenesis is part of a masculinist conspiracy to rob women of their reproductive powers; (3) ectogenesis is an unnatural technology that violates God's laws; (4) ectogenesis will destroy democracy, substituting for it a Brave New World in which state authorities selectively breed only those types of individuals likely to be maximally useful to society; and (5) ectogenesis will lead to organ farming.[42] Singer and Wells dismissed all but the first of these arguments as unfounded. They argued that women no less than men want to use reproductive technology; that ectogenesis is no more unnatural than most medical technologies; that the State has no interest in using an excessively costly technology to breed certain types of workers; and, as above, that most of the public would be appalled by the thought of growing fetuses as a supply of tissues and organs for adults.

Reflecting back on the arguments both for and against ectogenesis, Singer and Wells accepted *complete* ectogenesis as doing more overall social good than social harm. No longer will surrogate mothers and contracting couples be at odds with each and no longer will pro-life and pro-choice forces be at war. In contrast, they rejected *partial* ectogenesis as decidedly bad for society. They reasoned that adults who matter-of-factly "farm" embryos for replacement parts are not likely to have protective feelings toward vulnerable infants. Without such feelings, said Singer and Wells, a society is not likely to survive, let alone thrive.[43]

Although Singer and Wells established to their satisfaction that complete (as opposed to partial) ectogenesis is a morally permissible technology, their critics remain unconvinced. In opposition to them, philosopher David James noted that even if ectogenesis provides a better way to handle surrogacy arrangements than "renting" a living woman's womb, society should not spend scarce resources developing such a costly technology for a limited number of people.[44] In addition, feminist philosopher Christine Overall argued against Singer and Wells that women's right to an abortion is far more than the right to have one's fetus extracted from one's body. It is more fundamentally the right not to procreate, a point we noted in Chapter 6. When a woman seeks an abortion, she probably has fetal extinction and not merely fetal extraction as her goal. She simply does not want to procreate: to bring another life into the world.

In support of her position, Overall made four claims. First, keeping a fetus alive against the wishes of its biological mother violates that woman's reproductive autonomy. Although it is possible to free a biological mother from her gestational and rearing connections to her fetus by removing her fetus from her, it is not possible thereby to free her from her genetic connections to it. Because most biological mothers view abortion as a way to erase *all* their connections to the fetuses, anything less than the death of their fetus will fail to satisfy them.[45] Second, forcing a woman to submit to whatever abortion procedure is most likely to preserve the life of a fetus is "comparable to a compulsory organ 'donation' in which the patient chooses organ removal but does not agree to the subsequent salvaging and use of the organs."[46] Third, because of her close physical relationship to the fetus, "the biological mother is the most appropriate person—perhaps the only one—to decide the disposition of the fetus."[47] Fourth, limiting the biological mother's control over the disposition of the fetus "is yet another example of the takeover of reproduction from women."[48]

Overall's fourth concern about depositing women's unwanted fetuses in artificial wombs is echoed by feminist philosopher Anne Donchin. She claims that:

> . . . if extrauterine gestation were to become an established practice, would not many women be pressured to adopt it—'for the good of their baby'? For within the prevailing social framework, once the practice was established, it is unlikely that only intentionally aborted fetuses would be nourished in laboratories. Any other fetus considered 'at risk' for any reason would count as a potential beneficiary of laboratory observation and intervention.[49]

Donchin's observation is plausible. Ectogenesis would, in the minds of many, be the perfect solution to the so-called maternal–fetal conflict problem. Rather than seeking to designate crack-cocaine abusing pregnant women as fetal abusers and neglectors, for example, prosecutors would instead seek court orders to remove the fetuses from the wombs of these wayward mothers. Eventually, only women with "safe" uteri would be permitted to gestate their children. At the very best, one can, as Donchin does, imagine concerned women requesting physicians to transfer their fetus from them into a safer, albeit more artificial, environment.

VI. CONCLUSION

For those who view such speculations as fanciful, consider science reporter Sharon Begley's article, in which she points out, "[s]cientists now think that conditions during gestation, ranging from the torrent of hormones that flow from Mom to how well the placenta delivers nutrients to the tiny limbs and organs, shape the health of the adult that fetus becomes."[50] Begley does not think it is an accident that fetal programming has been the subject of two recent NIH conferences, both of which sought to establish connections between a variety of diseases and the conditions present in the womb during fetal gestation. Supposedly, there is growing evidence that individuals who have asymmetrical features, such as ears, fingers, and feet also have lower IQs. One theory to explain this correlation is that asymmetrical features may be tangible signs of stress which took place during pregnancy, and that whatever stress led to the asymmetrical features also could have affected the nervous system, causing impairments in the senses, memory, and cognition. Other studies indicate that the genes that affect the so-called stress response may "turn off" if a fetus is exposed to stress hormones (within the womb). Thereby, the growing child may be impaired in his or her ability to handle stress in adulthood. In the words of Dr. Peter Nathaniels, "The script written on the genes is altered by . . . the environment in the womb."[51]

Perhaps the most significant feature of Begley's article is its conclusion. There, Begley recollects the chapter in Huxley's *Brave New World* wherein he describes how fetuses develop in artificial wombs, the amniotic fluid adjusted with various ingredients depending on what type of child is desired.[52] Pondering this vision, Begley comments, "The quest for the secrets of fetal programming won't yield up such simple recipes. But it is already showing that the seeds of health are planted even before you draw your first breath, and that the nine short months of life in the womb shape your health as long as you live."[53]

Discussion Questions

1. Is a human embryonic stem cell more like an embryo or an ordinary somatic cell?
2. Who should be the decision-maker for surplus IVF embryos—the woman and man who provided the sperm and eggs, or the woman for whose womb the embryo was originally intended?

3. Are there any problems, including moral ones, with permitting the private sector and states to fund embryonic stem-cell research but not the federal government?

4. If the treatments and medications produced through embryonic stem-cell research are costly, who should have access to them and why? What if a treatment for Alzheimer's disease was discovered, but it cost $125,000 (or more)? Should Medicare cover this treat for everyone over 65?

5. Consider each of the following arguments/counterarguments for reproductive cloning. Where do you stand with respect to each point and why?

   a. Objection: Reproductive cloning is wrong because it violates human dignity by substituting the process of human replication for human procreation. Two no longer become one. Response: *But*, why must human beings procreate? Is anything inherently wrong with replicating?

   b. Objection: Reproductive cloning is wrong because it is probably very unsafe and costly. Response: *But*, someday cloning may become very safe and relatively inexpensive.

   c. Objection: Reproductive cloning is wrong because it threatens the clone's sense of individuality. Response: *But*, twins view themselves as individuals, and clones are simply twins separated at birth time by years instead of minutes.

   d. Objection: Reproductive cloning is wrong because it threatens the clone's autonomy. Response: *But*, parents need not try to get a clone to think and act in certain ways. They could instead let the clone develop as the clone wishes.

   e. Objection: Reproductive cloning is wrong because it leads to the objectification or instrumentalization of children. Response: *But*, parents need not view their clones (or naturally born children) as mere means to their own ends.

   f. Objection: Reproductive cloning is wrong because it undermines kinship, lineage, and family relations (cloning an existing or deceased child, cloning an unrelated third party, cloning one's self, and cloning one's parent). Response: *But*, what is wrong with transforming kinship, lineage, and family relations? They are far from perfect now.

   g. Objection: Reproductive cloning is wrong because it will lead to people selecting certain genetic characteristics. Response: *But*, people already do this in a variety of ways. They try to date and marry good-looking people. They try to eliminate harmful genetic diseases.

6. Do you think therapeutic cloning inevitably will lead to reproductive cloning? Why or why not?

7. Should reproductive cloning be banned, regulated, or freely permitted to develop?

8. Would you ever consider cloning yourself? Why or why not?

9. Where do you think reproductive cloning will be developed first? Why?

10. Wendy Wright asserts in this chapter that President Bush's stance on public funds for embryonic stem-cell research contradicts the Nuremberg Code. In what ways is she correct? How is she incorrect? Do you agree with President Bush's position? Why or why not?

Case Studies

1. In February, 2004, *Science* reported that two Korean researchers had created 200 human embryos by cloning human cells. Of these embryos, 30 survived to the blastocyst stage of more than 100 cells. During a press conference at a meeting of the American Association for the Advancement of Science in Seattle, one of the researchers, Woo Suk Hwang, stated: "Our goal is not to clone humans, but to understand the causes of diseases."[54]

    a. If reproductive cloning holds the promise of curing everything from juvenile diabetes to baldness, should the research remain banned?

    b. How can we be sure about Woo Suk Hwang's stated intentions? Can we assume that scientists always tell the public the truth?

2. In 2002, Dr. Hung-Ching Liu of Cornell University's Center for Reproductive Medicine and Infertility successfully prodded human embryos to grow onto artificial womb walls. The walls were constructed from extracted womb cells that were cultured *in vitro*. According to *Newsmagazine*, Dr. Liu stopped this experiment after 6 days, but intends to start a new experiment, this time for 14 days. Dr. Liu wants to proceed with her work because she thinks that women with "damaged uteruses" should be given the opportunity to "have their own baby in their 'own' womb."[55]

    a. What are some of the negative implications of the artificial womb?

    b. What are some of the positive implications of the artificial womb?

    c. Should Dr. Liu's research be encouraged or discouraged? Would you be in favor of banning it? Why or why not?

Endnotes

1. George Annas, *The Rights of Patients*, 2nd ed. (Carbondale and Edwardsville, IL: Southern Illinois University Press, 1989).

2. J. C. Polkinghorne, *Review of the Guidance on the Research Use of Fetuses and Fetal Material* (London: Her Majesty's Stationery Office, 1989).

3. Bonnie Steinbock, *Life before Birth: The Moral and Legal Status of Embryos and Fetuses* (New York: Oxford University Press, 1992).

4. Nicholas Wade, *Life Script: How the Human Genome Discoveries Will Transform Medicine and Enhance Your Health* (New York: Simon and Schuster, 2001), p. 125.

5. Endre Kelemen, "Recovery from chronic idiopathic bone marrow aplasia of a young mother after intravenous injection of unprocessed cells from the liver (and yolk sac) of her 22m. CR-length embryo: a preliminary report," *Scandinavian Journal of Haemotology* 10 (1973): 305–328.

6. LeRoy Walters, "Fetal research," in Warren T. Reich (ed.), *Encyclopedia of Bioethics* (New York: MacMillan Press, 1995), p. 857.

7. National Institutes of Health, *Report of the Human Embryo Research Panel* (Bethesda, MA: NIH, 1994).

8. Sharon Begley, "Cellular divide," *Newsweek Magazine* (July 9, 2001): 25–26.

9. Hollister H. Hovey, "Geron hopes to stage stem-cell tests in humans starting next year," *The Wall Street Journal* (March 17, 2004), *http://www.stemcellfunding.org/fastaction/news.asp?id=812* [accessed March 20, 2004].

10. Hollister H. Hovey, "Geron hopes to stage stem-cell tests in humans starting next year," *The Wall Street Journal* (March 17, 2004).

11. Andis Robeznicks, "States take action on cloning, embryonic research," *American Medical News*, 46, no. 24 (June 30, 2003): 14.

12. John A. Robertson, "Ethics and policy in embryonic stem cell research," *Kennedy Institute of Ethics Journal*, 9, no. 2 (1999): 125.

13. Charles Krauthammer, "Mounting the slippery slope," *Time Magazine* (July 23, 2001): 80.

14. Katharine Q. Seelye, "Bush backs federal funding for some stem cell research," *New York Times* (August 10, 2001): sec. B, 8.

15. Justin Gillis and Rich Weiss, "NIH: few stem cell colonies likely available for research of approved lines, many are failing," *The Washington Post* (March 3, 2004), *http://www.stemcellfunding.org/fastaction/news.asp?id=795* [accessed March 30, 2004].

16. Claudia Kalb and Debra Rosenberg, "Stem cell division," *Newsweek* (October 25, 2004): 47.

17. Ibid., p. 45.

18. Laurie Goodstein, "Abortion foes split over Bush's plan on stem cells," *New York Times*, 150, no. 51843 (August 12, 2001): 1.1.

19. Claudia Kalb and Debra Rosenberg, "Stem cell division," *Newsweek* (October 25, 2004): 46.

20. Ibid.

21. Theresa Tamkins, "State may fund stem cell work if budget passed; New Jersey will be first U.S. state to invest in cell research," *The Scientist* (February 25, 2004), *http://www.stemcellfunding.org/fastaction/news.asp?id=790* [accessed March 30, 2004].

22. Terri Somers, "California to soon take the lead in stem cell research," *The San Diego Union-Tribune* (November 4, 2004), *http://www.signonsandiego.com/news/business/biotech/20041104-9999-1b4stems.html* [accessed December 9, 2004].

23. Claudia Kalb and Debra Rosenberg, "Stem cell division," *Newsweek* (October 25, 2004): 47.

24. The Weldon–Stupak Bill, Human Cloning Prohibition Act of 2001 17.HR2505, To amend title 18, United States Code, to prohibit human cloning (August 3, 2001). See *http://thomas.loc.gov/cgi-bin/query/D?c107:1:./temp/~c107XE84jY::* [accessed October 24, 2005].

25. See *http://www.camradvocacy.org/fastaction/comparison.asp* [accessed March 30, 2004].

26. Alice Park and Christine Gorman, "Inside the Korean cloning lab," *Time Magazine* (May 30, 2005): 55–56.

27. Nicholas Wade, "Stem cell test tried on mice saves embryo," *The New York Times*, (October 17, 2005): A1.

28. George Annas, *Scientific Discoveries in Cloning: Challenges for Public Policy: Hearing Before the Subcommittee on Public Health and Safety of the Senate Committee on Labor and Human Resources*, 105th Congress 20–21 (1997): 43.

29. John A. Robertson, "Liberty, identity, and human cloning," *Texas Law Review*, 76, no. 6 (May 1998): 1410.

30. National Bioethics Advisory Committee, *Cloning Human Beings: Report and Recommendations of the National Bioethics Advisory Commission*, 104, (1997): 22.

31. John A. Robertson, "Liberty, identity, and human cloning," *Texas Law Review*, 76, no. 6 (May 1998): 1415.

32. Ibid., p. 1416.

33. Ibid., p. 1419.

34. Peter Singer and Deane Wells, *Making Babies: The New Science and Ethics of Conception* (New York: Charles Scribner's Sons, 1985), p. 118.

35. Ibid.

36. Ibid.

37. Ibid., p. 117.

38. John A. Robertson, "Embryo research," *Law Review Western Ontario*, 24 (1986): 15–37.

39. "Excerpts from decision by New Jersey Supreme Court in the baby M case," *New York Times* (February 4, 1988): sec. B, 6.

40. Peter Singer and Deane Wells, *Making Babies: The New Science and Ethics of Conception* (New York: Charles Scribner's Sons, 1985), pp. 120–124.

41. Ibid., pp. 124–26.

42. Implied in Peter Singer, "Talking life: the embryo and the fetus," *Writings on an Ethical Life* (New York: Harper Collins, 2000), pp. 160–64.

43. Peter Singer and Deane Wells, *Making Babies: The New Science and Ethics of Conception* (New York: Charles Scribner's Sons, 1985), pp. 120–124.

44. David N. James, "Ectogenesis: a reply to Singer and Wells," *Bioethics*, 1, no. 1 (1987): 90–95.

45. Christine Overall, *Human Reproduction: Principles, Practices, Policies* (Toronto: Oxford University Press, 1983), p. 67.

46. Ibid., p. 67.

47. Ibid., p. 68.

48. Ibid., p. 69.

49. Anne Donchin, "The growing feminist debate over the new reproductive technologies," *Hypatia* 4, no. 3 (Fall 1989): 144.

50. Sharon Begley, "Shaped by life in the womb," *Newsweek Magazine*, 134, no. 13 (September 9, 1999): 51.

51. Ibid.

52. Ibid., p. 57.

53. Ibid.

54. Michael D. Lemonick, Dan Cray, Donald Macintyre, Eli Sanders, and Sora Song, "Cloning gets closer: how a team cloned human cells to fight disease—and why that's revolutionary," *Time Magazine* (February 23, 2004), *http://www.time.com/time/archive/preview/0,10987,993421,00.html* [accessed November 8, 2004].

55. Celeste McGovern, "A womb with a view," *Newsmagazine*, Alberta Edition, 5, vol. 29 (March 4, 2002), p. 56.

chapter ten

The Aging Process and Long-Term Health Care

I. INTRODUCTION

Currently, black, non-Hispanic males have the lowest average life expectancy rates and non-Hispanic Asian females have the highest.[1] Married couples outlive single individuals; older siblings outlive younger ones; and women who have had children outlive women who have not had children. People with college degrees live about 6 years longer than people with only high school degrees; and people who participate in some form of organized religion live more years than those who do not.[2] The good news is that, in the near future, most Americans should be able to live well into their eighties provided that they remain optimistic and engaged in life, regularly exercise, eat a healthy diet, do not smoke, and have at least some relatives who have lived into their eighties or even nineties.[3] Indeed, projections indicate that by the year 2025 life expectancies at birth will be 77.8 for white, non-Hispanic males and 83.6 for white, non-Hispanic females; 73.6 for black, non-Hispanic males and 80.5 for black, non-Hispanic females; 80.0 for males and 86.1 for females of Hispanic origin; 78.4 for non-Hispanic American Indian males and 86.5 for non-Hispanic American Indian females; and 82.4 for non-Hispanic Asian males and 87.7 for non-Hispanic Asian females.[4] Moreover, projections indicate that by 2025, there will be at least one million American centenarians,[5] and that by 2040, there may be as many as four million American centenarians.[6]

An aging population is not only a national phenomenon, it is a global phenomenon. The United Nations predicts that the world's elderly population (defined as people aged 60 and over) will be larger than the world's youth population (defined as people aged 14 and under) for the first time ever in 2050.[7] By the middle of the twenty-first century, 10% of Africans, 25% of Asians, 35% of Europeans, 20% of Latin Americans, 30% of North Americans, and 25% of Oceanians will be 60 years old or older.[8] Although reports of increased longevity are usually met with rounds of applause, living longer is not necessarily an unalloyed blessing. Making it to 100 years or older sounds wonderful; but if centenarians are beset by multiple aches and pains, poor hearing and vision, incontinence problems, lack of mobility, little or no companionship, diminished mental functioning, and severe bouts of depression, they may have second thoughts about the desirability of increased longevity. The fact that some people age well and live vibrantly through their seventies, eighties, and even nineties does not mean that all or most people do so. Therefore, it is important to confront the aging process realistically, hoping for the best even as we prepare ourselves for the worst.

II. The Aging Process

Aging is both a biological and a psychological process. Chronologically, two people can be of the same age; yet one person's body and mind may be in far better health than those of the other for a variety of genetic and environmental reasons. But just because some individuals are in better shape than other individuals, it does not mean that they will perceive or experience themselves as so. For example, I know a married couple who are both 65 years old. The husband, who is healthier and younger looking than his wife, acts like an old man, whereas his wife, who has some significant health problems and looks every one of her 65 years, is a dynamo. Her mottos are "mind over matter" and "you're only as old as you think you are." Clearly, if we wish to understand the aging process, its psychological and subjective dimensions as well as its biological and objective dimensions must be fully appreciated.

A. A Biological View of the Aging Process

Although it is very difficult to describe the biological process of aging in a manner that neither oversimplifies nor overcomplicates it, reporter Geoffrey Cowley manages to accomplish this feat. He divides the aging process into four life stages: "the first years of growth; the early years of adulthood; the joys of middle age; and the inevitable decline of old age."[9] As we shall see, each one of these stages poses distinct challenges to the individual who lives through it.

Cowley describes the first years of growth as ones in which we experience the resilience of the human body. As young children, we play hard, run swiftly, and sleep soundly. Our tissues, muscles, and bones grow easily. During adolescence, our hormones begin to surge, wildly sometimes, signaling our readiness to reproduce. Girls' hips and breasts get fatter; and boys' muscles swell as their voices deepen.

Even better than the first years of our growth, says Cowley, are our twenties, during which our metabolism works efficiently, our bodies are strong, and our flexibility and energy levels are at a peak. On the whole, we feel alive, even invincible. But as we enter our thirties, we sense that we are less strong than we used to be; and by age 40 we realize that we look more like our parents than our children. Our wrinkle lines, graying hair, minor memory lapses, small vision problems, and hearing losses betray our middle age. Women begin to lose their reproductive powers as they enter menopause, and both men's and women's metabolism begins to slow down. Pounds creep on our bodies, as we discover that we cannot count on exercise to offset the calories we consume. By age 50, we begin to feel our mortality. We start to lose our steam, even though some of us will remain active until age 80, 90, or even 100. A few of us will even live past 100 years of age, but none of us is likely to live past year 120, which seems to be the maximum life span for humans.[10]

B. A Psychological View of the Aging Process

Even if science and medicine enable us to defy our present biological limits so that we can live more than 120 years, we will probably still experience psychological problems as we age and get closer to the moment of death. Whatever fears and/or hopes we now have about dying around age 80 will be present when we die around age 130 or more.

In *The Fountain of Age*, Betty Friedan claims that aging has two faces in the United States. One face of aging is quite ugly. Aging individuals are portrayed as falling victim to one chronic disease after another and losing a bit more of their minds each day. According to this view of aging, growing old is about becoming so dysfunctional that one no longer has anything valuable to contribute to society. To be old is to be spent. Friedan thinks this view of aging is unnecessarily harsh and in large measure false. Instead of presenting aging as a disintegrating process, Friedan presents it as an integrating process, a major opportunity to live intensely and meaningfully, a chance to become one's truest self.

Invoking psychologists such as Carl Jung, Abraham Maslow, and Erik Erikson, Friedan offers a challenging and ennobling vision of old age. She makes repeated use of Erikson's stages-of-life theory in which he assigns a particular achievement to each stage of life. The infant must learn how to trust; the growing child must achieve a certain range of competences (activities of daily living); the adolescent must resolve his or her identity crises; the young adult must decide how social or isolated he or she wishes to be; the middle-aged person must decide whether to pursue new projects or keep doing the same old ones until retirement; and the old-aged person must write a fitting conclusion to the book of life, a final chapter which brings together all of his or her successes and failures, joys and sorrows into a meaningful whole.[11]

Friedan uses herself as an example of an aging person striving to become whole. On an Outward Bound group-adventure trip, Friedan refused to descend a 300-foot cliff, despite the fact that everyone else in the group gave the task their best shot, succeeding more or less adroitly "to rappel down" the cliff. Realizing that her body could not successfully "rappel," Friedan was content to watch her traveling companions push themselves to their personal physical limits. She did not need to add "rappelling" to her list of accomplishments. Friedan turned her arguable defeat at rappelling into a personal victory, commenting that the best part of old age is "the amazing lightness and solidity of no longer feeling the need to prove oneself, to be the best, to outdo the others, to compete—and of being able to fail. What does it really matter?"[12]

Friedan's positive view of old age is echoed by many scientists and health care professionals. They maintain that science and medicine can help people in their sixties, seventies, eighties, and even nineties lead not simply longer lives but better lives. In addition, they stress that "in the past century, the focus was on improving the health of infants and children"[13] so that most people could reach middle age. In contrast, the focus of this century, at least in most developed nations, is to slow down or even stop disease processes so that most people can reach a very ripe old age. No longer are Americans, aged 45–65, willing to look at themselves as "over-the-hill" individuals—on the contrary. Because they know that even relatively simple lifestyle changes such as eating a healthy diet, exercising regularly, not smoking, not drinking alcohol to excess, and minimizing their stress levels can add several high-quality years to their overall life span, an increasing number of middle-aged Americans are taking better care of themselves. For example, over one-half of Americans over age 45 now exercise at least three times a week, most of them walking (56%), but others going to fitness centers where they use exercise machines (15%) or take strength training classes (16%).[14]

Living a healthy lifestyle contributes to a longer and healthier life, but so does staying connected to other people. Recent studies demonstrate that socializing with friends and family members keeps a person young. So too does minimizing stress levels, seeking treatment for depression, and keeping mentally active. Significantly, many researchers believe that resilience is the factor that best explains centenarians' longevity.[15] Optimistic people are more likely than pessimistic people to live longer, healthier, and, certainly, happier lives, according to Michael Craig Miller, M.D. He notes:

> . . . Pessimistic people tend to suffer higher blood pressure, a weakened immune system and slower recovery after major surgery. Optimists often have a number of qualities that help them adapt and persevere. They are calm, prudent, levelheaded, resilient. They do not underestimate real risks or discount the advantages of long-term planning. They manage misfortune by being flexible and creative, and by tolerating unpleasant feelings.[16]

One 93-year-old, wheelchair-bound optimist told *Newsweek* reporters that she viewed her wheelchair as a golden opportunity to get desirable attention.

In her experience, her wheelchair did not close doors; rather, it opened them. She was as happy as she had ever been.

Over and beyond taking the steps described above, some Americans are resisting aging by more aggressive means. In 2003, more than two million Americans over the age of 50 had elective cosmetic surgery,[17] with the most popular procedure being eyelid surgery.[18] In addition, aging women use every manner and fashion of skin cream and lotion to reduce their face wrinkles and shore up their sagging skin. So important is babylike skin to some aging women that they willingly pay anywhere from $700 to $3000 for acid or laser peels of their own well-worn skin.[19]

Although acid and laser skin peels are not entirely risk-free, they are probably less risky than the injections of Botox and collagen many women get to plump up their lips and firm their cheeks. Certainly, they are not nearly as risky as the antiaging remedies that unorthodox "doctors" offer wealthy people at spa-like clinics in the Alps and other popular travel destinations. A particularly questionable Alpine fountain-of-youth treatment consists in injecting live-cell, sheep-fetus extracts into men and women. Not only are these "sheep shots"[20] not cheap shots, they very likely are inefficacious and unsafe shots. Yet some people are so eager to look young, that they let literal violence be done to their bodies. For them, looking old is worse than being dead.

III. ANTIAGING MEDICINE

Because most people fear old age and want to avoid death for as long as possible, a newly created group of specialists called **biogerontologists** seek ways to make old age as pleasant as possible and even to extend the life span. Importantly, these biogerontologists fall into one of three groups, with progressively more ambitious goals.

The first group of biogerontologists have relatively modest goals. Their efforts to control aging are limited to warding off the diseases and disabilities associated with old age as long as possible. In other words, they want people to live healthy and happy lives until *very* shortly before they die. They also want all people, and not just privileged and lucky people to be able to live into their nineties and hundreds.

The second group of biogerontologists have more ambitious goals. They want to do more than ward off the infirmities associated with growing old. They also want to "increase the mean and maximal human life span by about forty percent, which is a mean age at death of about 112 years for Caucasian American or Japanese women, with an occasional winner topping out at about 140 years."[21] Among these biogerontologists are those who maintain that **extreme calorie restriction** is the key to living past the 120 mark. Studies show that some animals live up to 40% longer if they are fed 30%–60% fewer calories than they would normally consume. The bone mass, skin thickness, brain activity, and immune function of skinny animals is better than that of fat animals. Moreover, skinny animals appear better able to resist the effects of high temperatures, toxic chemicals, and traumatic injuries than fat animals.[22]

Although researchers have not attempted a full-scale, extreme caloric restriction study on human subjects for fear of harming them, some people have nevertheless decided to voluntarily consume no more than 1,200 calories a day. Extreme caloric restrictors admit that their diets leave them feeling hungry most of the time. Yet they are willing to forsake the pleasure of food in order to (possibly) secure several years of additional life. Scientists used to theorize that people who eat near starvation diets live longer than those who eat normal diets because their metabolic rate plummets and/or their development delays; however, they now think that extreme calorie restriction either protects the body's much needed insulin response[23] or reduces the production of harmful free radicals that "foster everything from cataracts to vascular disease."[24]

Because eating literally only enough to keep oneself alive is a regimen unlikely to strike the fancy of most Americans—addicted as we are to supersized portions of fatty and sugary foods—researchers are determined to find less onerous ways to extend the human lifespan. One alternative approach involves **genetic manipulation**. Scientists have already triggered a specific double gene mutation in roundworms that enables these lowly creatures to live six times longer than they would otherwise live. Commenting on this accomplishment, science reporter Nicholas Wade notes that if the equivalent of the roundworm's double gene mutation could be effected in human beings, most people in developed nations could live to 480 years; and some of them could even live to 720 years, "just 249 short of Methuselah's record."[25]

Living as long as Methuselah might be enough to satisfy most people, in the way of life. But because human beings are different from round worms, it is doubtful that the aging process works the same in human beings as it does in round worms. Most scientists think it is highly unlikely that only a few genes control the human aging process. Moreover, they claim that even if such genes did exist, manipulating them would be a two-edged sword because evolution theory operates on the assumption that a gain in longevity requires a loss in fertility.[26]

One empirical study that gives credence to the increased-longevity–decreased-fertility assumption goes back a half-century. Anatomist James Hamilton conducted a study on mentally disabled men in a Kansas State institution in the 1940s and 1950s. Whereas most of the men in the institution lived only to age 56, the ones who had been castrated typically lived to age 69. Hamilton speculated that although a lack of testosterone may limit a man's sexual prowess and athletic stamina, it may also add a significant number of years to his life.[27] By parity of reasoning, a lack of estrogen limits a woman's ability to get pregnant and bear children, but it may also enable her to live to a ripe old age.

Helping people lead very long lives is not enough for a third group of biogerontologists, however. They want to be able to control the aging process so that people can look and feel young, no matter how old they are. These biogerontologists view cloned embryonic stem cells as tiny fountains of youth. They want to use them to grow replacement muscles, tissues, organs, and neurons for people. Their ultimate goal is to create a new type of human being, a so-called **transhuman**. Unlike members of the old human species, members of the new posthuman species would not be "condemned" to disintegrate and die. In principle, they could live forever or at least for as long as they wanted.[28]

Not surprisingly, health care ethicists have mixed views about the antiaging strategies described above. In general, they accept proposals to help people live well until they die, and reject proposals to extend the median human life span to Methuselian lengths and/or to create posthumans. Yet even if most health care ethicists think that immortality is an inappropriate goal for antiaging medicine, there are a few who do. Among them is John Harris. He argues that because we cannot stop science's progression towards securing "immorality" for us, "[w]e should start thinking now about how we can live decently and creatively with the prospect of such lives."[29] We might have to develop some sort of system whereby volunteers give up their "immortal" lives to make room for new life coming into existence, for instance.

IV. AGING AND THE GROWING NEED FOR LONG-TERM CARE

Whether or not we favor efforts to transform humans into posthumans, for the foreseeable future, we are likely to remain all too *human*. Specifically, most of us will need some type of home-based or community-based care during our aging process.[30] In addition, 43% of us will probably need to enter a skilled nursing home sometime during our lifetime, 55% of us for only about one year, but 21% of us (mostly white, non-Hispanic women) for 5 years or more.[31]

Defining **long-term care** and its many modalities is not a simple process. According to Rosalie and Robert Kane, long-term care exists in the territory which borders on the boundary between health care services and social services.[32] In other words, aging people need both aggressive medical care— surgeries, drugs, wound care, and so forth—and help with **activities of daily living**—specifically, toileting, bathing, dressing, getting in and out of bed, money management, meal preparation, shopping, and housecleaning. My own father is a case in point. He is in his eighties, bedridden, afflicted with heart disease, diabetes, and arthritis, but retaining all his mental and sensory faculties (seeing, hearing, tasting, and the like). Over the past 5 years, he has had to be hospitalized for acute conditions related to one or the other of his diseases three times. Subsequent to each of these hospitalizations, one of which lasted 3 months, he has had to spend anywhere from 2 to 4 months in a skilled nursing home for rehabilitation. At present, my father is well enough to reside in his own home, but not without considerable help from me, my two sons, and a paid helper. Overall, my father's health is good. Medications effectively control his heart condition, arthritis, and diabetes. Because my father sees and hears quite well, and because his mind is sharp as a tack, he reads about two books a week, watches his favorite television shows, plays computer games, solves incredibly difficult math puzzles, debates public policy issues with anyone who stops by his home, and makes his wishes known (all too well sometimes). My father needs help with almost every activity of daily living, however, because he has lost his ability to walk. The only officially classified activity of daily living he is able to perform is money management, a task that is distressing to him only insofar as his personal savings have dwindled to less than a few thousand. If my father's health status remains stable, he could probably enjoy several more years in his home, assuming that I and others are able to continue helping him at the same level we do now. Unfortunately, I cannot predict how long we will be able to provide him with this care. There may come a day when it will no longer be possible for us to give my father the care he needs in the home he loves.

A. Long-Term Home Care

Focusing on the case of my father serves as a transition to a more general discussion of home care. In all, 80% of **home care** is provided by unpaid family members and friends, the bulk of whom are women.[33] On the average, female caregivers provide assistance from 1 year to 4 years, but it is not atypical for a female caregiver to provide care to a loved one for 5 or more years.[34] About one-third of female caregivers work outside their own home in the public sector, but because caring for a family member with disabilities is usually a very demanding and time-consuming task, many female caregivers find they must give up or substantially reduce work outside the home.

Although providing home care to family members is often emotionally and spiritually rewarding, it can also be draining and demoralizing, particularly if familial caregivers have children and/or a spouse, their own health problems, limited financial assets, and other heavy responsibilities. **Familial caregivers** report a wide range of positive and negative feelings about their service such as being loved (96%), appreciated (90%), proud (84%), worried (53%), frustrated (37%), sad or depressed (28%), and overwhelmed (22%).[35] Studies indicate that familial caregivers use prescription drugs for insomnia, anxiety, and clinical depression about two to three times more often than familial noncaregivers.[36]

Although familial caregivers sometimes think that unless they provide care to their loved ones no one else will, there are ways for familial caregivers to get help caring for the nonmedical as well as medical needs of their loved

ones. Some familial caregivers turn to a variety of charitable and civic organizations for help. Others turn to federal and state authorities for assistance.
Indeed, in the 1990s, public monies for home care were provided for both
medical services and nonmedical services such as home-delivered meals,
respite care for familial caregivers, adult daycare, transportation, housekeep-
ing, and personal care.[37]

As much as familial caregivers and those for whom they care may welcome some public assistance, using such help presents its own set of problems.
Federal and state employees do not set their clocks to serve the schedules
and preferences of the people whom they serve. Rather, they set their clocks
to the rhythm of government requirements and regulations. Moreover, as
soon as familial caregivers open their loved one's private home to the public
eye, they subject themselves to a level of scrutiny and supervision to which
they may not be accustomed. Misunderstandings may occur. For example,
because **elder abuse** (physical, psychological, financial, neglect) is a growing
problem in the United States, familial caregivers may find themselves asked
some uncomfortable questions. Specifically, they may be asked about loved
ones' cuts, bruises, burns, weight loss, and the like. Although it is not unusual for familial caregivers to "guilt trip" or seek to control their loved ones'
behavior in some way or another, most familial caregivers do not intentionally harm them. Indeed, experts estimate that only 5% or less of familial caregivers actually physically abuse, verbally assault, and or deliberately neglect
those for whom they care.[38] Yet, no matter how accurate these statistics are,
many publicly paid health care providers feel it is part of their job to be on
the alert for familial caregivers who may be mistreating their loved ones. Ac-
cusations may be made on the basis of little solid evidence and familial caregivers may rue the day they asked for public assistance.

Another source of tension and stress between familial caregivers and
publicly paid home care providers is disagreement about what is best for
the person needing care. For example, publicly paid home care providers
may think it is in the best interest of a diabetic client to adhere to a very low
carbohydrate diet, a diet that familial caregivers as well as the client may find
overly restrictive. When told they should stop giving foods such as potato
chips and donuts to their loved ones, familial caregivers may protest that
their mom is 92 years old and failing, and that one of her few remaining pleasures in life is eating "junk food." A small gain in health for mom—an extra
month or two of life—is simply not worth denying mom her treat foods.
Unimpressed by such reasoning, publicly paid home care providers may
chide familial caregivers. They may say something like, "You don't want
mom to get worse, do you?," to which familial caregivers may retort, "Just
because mom is old does not mean she has no will of her own." If a 50-year-
old diabetic is free to follow or not follow the diet prescribed for him, why
should not the same freedom be accorded to the 80-year-old diabetic? Is autonomy only to be respected if one is young?

Exchanges such as the one described above are part and parcel of familial caregivers' negotiations with privately paid as well as publicly paid home care providers. A veritable home care industry has sprung up over the last 15 years, providing a range of unskilled and skilled services depending on a care recipient's needs. Some home care recipients require 24-hour-a-day care, but most of them require only a quarter or less of that amount of time. To the degree that home care is nonmedical, it is usually paid for out-of-pocket. Thus, clients are often willing to settle for low-quality home care services because such help is all they can afford.

Although many **privately paid home care providers** have an excellent work ethic, good skills, and sterling characters, a few work in the home care industry simply because it is the only kind of work they can find or do. For the most part, privately paid home care providers earn minimum wages, work undesirable hours, have few, if any, benefits, and must be willing to work for all sorts of clients in all sorts of homes and neighborhoods. Some privately paid home care providers find themselves assisting very unpleasant or even abusive clients. Others find themselves tending very ill clients with oozing wounds and seeping bodily orifices. Yet other paid home care providers are asked to provide services in unclean homes or in homes located in unsafe neighborhoods.

Adding to privately paid home care providers' burdens is the fact that as their industry grows, it is subjected to "increased competition, oversight, and regulation."[39] Not surprisingly, responsible privately paid home care providers want to be sure that those for whom they care are *able* as well as *willing* to live at home. They fear that if any harm befalls a care recipient, they (and/or their agency) will be blamed and even held legally liable for the harm. Thus, many privately paid home care providers seek to control care recipients' autonomy in order to assure their safety. For example, one of my father's first home helpers, whom I eventually discharged, would not let him use his walker to get to and from the toilet. She insisted that it was safer for him to defecate and urinate in a bedpan or a diaper. My father and I objected, insisting, first, that the bathroom was less than 10 feet from his bed and, second, that she could walk with him as far as the bathroom. But she did not like our solution to my father's problem. I suspected that her convenience rather than concerns about my father's safety were her real reason for not wanting him to go to the bathroom.

B. Long-Term Care in Assisted-Living Residences

Not everyone who requires long-term care is able and/or willing to secure adequate care in their own home. For example, an 88-year-old widow with no children may have siblings whose need for care is just as great as her own. In addition, a significant number of people who need help may not want their loved ones to provide it. For example, a couple in their seventies may not want their middle-aged children interfering with their lives; or a husband may not want his wife jeopardizing her own health and well-being to care for him at home. Although such persons have, as we just discussed, the option of hiring privately paid home care providers to assist them, they may not have enough money to pay for adequate help or they may discover that the help they hire is not all that helpful. Regrettably, many care recipients find themselves continually hiring and firing privately paid health care providers for lack of compatibility, tardiness, absences, poor performance of duties, or even abuses that range from theft to withholding certain levels of care from them in order to control their behavior. Therefore, to resolve one or more of the problems just mentioned, a significant number of people leave their private homes and move into an alternative residential setting.

Among these alternative residential settings are those called **assisted-living facilities**. Typically, these facilities meet the nonmedical as well as medical needs of aging persons who do not need to be in a skilled nursing facility, but who are unwilling and/or unable to get the help they require to live safely in their own homes (assuming that they have a home). Rightly or wrongly (more likely, wrongly), the term "assisted-living facility" is increasingly used as a generic term to designate both licensed and unlicensed residences, ranging from basic-service housing (retirement homes, personal care homes, board and care facilities) to continuing care retirement communities which combine housing, health care, and social activities and events.[40] Not surprisingly, people with low incomes tend to live in residences that provide few services, and people with high incomes tend to live in residences that provide many services catering to their specific likes and dislikes.

Although Medicaid provides limited subsidies to a significant number of people living in basic "board and care" facilities, the amount provided varies widely from state to state. Importantly, public monies are not used to help defray the costs of middle-class and upper-class people who live in full-service **continuing care retirement communities**. Thus, it is not that difficult for individuals to exhaust their life savings relatively swiftly. Even a $500,000 nest egg can be spent in under a decade.

In the past, continuing care retirement communities charged their residents a very large entry fee (in hundreds of thousands), with the understanding that if monies were left over when the residents left the community or died, the monies would not revert back to the residents or their heirs but would remain with the facilities. But this arrangement ultimately proved unsatisfactory to everyone involved. Specifically, when residents died only a short time after paying their huge tabs to the community, their heirs were likely to protest that their parents (and they) had been "ripped off!" Similarly, when residents who entered the community at age 65 or so "failed" to die by age 90 or so, the community felt cheated, obligated as it was to pay for years of care it had not factored into its bottom line. Thus, both profit-driven communities and residents currently favor a "pay-as-you-go" monthly method of billing, just in case residents live for less or more years than was initially anticipated. For example, in the 1990s, one continuing care retirement community offered the following three levels of care to residents: (1) "independent living" in a studio apartment for residents who need no help for $2,000 a month; (2) "assisted living" for residents who need help with one or more tasks of daily living for $2,400 a month; and (3) "nursing-home" care for residents who are incontinent, need to be fed, are demented, and/or require intensive rehabilitation for $3,000 a month.[41] No doubt, these costs are considerably higher nowadays, a fact that explains why so many residents of continuing care communities are now "praying" their money "doesn't die" before they do.[42] They leave in fear of being forced to move from the only home they know to a state-subsidized facility not to their liking.

C. Long-Term Care in Nursing Homes

Despite the increasing popularity of assisted-living residences, including continuing care retirement communities, most people 65 years old or older who need nursing care and/or continual care supervision receive it in a **nursing home**. As we noted above, over 40% of elderly Americans will probably enter a nursing home sometime during their life; and if they have personal funds, their out-of-pocket bill will be large. As of 2004, the annual average cost of a nursing home for a 1-year stay was $57,700,[43] and most experts fear that this cost is bound to rise.

Because it is no secret that U.S. nursing homes are not always as high quality or well-staffed as they should be,[44] the decision to enter a nursing home is often made reluctantly. Sometimes care recipients decide to enter a nursing home because they no longer want to impose themselves and their burdens on familial caregivers. Just as often, however, familial caregivers make the nursing home transition decision. They initiate a conversation with the care recipient that runs something like the following: "This arrangement just isn't working any more. . . . It's getting too hard for everyone including yourself . . . you need more care than we can provide, and we are getting very worried about your safety and health . . . what's more, we just don't have the money to hire 24-hour-a-day home care help for you . . . it's probably time to move to a place where professionals can care for you . . . ." Of course, familial caregivers are not always of one mind when it comes to decisions about proper care for their aging loved ones. They may get into serious arguments about placing mom or dad in a nursing home where they might not only get worse care than the makeshift, "unprofessional" care they received at home but also have to deal with a wide range of people, some of them quite annoying, disconcerting, or even repulsive.

Nursing home residents run the gamut from "live-wire," totally "with-it" folks to individuals desperately clinging to life. Although it is difficult to sort nursing home residents into precise categories, at least three types of individuals reside in the typical nursing home. First, there are the residents who need only short-term rehabilitation for a specific medical condition or long-term assistance with several activities of daily living. Most of these residents are both mentally alert and physically able to get around, albeit in wheelchairs, on walkers, or with canes. Nursing home staff members plan activities that usually consist in game playing "sing-alongs," and arts and crafts for these residents. They also schedule entertainment programs (typically church or school choirs) and lectures (typically local ministers, celebrities, or educators) for them.

Not all mentally alert nursing home residents want to participate in the activities and programs the nursing-home staff schedules, however. Some of them regard these activities and programs as boring, "syrupy-sweet," and/or childish. Nevertheless, at some nursing homes, the staff hounds *all* mentally-alert residents to "join the fun," implying that nonparticipants are uncooperative "sour pusses" who think they are better than other folks. Pressured into being good sports, many mentally-able residents attend programs and engage in activities they do not enjoy. They do so simply to avoid the staff's disapproval.

In contrast to the individuals in the first category of nursing home residents, a second category of residents are clearly mentally dysfunctional in one way or another. Many people in nursing homes suffer from either senile dementia or **Alzheimer's disease**, a mind-robbing condition that is difficult to diagnose until it has progressed for sometime. In fact, during the first stage of Alzheimer's disease, its victims manifest symptoms no worse than forgetfulness, losing interest in formerly absorbing hobbies and favorite activities, and increasingly poor judgment that leads to wearing inappropriate clothes, for example.[45] It is only during its second stage that Alzheimer's disease clearly reveals itself as a "mind stealer." Over a period that lasts anywhere from 2 to 8 years, Alzheimer's disease victims become unable to recognize even close family members and dear friends. Many of them begin to wander aimlessly, frequently getting lost. In addition, the personality of many Alzheimer's disease patients starts to change, most usually for the worse. They may become sleepless, paranoid, delusional, or even violent. Bad as stage two of Alzheimer's disease is, stage three is even worse, however. Over the course of 2 to 3 years, Alzheimer's disease victims gradually become unable to remember past events, to process new information, or to engage in meaningful conversations. Toward the end of their lives, Alzheimer's disease victims become incontinent, incapable of eating or even swallowing naturally, and entirely bedridden.

Sadly, stage-three Alzheimer's disease victims are not the only totally bedridden residents in many nursing homes. A third category of residents, who suffer from a variety of diseases that systematically destroy their bodies and minds, lay in beds, barely alive. Most of these individuals are in the end stages of a disease, or so weakened by the aging process that they can no longer move. Category one residents look at category three residents with alarm, fearful that their fate will soon be their own.

Arguably, it is less than desirable to house people who are mentally alert and/or physically able with people suffering from advanced Alzheimer's disease or people on the verge of dying. And certainly, it is less than realistic to expect nursing home staff to meet the disparate needs of three distinct categories of nursing home residents. For these reasons and others, nursing homes are beginning to specialize. For example, a significant number of nursing homes now serve only residents with Alzheimer's disease, because the things that people with this affliction usually enjoy are often the things that people without this affliction view as "demeaning" or "nutty." Specifically, hugging dolls and teddy bears seems to provide special comfort to many persons with Alzheimer's disease. So too does watching children's programs. Indeed, in his moving account of his wife's descent into the depths of Alzheimer's disease, the husband of the brilliant philosopher and writer Iris Murdoch describes how, towards the end of her life, Iris could not get enough of "Teletubbies," a British cartoon show for toddlers.[46] Responding to critics who think that persons with Alzheimer's disease do not have lives worth living, Joanne Koening-Costa, President of the Alzheimer Consulting Association in Framingham, Massachusetts, told a news reporter that, for all she knew, Alzheimer's disease patients, who spent their days hugging stuffed animals, might be immersed in feelings of loving and being loved.[47]

D. Long-Term Care Costs

1. Medicare and Medicaid Coverage

Throughout this chapter, reference has been made to the high costs of long-term care, but these costs deserve more than passing mention. Relatively few people can pay out-of-pocket for more than a year or two of care in a nursing home, and yet only about 4%–5% of Americans have long-term care insurance.[48] Many people assume that **Medicare** will pay for their long-term care when, in point of fact, Medicare pays for no more than 100 days of care in a skilled nursing home following a hospitalization. In addition, it covers some physician-authorized home health care, but only for "skilled nursing, therapeutic services, durable medical equipment, and short-term care by home health aides, provided that the services are related to acute health conditions."[49]

The main source of funding for long-term care is **Medicaid**, the welfare program that pays for medical assistance for qualified individuals and families with low incomes and limited resources. Medicaid pays the bills for about three-fifths of the individuals in nursing homes.[50] It also pays the bills for about one-fourth of home care and community-based care.[51] Unlike Medicare, which is funded and administered solely by the federal government and which provides uniform benefits to all U.S. citizens over the age of 65, Medicaid is funded by state governments as well as the federal government. Each state is permitted to set its own eligibility standards for Medicaid; determine the type, amount, length, and scope of provided services; set its payment rates; and administer its own programs.[52]

Because the federal government's subsidies for Medicaid are quite limited (a fact we will discuss in greater length in Chapter 13), and because some states are far more reluctant than others to use state monies for Medicaid, there are severe inequities in the cost, quality, and accessibility of long-term care in the United States. Moreover, just because someone is poor enough to qualify for Medicaid and disabled enough to need a bed in a skilled nursing home, it does not mean that he or she will be able to secure a Medicaid bed. Nursing homes cannot always afford to set aside a large number of their beds for Medicaid and Medicare patients. It is not financially feasible for them to do unless they are able to shift their uncompensated Medicaid costs unto the bills of private-pay residents.

Qualifying for Medicaid requires people with assets to pay for their care out-of-pocket until they spend their monies down to a very low sum, usually $2000 or so. Not surprisingly, people who have spent their lives trying to amass monies to pass on to their heirs have a hard time resigning themselves to giving all these monies to nonfamilial caregivers. They lament the fact that they have become a burden to their loved ones. Thoughts such as this one tempt some people of means to shelter their assets in "protected investments" such as trusts and annuities[53] and/or to give their monies as outright gifts to family members and friends once they reach a certain age. Although sheltering assets may make good financial sense, it is doubtful that this practice is morally justifiable. Wealthy people who shelter their assets for their heirs to enjoy "are able to take advantage of a program for the poor [Medicaid] without actually being poor themselves."[54] Aware that people of means are abusing Medicaid, federal and state governments are increasingly passing legislation that precludes people "who transfer assets within twenty-four months of applying to Medicaid from becoming eligible for Medicaid benefits."[55]

2. Long-Term Care Insurance

As mentioned above, very few people have **long-term care insurance**. It is not a routine part of most standard employer-provided health care insurance policies, although some employers offer it as an out-of-pocket add-on. One of the main reasons that people do not purchase long-term care insurance, over and beyond the fact that they think they will not need it, is that it is quite expensive, particularly if it is purchased when one is already elderly. Whereas a 40-year-old male may have to pay $400 a year for long-term health care insurance, a man or woman over age 70 may have to pay $3000.[56]

Unless they cost at least as much as the policies described above, few long-term care policies are generous enough to cover all of a person's long-term care needs; and most of them cannot be used unless they are properly triggered. Typically, there are three **benefit triggers** for long-term care. The first one is physical impairment. Although most long-term care policies provide care only if a person needs substantial assistance with at least two activities of daily living (for example, getting in and out of bed and using the toilet), some of the higher-cost ones provide long-term care as soon as an individual thinks he or she needs "standby assistance."[57] A second benefit trigger for long-term care is mental incapacity measured in terms of failure to pass certain mental-functioning tests. Not surprisingly, the high incidence of Alzheimer's disease in the United States, coupled with the high costs of caring for someone with Alzheimer's disease (typically, $174,000 from the time of diagnosis to death), has generated much interest in Alzheimer's disease-specific long-term care policies, which, as one might expect, are quite costly.[58] The third benefit trigger for long-term care is physician-certification that such care is necessary, irrespective of whether a certain type of physical impairment and/or mental incapacity is present. Policies with physician-certification clauses are particularly costly, however and most long-term care insurance providers are not willing to underwrite them. The possibilities of abusing such policies are many. For example, a physician may certify a patient as in need of long-term care simply because the patient is lonely and would like daily companionship.

3. Long-Term Care and Age-Based Rationing

Because the need for long-term care is so obvious, many critics of the status quo recommend that Medicare include long-term care among its standard benefits. But expanding Medicare to include long-term care for all Americans—the cost of which was $106.5 billion in 1995—[59] would probably require the federal government both to increase taxes substantially and to reduce some of the benefits Medicare currently provides. In this connection, health care ethicist Daniel Callahan has stressed that the U.S. government cannot provide all its citizens with universal health care coverage unless it sets this coverage "within a context of limits—limits to an extension of old age and to the pursuit of individual care."[60] As Callahan sees it, the U.S. government should fund, first, those modes of health care that are most likely to have the greatest positive impact on mortality and morbidity rates. Callahan specifically recommends that the U.S. government spend sparingly on "general, advanced forms of medical care or restoration (e.g., advanced surgery, cancer chemotherapy, extensive rehabilitation)"[61] and on "the provision of highly advanced, technological medical therapy (e.g., dialysis, open-heart surgery, organ transplants, total parenteral nutrition)."[62] Instead he urges the U.S. government to spend most of its health care dollars on the following:

> the provision of caring in its most basic forms: the (topical) relief of pain; hospice or comparable care for the dying; nursing or home care and companionship for the elderly and otherwise frail; simple mental health programs for the mildly disturbed; basic and decent home and institutional care for the chronically ill, the demented, the disabled, the retarded, the severely mentally ill—all those powerless to care for themselves.[63]

Callahan's prescription for long-term care seems promising. It meets the needs of aging people without expecting them to spend every penny of their life savings on health care or strangling them in bureaucratic webs that choke the dignity out of them. It is important, however, to stress that, in the end, Callahan requires aging people to pay with their lives for government-subsidized long-term care. As he sees it, when it comes to access to costly medical technologies, drugs, and surgeries, the old should step aside for the young. It is not, in his estimation, morally wrong to ration health care on the basis of age—to refuse, for example, to provide people in their eighties with 6-figure organ transplants or (in the future) gene therapies.

Calls for **age-based rationing of health care**, such as Callahan's, are not met with universal approval, however. Opponents of age-based rationing claim that because people cannot control their chronological age any more than they can control their genetic composition, it is just as wrong to discriminate against someone on account of their age as on account of their race or sex. If it is wrong to deprive someone of an organ transplant simply because he is *African-American* or simply because she is *female*, then it is equally wrong to deprive someone of an organ transplant simply because he or she is *elderly*. Ageism is as reprehensible as racism or sexism.[64] Moreover, opponents of age-based rationing argue that if any group of people deserve care, including health care, it is the elderly, because of all they have done for others throughout their entire lives.

Although advocates of age-based rationing agree that ageism is wrong, they insist that an age-based rationing policy is not necessarily "ageist"—that is, a policy that *unfairly* discriminates against the elderly. For example, Callahan roots his defense of age-based rationing of health care in natural law and communitarian traditions. He argues that upon reaching the end of one's natural life, one should no longer be a candidate for aggressive medical treatment that primarily aims to extend one's life a few days, weeks, months, or even years. Callahan does not assign a precise numerical value to a natural life span, though he suggests that nature begins to have its way with most of us when we hit our eighties. Rather, he emphasizes that a natural life span is correlated with one's **biographical age** rather than with one's **chronological age**.[65] We are each writing our own stories, and there comes a time when there is not much new to tell—when we simply keep repeating ourselves in a futile effort to stave off the inevitability of death. Like books, people's lives have a beginning, middle, and end. When the end draws near, a person should have the wisdom to dot the "i's" and cross the "t's" of his or her life. Enough *is* enough.

Although few of us look forward to death, Callahan believes that most of us can distinguish between what he terms a tolerable death[66] and what might be termed an intolerable death. A tolerable death is a death that occurs when one has accomplished most of what life has to offer, and has fulfilled most of one's major obligations to family, friends, colleagues, and so forth. It is a death that does not prompt us to rage and despair at human finitude. Thus, when an 85-year-old, widowed professor emeritus with severe Alzheimer's disease dies, we do not feel as cheated as we do when a 30-year-old assistant professor, who has just published her first book and given birth to her first child, dies of unexpected complications subsequent to a caesarean section. The former death strikes us as tolerable, indeed merciful; the latter one as intolerable, even cruel.

Having distinguished between tolerable and intolerable deaths, Callahan argues that there is something disproportionate—in fact, wrong—about aggressively treating 80-year-olds with everything in the medical cabinet, no matter how expensive or unproven, so that they can live a little longer, when many young people die prematurely and unnecessarily because they lack access to basic health care. Callahan reasons that because the U.S. health care system cannot fund everything for everyone, it is time for older Americans to forego costly end-of-life treatments so that younger Americans can be assured of basic health care.

V. CONCLUSION

Hiding between the lines of Callahan's reasoning is the notion of a duty to die, a duty we shall discuss in Chapter 11. Callahan thinks the old should make room for the young, even though doing so requires that they stop searching for quasi-immortality on earth. Interestingly, his point is joined by the more pragmatic points health care ethicist and physician Leon Kass has raised against the life-extending projects discussed earlier in this chapter. Kass points out that if most of us lived to the age of 120 and were fairly vigorous up to the point of our death, the effects on the size and distribution of our population would be enormous. In addition, the effects on "work opportunities, retirement plans, new hiring and promotion, social security, housing patterns, cultural and social attitudes and beliefs, the status of traditions, the rate and acceptability of social change, and the structure of family life" would be overwhelming.[67] Unemployment is already a problem and would become an even greater problem if everyone over the age of 65 held on to their positions until the age of 95 or so; and if the government forced people to retire at the age of 65, how would retirees support themselves for decades in view of the fact that the Social Security system is already falling apart, and families no longer feel a strong obligation to take care of their elderly members?

Significantly, Kass's main argument against extending the lifespan is that corporeal immortality is not one of the proper goals of medicine.[68] He notes that our culture is a particularly death-denying and death-fearing one, and that if we felt as good at age 120 as we did at age 30, we would find death even more intolerable than we presently do. We would insist even more adamantly than some of us do now that researchers find some way to prolong our lives for ever longer periods of time. Therefore, Kass claims that the current aging process, as bumpy as it is, is the best possible preparation for death. He quotes the philosopher Montaigne:

> I notice that in proportion as I sink into sickness, I naturally enter into a certain disdain for life. I find that I have much more trouble digesting this resolution when I am in health than when I have a fever. Inasmuch as I no longer cling so hard to the good things of life when I begin the use and pleasure of them, I come to view death with much less frightened eyes. This makes me hope that the farther I get from life and the nearer to death, the more easily I shall accept the exchange . . . If we fell into such a change [decrepitude] suddenly, I don't think we could endure it. But when we are led by Nature's hand down a gentle and virtually imperceptible slope, bit by bit, one step at a time, she rolls us into this wretched state and makes us familiar with it; so that we find no shock when youth dies within us, which in essence and in truth is a harder death than the complete death of a languishing life or the death of old age; inasmuch as the leap is not so cruel from a painful life as from a sweet and flourishing life to a grievous and painful one.[69]

In other words, as interpreted by Kass through Montaigne, aging enables us to look at death as a friend of sorts. In particular, writes Kass, the older we get, the more we are able to view death as a liberator. After a while, life gets boring. There are only so many activities we wish to pursue, and only so many times that we can do them, until they no longer excite or interest us. Likewise, there are only so many human relationships we wish to forge. It is very meaningful to create and maintain one family—even two families, as happens after some divorces or deaths—but it is not clear how many of us would like to do this three or four times. Finally, and most importantly, says Kass, death helps us be serious about life:

> . . . To know and to feel that one goes around only once, and that the deadline is not out of sight, is for many people the necessary spur to the pursuit of something worthwhile. To number our days is the condition for making them count, to treasure and appreciate all that life brings. Homer's immortals, for all their

eternal beauty and youthfulness, live shallow and rather frivolous lives, their passion only transiently engaged, in first this and then that. They live as spectators of the mortals who by comparison have depth, aspiration, genuine feeling, and hence a real center to their lives. Mortality makes life matter.[70]

Perhaps Kass is right. Immorality may not be all that it is cracked up to be. Death may be a friend, after all.

Discussion Questions

1. What are the social, economic, and political forces that come to bear on older adults' images of well being?
2. Do you have a positive or negative view of aging? Explain why.
3. Are you in favor of extending average life expectancy to 120 years or more? Why or why not?
4. Do you think medicine should attempt to make people "immortal"? How long do you want to live and why?
5. Is the U.S. health care system adequately prepared to handle the aging U.S. population? Will it be able to handle the health care needs of the Baby Boom Generation?
6. How would you reform Medicare and Medicaid to be more responsive to the needs of aging Americans?
7. Do you think it is fair to ration health care on the basis of age? Why or why not?
8. What plans do you (your parents) have for retirement)? Do you think you will be able to afford them? What happens if you get very ill after you retire? Can you envision yourself living relatively happily in a residential care community? Would you do so in a nursing home?

Case Studies

1. Mrs. B, a 74-year-old diabetic who is partially blind, has lived in a nursing home for 10 years. Medicaid pays her bills. She likes the home, where she has made many friends. However, the state is trying to save money by caring for its elderly medical patients at the lowest possible cost. It needs to transfer as many patients as possible from nursing homes to less costly facilities that offer only custodial care and are not required to provide medical care.

An arbitrary grading system has been established to evaluate nursing home patients to determine their suitability for transfer. Patients are assigned a certain number of points according to their ability to dress, feed, clothe themselves, and the like. If the number of points the patient receives is higher than a designated total, officials deem that the patient can be transferred without any harmful effects.

When she is evaluated, Mrs. B receives more than the designated number of points. The decision is made to transfer her. She is not consulted, nor is she given a voice in the decision. She is simply moved—forcibly and against her wishes—to a custodial care institution. The evaluation does not take into account the psychological impact of the move on Mrs. B who is, for all practical purposes, being exiled from a home she loves.

a. Is the state's conduct ethical?

b. Because it has assigned a higher priority to other areas of medical care for funding, does the state have the right to disregard individual patients' wishes concerning the location of their care?

c. Should age have a significant role in this decision and allocation of resources?

2. Mrs. A, who is 70 years old, suffers from respiratory difficulty. The last time she was in the hospital she nearly died. She has severe emphysema, and when she developed a cold, her deterioration was so rapid that only artificial respiration in the emergency room saved her life. She spent 4 weeks in the Intensive Care Unit and required constant care from the medical staff. It was extremely difficult to wean her from the respirator. After she was discharged, she remained short of breath even while simply sitting in her wheelchair. Now, several months later, she has contracted another cold, and has been admitted to the hospital for a fifth time in a 5-year period. Dr. X initially manages to treat her without resorting to the ICU and a respirator. However, Mrs. A's condition worsens, and it becomes obvious to Dr. X that she will die before morning if she is not given a respirator.

Regrettably, hospital policy requires that respirators be used only in the ICU, where the required supporting staff and facilities are available. There is only one bed open in the ICU. The staff likes to save one bed for an emergency. Dr. X is disinclined to admit Mrs. A to the ICU, but he is well aware that her solicitous sons will probably insist that he admit her.

a. What should the physician do? Is he simply letting Mrs. A die or actively contributing to her death?

b. Who should make the final decision in this case—Mrs. A's sons, the physician, or the hospital administrators?

c. Would there be a hesitancy to admit Mrs. A to the ICU if she were age 16 rather than age 70?

3. Rosemarie, a well-educated bioethicist who is a widow with two sons and the only daughter of a 77-year-old widower, seeks with her father some way to get around the Medicare/Medicaid system. Dad worked hard all his life as a baker and wants his daughter and two grandchildren to enjoy

his modest legacy. Rosemarie and her dad "cook-up" the following recipe. Dad will transfer all of his assets to her now. Then Rosemarie and he will cross their fingers and hope that dad does not need serious, institutional care for the next 30 months (the point after which he will be eligible for Medicaid without any officials "looking back").

Rosemarie has some qualms about this procedure. She knows that if "push comes to shove," she will see to it that her father gets the best care possible, even if she is forced to spend the legacy she wishes to pass on to her sons. She would prefer not to jeopardize her and her sons' relatively-good style of life, however. It bothers her that because she knows how the system works, she can secure benefits that other people, who do not know how the system works, cannot. She wonders whether she and her father are violating the principle of justice by having him transfer his assets to her now.

a.   What would you do if you were in Rosemarie's position?

b.   Should adult children be legally obligated to pay for their indigent parents' health care bills?

Endnotes

1. Richard Saul Wurman, *Understanding Healthcare* (Newport, RI: Top, 2004), p. 9.
2. Richard Corliss and Michael D. Lemonick, "How to live to be 100," *Time Magazine* (August 30, 2004): 38–46.
3. Ibid.
4. U.S. Census Bureau, "Projected life expectancy at birth, middle series," *U.S. Census* (January 13, 2000), *http://www.census.gov/population/documentation/twps0038/tabC.txt* [accessed April 6, 2005].
5. Claudia Wallis, "How to live to be 120," *Time Magazine* (March 6, 1995): 85.
6. Ibid.
7. "Will you still feed me?," *New York Times* (April 28, 2002): A16.
8. Ibid.
9. Geoffrey Cowley, "The biology of aging," *Newsweek Magazine*, Special Edition, Health for Life (Fall/Winter 2001): 16–18.
10. Richard Saul Wurman, *Understanding Healthcare* (Newport, RI: Top, 2004), p. 9.
11. Betty Friedan, *The Fountain of Age* (New York: Simon and Schuster, 1993), p. 122.
12. Ibid., p. 326.
13. Barbara Kantrowitz, "Health for life: the new keys to women's health," *Newsweek Magazine*, Special Edition, Health for Life (Fall/Winter 2001): 6.
14. "By the numbers: a *Newsweek* poll on aging," *Newsweek Magazine*, Special Edition, Health for Life (Fall/Winter 2001): 9.
15. Geoffrey Cowley, "How to live to 100," *Newsweek Magazine* (June 30, 1997): 67.

16. Michael Craig Miller, quoted in Susan H. Greenberg and Karen Springen, "Keeping hope alive," *Newsweek Magazine*, Special Edition, Health for Life (Fall/Winter 2001): 63.

17. "More than 8.7 million cosmetic plastic surgery procedures in 2003—up 32% over 2002," *American Association of Plastic Surgeons* (February, 2005), *http://www.locateadoc.com/articles.cfm/search/1225* [accessed March 8, 2005].

18. Ibid.

19. Peg Tyre, "Turning back the clock," *Newsweek Magazine*, Special Edition, Health for Life (Fall/Winter 2001): 49, 51.

20. Melinda Beck et al., "Peddling youth over the counter," *Newsweek Magazine* (March 5, 1990): 51.

21. Richard A. Miller, "Extending life: scientific prospects and political obstacles," *The Milbank Quarterly*, 80 (2002): 164.

22. Michael D. Lemonick, "Eat less, live longer," in: Corliss and Lemonick, "How to live to be 100," *Time Magazine* (August 30, 2004): 38–46.

23. Geoffrey Cowley, "The biology of aging," *Newsweek Magazine*, Special Edition, Health for Life (Fall/Winter 2001): 18.

24. Ibid., p. 17.

25. Nicholas Wade, *Life Script: How the Human Genome Discoveries Will Transform Medicine and Enhance Your Health* (New York: Simon and Schuster, 2001), p. 152.

26. Ibid., p. 152.

27. Geoffrey Cowley, "The biology of aging," *Newsweek Magazine*, Special Edition, Health for Life (Fall/Winter 2001): 19.

28. Francis Fukayama, *Our Posthuman Future: Consequences of the Biotechnology Revolution* (New York: Farrar, Straus, and Giroux, 2002).

29. John Harris, "Intimations of immortality," *Science*, 288 (2000): 59.

30. Nancy Wilson, "Long-term care in the United States: an overview of the current system," in: Laurence B. McCullough and Nancy L. Wilson (eds.), *Long-Term Care Decisions: Ethical and Conceptual Dimensions* (Baltimore: Johns Hopkins University Press, 1995), p. 39.

31. Ibid.

32. Robert A. Kane and Rosalie L. Kane, *Long-Term Care: Principles, Programs, and Policies* (New York: Springer Publishing Company, 1987), p. 4.

33. American Association of Retired Persons, *Working Caregivers: National Survey of Caregivers Final Report* (Washington, DC, 1989).

34. Robyn Stone, Gail Cafferata, and Judith Sangl, "Caregivers of the frail elderly: a national profile," *Gerontologist* 27 (1987): 616–626.

35. Cited in Richard Saul Wurman, *Understanding Healthcare* (Newport, RI: Top, 2004), p. 236.

36. Ibid.

37. Ibid., p. 236.

38. Karl A. Pillemer, "Risk factors in elder abuse: results from a case-control study," in: Karl A. Pillemer and Rosalie S. Wolf (eds.), *Elder Abuse: Conflict in the Family* (Dover, MA: Auburn House, 1986).

39. Nancy Wilson, "Long-term care in the United States: an overview of the current system," in: Laurence B. McCullough and Nancy L. Wilson (eds.), *Long-Term Care Decisions: Ethical and Conceptual Dimensions* (Baltimore: Johns Hopkins University Press, 1995), p. 52.

40. Ibid., p. 51.

41. Tamar Lewin, "As alertness outlives vigor, new kinds of care for the old," *New York Times* (December 2, 1990): 24.

42. Ibid.

43. Richard Saul Wurman, *Understanding Healthcare* (Newport, RI: Top, 2004), p. 304.

44. Robert Pear, "U.S. recommending strict new rules at nursing homes," *New York Times* (July 23, 2000): 1.

45. Christine Gorman, "The three stages of Alzheimer's," in: J. Madeleine Nash, "The new science of Alzheimer's," *Time Magazine* (July 27, 2000): 57.

46. Robert McCrum, "Second thoughts," *New York Times Book Review* (October 3, 1999): 9.

47. Cited in Claudia Calb, "Coping with the Darkness," *Newsweek Magazine* (January 31, 2000): 53.

48. Robert Binstock, Leighton Cluff, and Otto Von Mering (eds.), *The Future of Long-Term Care: Social and Policy Issues* (Baltimore: Johns Hopkins University Press, 1996).

49. Nancy Wilson, "Long-term care in the United States: an overview of the current system," in: Laurence B. McCullough and Nancy L. Wilson (eds.), *Long-Term Care Decisions: Ethical and Conceptual Dimensions* (Baltimore: Johns Hopkins University Press, 1995), p. 45.

50. Joshua Wiener and Laurel Illston, "Health care financing and organization for the elderly," in: Robert Binstock and Linda George (eds.), *Handbook of Aging and the Social Sciences*, 4th ed. (San Diego: Academic, 1996).

51. American Association of Retired Persons, Public Policy Institute, *The Costs of Long-Term Care* (Washington, DC: American Association of Retired Persons, 1994).

52. Richard Saul Wurman, *Understanding Healthcare* (Newport, RI: Top, 2004), p. 302.

53. Leslie C. Walker and Brian Burwell, "Access to public resources: regulating asset transfers for long-term care," in: Leslie C. Walker, Elizabeth H. Bradly, and Terrie Wetle (eds.), *Public and Private Responsibilities in Long-Term Care* (Baltimore: Johns Hopkins University Press, 1998), p. 167.

54. Robert H. Binstock, "The financing and organization of long-term care," in: Leslie C. Walker, Elizabeth H. Bradly, and Terrie Wetle (eds.), *Public and Private Responsibilities in Long-Term Care* (Baltimore: Johns Hopkins University Press, 1998), p. 10.

55. Leslie C. Walker and Brian Burwell, "Access to public resources: regulating asset transfers for long-term care," in: Leslie C. Walker, Elizabeth H. Bradly, and Terrie Wetle (eds.), *Public and Private Responsibilities in Long-Term Care* (Baltimore: Johns Hopkins University Press, 1998), p. 170.

56. Richard Saul Wurman, *Understanding Healthcare* (Newport, RI: Top, 2004), p. 304.

57. Ibid.

58. Geoffrey Cowley, "Alzheimer's: unlocking the mystery," *Newsweek Magazine* (January 31, 2000): 48.

59. Robert H. Binstock, "The financing and organization of long-term care," in: Leslie C. Walker, Elizabeth H. Bradly, and Terrie Wetle (eds.), *Public and Private Responsibilities in Long-Term Care* (Baltimore: Johns Hopkins University Press, 1998), p. 5.

60. Daniel Callahan, *What Kind of Life: The Limits of Medical Progress* (New York: Simon and Schuster Inc., 1990), p. 175.

61. Ibid., p. 177.

62. Ibid.

63. Ibid., p. 176.

64. American Psychological Association, "Resolution on ageism," *APA Online* (February 22, 2005), *http://www.apa.org/pi/aging/ageism.html* [accessed March 9, 2005].

65. Daniel Callahan, *Setting Limits: Medical Goals in an Aging Society* (Washington, DC: Georgetown University Press, 1995).

66. Ibid.

67. Leon Kass, *Toward a More Natural Science: Biology and Human Affairs* (New York: Free Press, 1985), p. 304.

68. Ibid., pp. 162–164.

69. Ibid., p. 307.

70. Ibid., p. 309.

chapter eleven

Euthanasia, Assisted Suicide, and Palliative Care

I. INTRODUCTION

End-of-life health care decision-making is a process that concerns not only patients but also patients' family members and friends, health care professionals, health care policy makers, and the public at large. Members of hospital-based ethics committees report that most of the cases they consider involve decisions about starting, continuing, and/or stopping treatment for patients who have entered the dying process. As in the past, people today, be they patients or health care professionals, have a difficult time facing death and the pain and suffering that often accompanies it. Some people hold on to life for as long as possible. They are willing to submit to any treatment, no matter how onerous or experimental, if it promises to extend their days on earth. But other people are just as glad to relinquish themselves to the forces of death. They have no interest in fighting what they know is an impossible-to-win war. They would much prefer to slip away gently into the night. Thus, it is no surprise that discussions about refusing treatment, euthanasia, suicide, assisted suicide, palliative care, and hospice care have a long and rich history in the realm of health care. In fact, many contemporary debates about the **right to die** and, more controversially, the **duty to die** bear a striking resemblance to the ancient Greeks' debates about the rights and responsibilities of dying persons.

II. TYPES OF EUTHANASIA

Euthanasia (which in Greek means "a good death" and in English means "an easy death") is a practice that is quite difficult to distinguish from suicide and even murder. Specifically, if I refuse life-saving or life-prolonging treatment in order to die immediately or relatively quickly, am I thereby committing suicide? Or am I simply saying "no" to medical treatment that has become incredibly burdensome to me, more of a torment than a treatment? Are health care professionals who withhold or withdraw treatment from me at my request or the request of my legally authorized surrogate(s) simply honoring my right to refuse treatment, or are they instead killing (murdering) me? If I take more active steps to hasten my death by refusing to eat or drink, am I committing suicide? If a health care professional provides me with adequate pain medication that may, as an unintended side effect, hasten my death, is he or she assisting my suicide (assuming that he or she knows of my desire to die sooner rather than later)?

Questions such as the ones just posed have led health care ethicists to distinguish between **passive euthanasia** on the one hand and **active euthanasia** on the other. Whereas active euthanasia or killing (an act of commission) is forbidden by legal and medical authorities, passive euthanasia or letting die (an act of omission) is permitted. Although the passive/active euthanasia distinction is recognized in most contemporary medical codes and entrenched in Anglo-American law, it is the object of increasing criticism. According to many contemporary thinkers, it is not the *manner* of causing death (withdrawing a ventilator as opposed to giving a lethal injection) which makes euthanasia a good or bad practice, but the *reason* for which death is caused. Was it the intention of the health care professional to end a patient's unbearable pain or suffering, or was it instead to eliminate the life of an obnoxious or indigent patient?

A. Passive Euthanasia

Passive euthanasia or letting die usually involves an instance of withdrawing or withholding a life-sustaining treatment from a patient. In general, health care ethicists maintain that there are three types of passive euthanasia: voluntary, nonvoluntary, and involuntary. Although these three varieties of letting die share many features in common, each of them is different enough to merit separate consideration.

1. Voluntary Passive Euthanasia

Typically, **voluntary passive euthanasia** occurs when *competent* adult patients ask their health care professionals to withhold or withdraw one or more life-sustaining treatments from them. For example, were I in a very advanced stage of ovarian cancer, I might ask my physician to enter a do-not-resuscitate (DNR) order for me, or ask him/her to remove my feeding tube. Whether it is more appropriate to describe my requests as a simple refusal of treatment rather than voluntary passive euthanasia is an open question, however. The answer to it probably depends on my primary reason for requesting a withholding or withdrawing of a treatment from me. Is my request based more on the fact that I find the treatment burdensome, even noxious, or on the fact that I just want to die and am eager to hasten the process?

a. The Karen Ann Quinlan Case

Voluntary passive euthanasia also includes cases in which *incompetent* adult patients communicate their treatment wishes indirectly through their previously written and/or oral statements. For example, in the 1970s the **Karen Ann Quinlan** case dominated the public media's attention. As the result of ingesting a potent combination of alcohol and barbiturates, 21-year-old Quinlan lapsed into what is today known as a **persistent vegetative state (PVS)**. She would, according to her attending health care professionals, never regain consciousness; her coma was irreversible.

As the months dragged on, Quinlan became less discernibly human as she wasted away into a 70-pound "vegetable," a gnarled twist of human flesh with no hope of recovery, sustained by a respirator and a feeding tube. When Quinlan's father requested that his daughter's respirator be turned off, a lower New Jersey court ruled against him on the grounds that no constitutional right to die exists, let alone one that permits a father to toll the bell for his daughter.[1] Although some people applauded the lower court's ruling as a victory for "life," most people seemed genuinely relieved when the New Jersey Supreme Court later overturned the lower court's ruling. It did so on the grounds that the constitutional right to privacy covers the decisions of formerly competent patients whose legal **surrogates** may speak for them when they can no longer speak for themselves.[2]

Significantly, Quinlan did not die after the respirator was removed from her body for two reasons. She continued to breath on her own, and the Quinlan family decided that, even in her condition, she would want her tube feedings to continue. Apparently, no one ever told Quinlan's family that artificial nutrition and hydration can be just as extraordinary and burdensome from a patient's perspective as artificial respiration is. Nor did anyone tell them that patients in a persistent vegetative state cannot experience the pangs of hunger and the sensations of thirst if their feeding tubes are withdrawn from them. They die painlessly, too unconscious to experience their body's disintegration.

b. The Nancy Cruzan Case

The Quinlan family's 1970s views about artificial food and hydration were still prevalent in the 1980s. For this reason, it was difficult for the family of another young woman in a persistent vegetative state to convince the courts that their loved one would not want to be kept alive by means of a feeding tube. As the result of a 1983 automobile collision, 24-year-old **Nancy Cruzan** lapsed into a persistent vegetative state. For over 7 years, Cruzan's parents watched their daughter, sustained by a feeding tube, turn into what they regarded as a living corpse. Knowing that their daughter would not want to go on living in such a debilitated state, Cruzan's parents requested that the staff of the Missouri Rehabilitation Center stop tube feeding her. When their request was denied, Cruzan's parents took their daughter's case to court. A lower court ruled in favor of discontinuing the tube feedings, but an appellate court, later affirmed by the Missouri Supreme Court, reversed the ruling. Relying on Missouri's living will statute, which permits the withdrawal of life-sustaining treatment only in cases in which individuals are hopelessly ill or injured *and* there is **clear and convincing** evidence that, were they able to speak for themselves, they would request such withdrawal, the Missouri Supreme Court determined that Cruzan's parents lacked such evidence.

Frustrated by the Missouri Supreme Court's decision, Cruzan's parents appealed to the U.S. Supreme Court. Although the U.S. Supreme Court did not overturn the Missouri Supreme Court's decision, it did emphasize that people have a Constitutional "liberty interest" to reject unwanted medical treatment, including feeding tubes. Later, when the state of Missouri withdrew from the case, Cruzan's parents went back to the same lower court where their ordeal had begun, this time with some of their daughter's friends who had not been able to testify the first time the case was heard. Cruzan's friends told the court that while she was alive, Cruzan told them she would not want to go on living if she were more like a "vegetable" than a full human person. The court found this testimony compelling, and ruled that, after all, there was "clear and convincing" evidence that Cruzan would want her feeding tube removed were she able to speak for herself. The Missouri Rehabilitation Center was instructed to remove Cruzan's feeding tube. She died 12 days later on December 26, 1990, nearly 8 years after the car accident that had robbed her of a meaningful life.[3]

c. The Robert Wendland Case

Cases such as the ones involving Karen Ann Quinlan and Nancy Cruzan are troublesome enough, but they are not nearly as contentious as cases that involve squabbling families who disagree about their loved one's end-of-life wishes. So confusing and acrimonious can such cases become that not only judges but also legislators may elect to enter the fray. Among the cases that best illustrate the results of such regrettable family feuds, court battles, and legislative maneuvers is the **Robert Wendland case**.

In September 1993, Robert Wendland had a serious automobile accident that left him comatose and totally unresponsive for several months. During this time, his wife, sometimes accompanied by their two children, visited him daily and made treatment decisions on his behalf. Wendland seemed to improve, and his health care professionals as well as his family reported that he was starting to interact with his environment. In fact, for a few months in 1995, Wendland was able to do such things as throw and catch a ball, operate an electric wheelchair with assistance, turn pages, draw circles, and respond to some simple commands. He remained unable to speak, however, and to master the use of an augmented-communication machine that pronounces the words "yes" and "no" when corresponding buttons are touched.

After several months, therapists decided to reduce the number and intensity of Wendland's physical and occupational therapy sessions. As they saw it, the sessions were unproductive. Subsequently, Wendland's cognitive status plateaued and then started to get worse. Although he remained alert enough to recognize (or appear to recognize) certain caregivers, his health care professionals were convinced he would never be able again to walk, talk, feed himself, or control his bowel and bladder functions, let alone make decisions for himself. As it became clearer to Wendland's wife, children, and brother that he was never going to get better, they began to ask themselves questions about his wishes. Based on earlier conversations they had had with him when he was well, they decided that Wendland would not want to be kept alive for years on end in a state of minimal consciousness. Wendland's wife then asked his health care professionals to remove his feeding tube; however, before they did so, they thought it best to consult the hospital's ethics committee.

After discussing Wendland's case, the hospital ethics committee decided that Wendland's feeding tube should be removed. At this point in the drama, Wendland's mother and sister, who had been left out of the decision-making loop, appeared on the scene unexpectedly and with dramatic consequence. They secured a temporary restraining order to prevent the feeding tube removal. As they saw the situation, Wendland could get better with proper care.

Fearing that her mother-in-law and sister-in-law would never let her husband die, Wendland's wife petitioned that she be appointed her husband's legal guardian. Wendland's mother and sister objected to her petition and got the court to appoint an independent guardian for Wendland who, to their shock, decided against further treatment for Wendland. After several court battles between Wendland's wife, children, and brother on the one hand, and Wendland's mother and sister on the other hand, the California Supreme Court ruled in favor of Wendland's mother and sister.

Importantly, the court found that neither of the two standards used in making treatment decisions for incompetent patients applied in the case of Wendland. These two standards are termed the **best interests standard** and the **substituted judgment standard**, respectively. Both of these standards are very complex, and there is sometimes great confusion about which one to use. In fact, so conflicted was the California Supreme Court about Robert Wendland's situation that it came to the conclusion that *neither* the substituted judgment standard *nor* the best interests standard applied in his case. The court reasoned that the substituted judgment standard, which requires the surrogate decision-maker to make the decision the formerly competent patient would make were he or she still competent, did not apply because the evidence Wendland's wife provided about her husband's treatment wishes was not "clear and convincing." In addition, the court reasoned that the best interests standard, which requires the surrogate decision-maker to make the decision that society as a whole would make in the case, did not apply because at present there is no clear societal consensus that supports withholding artificial nutrition and hydration from a patient who is *not* terminally ill, permanently comatose, or in a persistent vegetative state, and who has left *no* written directions for his or her own care.[4] For now, we must continue to operate on the assumption that life is in the best interests of nonterminal patients who are minimally conscious or suffer from mind-robbing conditions such as advanced Alzheimer's disease and advanced senile dementia.

d. The Terri Schiavo Case

Importantly, in ruling as it did about the Wendland case, the California Supreme Court left open the possibility that the best interests standard *might* be applicable in cases where, unlike Wendland, the patient *is* terminally ill, permanently comatose, or in a persistent vegetative state and has not left written directions; however, as the 2005 **Terri Schiavo** case demonstrated, "might" walks hand in hand with "might not." Terri Schiavo was left in a persistent vegetative state subsequent to a 1990 heart attack caused by a severe potassium imbalance. Her husband, Michael Schiavo, was appointed her legal guardian. Angered that his wife's physician had failed to notice her potassium imbalance shortly before her cardiac arrest, Michael Schiavo sued him and won a $750,000 settlement for her (which he put into a trust for her health care expenses) and a $300,000 settlement for himself.

After Schiavo's husband won the 1992 suit, Schiavo's parents, Robert and Mary Schindler, who had previously gotten along with their son-in-law, became alienated from him and unsuccessfully challenged his guardianship of their daughter. By 1994, it became clear to Schiavo's physicians that she was not going to get better. Subsequent to this prognosis, Schiavo's husband told the physicians that, under the circumstances, his wife would not want to be resuscitated if she had a heart attack. Later, in 1998, he petitioned a Florida court to remove the feeding tube that was keeping his wife alive. The Schindlers went ballistic. They accused their son-in-law of trying to kill their daughter because he had not only a relationship with another woman but also two children with her. Moreover, the Schindlers insisted that, "as a devout Catholic," their daughter would want to live no matter what, and that, truth be told, their daughter was not really in a persistent vegetative state, but instead in a minimally conscious state from which she could recover.[5]

Despite the Schindlers' protestations, a Florida appellate judge ruled that Schiavo's husband had provided clear and convincing evidence that, were she able to speak for herself, his wife would ask to die. The judge ordered that Schiavo's feeding tube be removed, whereupon the Schindlers appealed his decision to the Florida Supreme Court. To their dismay, the Florida Supreme Court refused to hear their appeal. Desperate to keep their daughter alive, the Schindlers filed a civil suit against their son-in-law. They alleged that he was lying about their daughter's treatment wishes. So serious were the Schindlers' allegations that a five-physician panel—two chosen by the Schindlers, two by Michael Schiavo, and one by a Florida appellate court—was appointed to determine whether Schiavo was truly in a persistent vegetative state as opposed to a state more akin to the minimally conscious state in which Robert Wendland had found himself.

After nearly a year went by, Schiavo's original case, together with the additional evidence provided by the five-physician panel case, came back to the judge that had first heard the case. He ruled that the physicians had satisfactorily established that Schiavo's condition was beyond medical remedy. Once again, he ordered physicians to remove Schiavo's feeding tube, but again his order was stayed. The Schindlers had filed a suit in a federal court to keep their daughter alive, and the governor of Florida, Jeb Bush (brother of U.S. President George W. Bush) had filed a brief in support of the Schindlers' suit.

Governor Bush's support notwithstanding, the federal court sided with the state court. Still, the Schiavo case did not end. On October 15, 2003, the Florida state legislature got into the fray. It passed **Terri's Law**, which authorized continuance of life-sustaining treatment for Schiavo. Michael Schiavo immediately contested the constitutionality of the law, and in 2004, a Florida state appellate judge ruled it unconstitutional, with the Florida Supreme Court concurring. The Schindlers then appealed this ruling to the U.S. Supreme Court, which refused to hear their appeal. Not ones to give up, the Schindlers decided to take their case to the U.S. Congress which quickly passed a presidentally signed bill requiring a federal court to hear the Schindlers' case. The court heard the appeal, but refused to order a tube reinsertion.[6] As Schiavo lay dying, right-to-life defenders and advocates for persons with disabilities joined forces. They surrounded the skilled nursing home in which she resided, protesting what they viewed as her "murder." Their protests notwithstanding, Schiavo died in March 2005.

Although the Schiavo case demonstrated how badly things can go when an incompetent person without a written advanced care directive has a squabbling family, or when courts and legislatures get overly or unnecessarily involved in the personal affairs of people, it had some positive consequences. Many people decided to execute advanced care directives, specifying their wishes about end-of-life care. Not surprisingly, many of these advanced care directives included a feeding tube clause. Reliable polls taken after the Schiavo case indicated that whereas 69% of the U.S. population would want their guardian to remove their feeding tube if they were in Schiavo's place, only 24% would not and 7% were unsure.[7]

2. Nonvoluntary Passive Euthanasia

a. Formerly Competent Patients

Unlike cases of voluntary passive euthanasia, which involve competent or incompetent patients whose treatment wishes are *known*, cases of nonvoluntary passive euthanasia involve incompetent patients whose treatment wishes are *not known*. Such a situation arises, for example, when a homeless person with no identification papers or a very old person with no living relatives, existing friends, or caretakers arrives unconscious in a hospital emergency department. Should he or she not regain consciousness and/or lapse into a persistent vegetative state or a minimally conscious status, health care professionals rely on the best interests standard to make treatment decisions on behalf of the patient. Not surprisingly, health care professionals sometimes seek court orders to support decisions to withhold or withdraw life-sustaining treatment from patients whose wishes are not known. In the main, courts are far more likely to use the best interest standard to stop life-sustaining treatment for incompetent patients who are terminally ill, permanently comatose, or in a persistent vegetative state than for incompetent patients who are *not* terminally ill, permanently comatose, or in a persistent vegetative state. Like ordinary U.S. citizens, most U.S. judges do not want to be perceived as people who, on the basis of their own *subjective* preferences, decide that someone else's life is *objectively* not worth living. In other words, most Americans remain very hesitant about making quality-of-life decisions for anyone other than themselves.[8]

b. Never Competent Patients: Adults and Infants

As we have just noted, cases that involve formerly competent patients whose treatment wishes are not known are very difficult to resolve. So too are cases that involve patients who have never been competent enough to make their own decisions. A case in point is the **John Storar** case.

1. The John Storar Case

At the time a decision had to be made about his health care, Storar was 52 years old and had a mental age of 18 months. His 77-year-old mother had previously given physicians permission to treat her son's bladder cancer with radiation therapy which proved unsuccessful. When the radiation treatments were discontinued, the physicians sought his mother's permission to keep transfusing him so that he could engage in the simple activities that gave him pleasure. Storar's mother told the physicians to stop transfusing her son because he hated the treatments which would lengthen his life by only 3–6 months. But they would not listen to her. Instead, they sought a court order to force the transfusions. Although a New York trial court agreed with Storar's mother, a higher New York court agreed with the physicians. Invoking the best interests standard, this higher court reasoned that were Storar an infant instead of a man in his fifties, the transfusions would be ordered because of their beneficial effects.[9]

2. The Joseph Saikewicz Case

The Storar case provides a contrast with the better-known **Joseph Saikewicz** case in which a Massachusetts court incorrectly used the substituted judgment standard to get results opposite to the ones in the Storar case.[10] Like Storar, Saikewicz had been severely mentally retarded since birth. At the time of his case, he was in his late sixties with the mental age of a toddler. He had no family and was suffering from leukemia, for which the only effective treatment at the time was chemotherapy with all its noxious and unpleasant side effects. Although Saikewicz would die without chemotherapy, and although most competent people in Saikewicz's condition would probably accept chemotherapy, Saikewicz's court-appointed guardian petitioned that he not be given the treatment. Invoking the substituted judgment standard, the Supreme Court of Massachusetts ruled that were Saikewicz competent, he would not want the chemotherapy on the grounds that he would experience its administration simply as something painful being done to him. But the fact of the matter is that, like Storar, Saikewicz had never been competent. Therefore, the court should have invoked the best interests standard in his case to arrive at results similar to the ones achieved in the Storar case. According to legal experts Hall, Ellman, and Strouse, the real reason the court ruled that Saikewicz would not want the chemotherapy is that no one really cared enough about him, and that physicians were reluctant to struggle with Saikewicz, a very large man, each time they had to administer the treatment.[11]

3. In Re Guardianship of Infant Doe

Another category of never competent patients is that of severely **imperiled newborns**. Some infants are born with such serious physical and mental disabilities that the best course of treatment may be to provide them with palliative care only rather than any aggressive treatment. But just because health care professionals and parents agree that an infant's disabilities are severe enough to warrant a course of palliative care only does not necessarily mean that this level of care serves the best interests of the infant. For example, in the 1982 case **In Re Guardianship of Infant Doe**, an infant was born in Indiana with Downs Syndrome and an esophageal blockage that made eating impossible. The infant's parents as well as attending physician decided against the surgery needed to remove the blockage. An Indiana court upheld their decision, and the infant died of starvation and dehydration 6 days after its birth. The public's reaction to Infant Doe's death was generally one of outrage. Although some people defended the decision, most people voiced the view that not operating on an infant with an esophageal blockage simply because it has Downs Syndrome, a condition which is compatible with a happy and meaningful life, is both discriminatory and wrong, and should not be permitted in a decent society.[12]

Largely as a result of the Infant Doe case, the federal government decided in 1983 to regulate withholding and withdrawing decisions for severely impaired newborns. Within months of Infant Doe's death, the Department of Health and Human Services (HHS) put the nation's hospitals on alert that section 504 of the **Rehabilitation Act of 1973** made it unlawful for any institution receiving federal money to withhold beneficial treatment from an infant with serious disabilities solely on account of its condition. Later, the HHS also required hospitals and other institutions treating handicapped infants to post conspicuous notices with a toll-free, 24-hour hotline number. Individuals who suspected mistreatments of infants with serious disabilities were encouraged to call the number so that HHS authorities could make an immediate, on-site investigation. Needless to say, health care professionals protested the intrusive way in which the federal government was handling the situation. Eventually, the U.S. Supreme Court struck down the initial HHS regulations as unwarranted government interference with parents' and health care professionals' treatment decisions.[13] The court's ruling did not preclude the HHS, however, from issuing more reasonable guidelines for withholding and withdrawing medically indicated treatment and nutrition from infants with serious disabilities.

At present, states are required to implement the **1984 and 1985 Child Abuse Amendments to the 1973 Rehabilitation Act**. According to these amendments, treatment may be withheld from an infant only if at least one of the following conditions hold:

1. The infant is chronically and irreversibly comatose;
2. The provision of such treatment would merely prolong dying, not be effective in ameliorating or correcting all of the infant's life threatening conditions; or otherwise be futile in terms of the survival of the infant or,
3. The provision of such treatment would be virtually futile in terms of survival of the infant and the treatment itself under such circumstances would be inhumane.[14]

Because these guidelines are subject to multiple interpretations, many hospitals rely on institutional ethics committees to advise parents and health care professionals about the moral appropriateness of withholding or withdrawing treatment from a severely impaired newborn. As it stands, the consensus view is that although the 1985 federal guidelines provide parents and health care professionals with some discretionary space, if a mistake about treating a severely imperiled newborn is to be made, it is better to err on the side of life than death. Thus, it is not surprising that many health care professionals are reluctant to withhold or withdraw life-sustaining treatment from a severely imperiled newborn unless they regard the treatment as not only inhumane but also virtually futile.

3. Involuntary Passive Euthanasia

Unlike the concept of nonvoluntary passive euthanasia which, though difficult to grasp, is plausible enough, the concept of **involuntary passive euthanasia** initially seems incoherent. After all, euthanasia is supposed to benefit individuals, not deprive them of lives they want to lead. And yet, in cases of so-called **medical futility**, a conflict may emerge between patients and/or families who want to continue life-sustaining treatment and health care professionals who want to stop it. Such a conflict arose in the 1987 **Helga Wanglie** case.[15] Wanglie's husband, maintained that, while still competent, his wife had told him she would want any and every treatment so long as there was even an ounce of life left in her. When Wanglie fell into a persistent vegetative state, however, her physicians gradually came to the conclusion that keeping Wanglie alive with technology's tools jeopardized the integrity of medicine itself.[16] They reasoned that physicians should not treat patients with remedies that provide no medical benefit. Disagreeing with the physicians, Wanglie's husband protested that there is more to life than securing medical benefits. He claimed that were his wife able to speak for herself, she would beg her physicians not to deprive her of the nonmedical benefit of continuing existence.

Because the physicians knew it would be difficult to get a court order permitting them to withdraw life support from Wanglie against her expressed will, they decided instead to contest her husband's guardianship of her. They argued that Wanglie's husband was not able to make good decisions for his wife, and that a guardian *ad litem* should be appointed to represent Wanglie's "true" best interests—presumably, to be allowed to die. To their surprise, the court found their argument unpersuasive. In fact, it ruled that Wanglie's husband was fully competent and the person best able to express his wife's treatment wishes. At this point in the court battle, Wanglie died. With her death, her physicians lost the option to legally test the issue that really concerned them; namely, whether health care professionals have a right not to provide patients with medically futile care even if patients demand it.[17]

Reaction to the Wanglie case was mixed. Some health care ethicists thought that, absent a thorough public discussion, health care professionals have no right to stop life-sustaining treatment that *they*, but not their patients, think is burdensome, pointless, or even inhumane. For example, Daniel Callahan, former Director of the Hastings Center, commented that:

> The debate on the meaning of 'futility' is still in its infancy: we have no clear sense of public values on these matters, no good figures on costs, no clear criteria for cost–benefit calculations, and no political process to allow physicians and lay people together to develop appropriate standards. There is no literature of any importance on the extent to which doctors should feel free to refuse to provide treatment they believe to be useless in the absence of common public standards for such refusal. Since it is possible—probably likely—that some will want to extend the notion of futility well beyond the persistent vegetative state to care of severe dementia and multi-organ failure, it is important that the discussion proceed carefully.[18]

Adding credence to Callahan's line of argument is the fact that, at present, health care professionals themselves disagree about when a life-sustaining treatment for a patient is medically futile. Some physicians claim that in order to count as futile, a medical treatment must have no chance of success; others associate futility with success rates as high as 13%.[19]

In contrast to Callahan and those who agree with him, lawyer Michael A. Rie maintains that it is possible for health care professionals to develop a consensus on the meaning of medical futility, and that patients have no right to demand medically nonbeneficial treatment from health care professionals. Patients' autonomy is not an absolute right in Rie's estimation. Certainly, it is not strong enough to require health care professionals to provide treatment they believe goes against the essential aims and purposes of medicine.[20]

Rie's views have recently gained ground over Callahan's views. Three states—Texas, Virginia, and California—have passed medical-futility laws. Texas's law is particularly explicit. It permits physicians to stop treatment over the family's and sometimes even the patient's previously stated objections provided the hospital ethics committee agrees. In addition, the family must be given 10 days to see if they can find some institution or individual(s) willing to keep their loved one alive.[21] Interestingly, at this point in the process, most families, at least in Texas, give in to physicians and let their loved one die. But there are exceptions. In a 2005 article, the *New York Times* cited one case in which a Texas judge gave a hospital permission to disconnect a 5-month-old's ventilator, over the fierce objections of his distraught mother, and another case in which the family of a 68-year-old patient found a nursing home willing to do what the hospital was not—namely, keep him alive on a ventilator.[22] Depending on how frequently hospitals invoke medical-futility laws that go against patient's as well as family's wishes, involuntary passive euthanasia may become increasingly common. Nature will be allowed to take its course even when patients wish to resist its decrees.

B. Active Euthanasia

If treatment decisions based on determinations of futility are controversial, **active euthanasia**, defined as the taking of immediate, direct steps to end a person's life (administering a lethal injection, for example), is even more controversial. As with passive euthanasia, there are three types of active euthanasia—voluntary, nonvoluntary, and involuntary—each of which demands separate consideration because of their specific complexities.

1. Voluntary Active Euthanasia

In **voluntary active euthanasia**, competent adult patients request their physician (or some other designated person) to directly and immediately end their lives because of their uncontrollable pain, enormous existential suffering, and/or because they do not want to burden others with their care no longer. At present, the only countries that have passed laws which permit both voluntary active euthanasia and physician-assisted suicide (to be discussed below) are the **Netherlands, Belgium, and Switzerland**.[23] Of these three nations' "right" to die laws, the Netherlands's law is the most developed one. It insulates physicians who follow its guidelines from criminal prosecution for murder. Among its guidelines are the following:

1. The patient's request must be voluntary in the sense of persistent, conscious, and freely made;
2. The patient must be clearly competent at the time of the decision, in no way demented or clinically depressed;
3. The patient's suffering, *as he or she experiences it*, must be 'perpetual, unbearable, and hopeless;'
4. The physician must consult with at least one other physician about (1)–(3);
5. The physician must submit a report to the government about the patient's medical history and request for voluntary euthanasia.[24]

After the physician and the patient meet the terms of the law, the physician typically injects a barbiturate to induce sleep, combined with curare to produce death.

Physicians in the Netherlands are not required to participate in active voluntary euthanasia and approximately 11% of Dutch physicians refuse to do so.[25] Active voluntary euthanasia is not legal in the United States and is regarded as murder. Moreover, the American Medical Association (AMA) officially opposes voluntary active euthanasia, even though some of its members—primarily younger ones—support it.[26] Like the AMA, the U.S. public is fairly split on the morality of voluntary active euthanasia with 49% in agreement, 39% in disagreement, and 16% unsure.[27]

a. Proponents of Voluntary Active Euthanasia

Proponents of voluntary active euthanasia stress that competent patients who are terminally ill, and who can no longer stand the burdens of their condition, should have the option of being euthanized. They stress that the availability of this option is not likely to cause large numbers of patients to take it—on the contrary. Only about 2% of all hospital deaths in the Netherlands are attributable to voluntary active euthanasia, for example.[28]

Another argument that may count in favor of voluntary active euthanasia is the seeming unfairness of the following state of affairs. Imagine two competent patients, both of them suffering to the same degree from advanced terminal ovarian cancer. One of the patients is on a ventilator, but the other is breathing on her own. Physicians may legally withdraw the ventilator from the first patient if she so requests, thereby permitting her to die. There is nothing physicians can legally do to help the second patient die more quickly, however, short of encouraging her not to eat or resorting to so-called **terminal sedation**.

As described by Dr. Timothy Quill, terminal sedation is a "radical" approach to eliminating some patients' otherwise uncontrollable suffering.[29] It consists of heavily sedating a patient with an intravenous infusion of barbiturates. Subsequent to the infusion of these drugs, the patient is under the equivalent of general anesthesia. He or she is unconscious, unable to communicate, and unable to eat or drink. Quill believes that terminal sedation falls under the rubric of the **principle of double effect** (see Chapter 2). Although the physician knows that terminal sedation will result in the patient not being able to eat or drink, the primary, intended purpose of the treatment is supposedly to relieve the patient's suffering. Therefore, the physician is not engaging in active euthanasia. But many people criticize Quill, accusing him of duplicity. As they see it, the primary, intended purpose of terminal sedation is to put the patient into a coma so that he or she can starve to death without experiencing any discomfort. Were the purposes of terminal sedation simply the relief of the patient's suffering and not killing the patient by means of starvation, the physician could order tube feeding along with the terminal sedation.

Finally, proponents of voluntary active euthanasia claim that the distinction between active and passive euthanasia does not make sense any more. As they see it, as soon as health care professionals decide to help a patient die, it makes no moral difference whether they "let" the patient die by withdrawing treatment or whether they "kill" the patient with a lethal injection. In fact, if health care professionals want to help a patient escape a life of unbearable pain/suffering, voluntary active euthanasia may be preferable to voluntary passive euthanasia. Under certain circumstances, helping someone die *quickly* seems far more merciful than helping them die *slowly*.[30]

b. Opponents of Voluntary Active Euthanasia

Opponents of voluntary active euthanasia concede that some patients' autonomy may be blocked when physicians, regulated by law, refuse to honor their requests to be euthanized. However, they maintain that U.S. law should continue to ban voluntary active euthanasia for at least two reasons. First, permitting physicians to act as the agents of death may seriously undermine the traditional healing and life-protecting mission of the health care professions. Comments Willard Gaylin, M.D.:

> . . . if physicians become killers or are even licensed to kill, the profession—and, therewith, each physician—will never again be worthy of trust and respect as healer and comforter and protector of life in all its frailty.[31]

Second, legalizing voluntary active euthanasia in the cultural context of the United States may cause some patients to choose death over life in order to save money, or to be less of a burden on family members, friends, and/or health care professionals. Indeed, we increasingly hear that, under certain circumstances patients have not only a **right to die** but also a **duty to die**. This is the view of philosopher Donald Hardwig. He claims that if a patient is seriously draining others, particularly family members of their physical, emotional, and financial resources, "there can be a duty to die before one's illnesses would cause death, even if treated only with palliative measures. In fact, there may be a fairly common responsibility to end one's life in the absence of any terminal illness at all . . . there can be a duty to die even when one would prefer to live."[32]

2. Nonvoluntary Active Euthanasia

In **nonvoluntary active euthanasia**, physicians (or other health care professionals, family members or friends) make the decision to terminate the lives of incompetent patients who they *think* are in enormous unrelieved pain or suffering. Proponents of this practice claim that the value of mercy demands such an option. They reason that the fact that an incompetent patient cannot express his wish to be euthanized should not condemn him to suffer the pain from which a competent patient can request liberation. In contrast, opponents of this practice reason that even if it is justifiable to actively euthanize an infant who is the victim of an incredibly painful, terminal disease, it is not justifiable to actively euthanize an incompetent adult patient suffering from an advanced, though nonterminal case of Alzheimer's disease on the grounds that "we" know he or she wants to die. They call attention to the fact that although Dutch physicians are supposed to euthanize only competent patients, reports indicate that anywhere from 1,000 to 2,000 cases of nonvoluntary active euthanasia occur in Dutch hospitals every year.[33]

Whether these reports are entirely accurate or not is not known. But some Dutch physicians have provided anecdotal support for the claim that a number of well-meaning Dutch physicians take the step from voluntary to nonvoluntary active euthanasia as a matter of fact. For example, a physician willingly admitted that in her hospital, about 30 patients a year were put in a fatal morphine coma without directly requesting that they be killed. Because these patients were, in the estimation of their health care professionals, leading lives no rational person would choose to live, their health care professionals took it upon themselves to end their supposed misery.

A notorious instance of nonvoluntary active euthanasia in the United States was the 1988 case of **Debbie**. In the *Journal of the American Medical Association*, an unnamed physician described how, when he was still a resident, he lethally injected a young woman suffering from the ravages of ovarian cancer. He justified his action on the grounds that, when he answered her page call, Debbie said, "Let's get this over with."[34] Not only was public reaction to the Debbie case largely negative, so too was that of the medical community. Because the unnamed physician was not Debbie's attending physician and had no personal insight into her values or modes of self-expression, her words, "Let's get this over with," may have meant something quite different from "Kill me now and ask questions later." Perhaps all Debbie meant to say was, "Let's get this pain-medication injection over with. I hate shots."

3. Involuntary Active Euthanasia

In **involuntary active euthanasia**, physicians (or other health care professionals, family members, or even state authorities) make a decision to terminate the life of a competent patient who does not wish to die. **Murder** is the proper synonym for this form of "euthanasia." The worst example of it occurred during the Nazi era in Germany. German physicians killed nearly 90,000 patients, most of them of Aryan stock because of presumed mental or physical "inferiority."[35] No matter how much some U.S. health care professionals support voluntary and even nonvoluntary active euthanasia, none of them support involuntary active "euthanasia."

III. PHYSICIAN-ASSISTED SUICIDE

Closely related to active euthanasia is **physician-assisted suicide**. The difference between physician-assisted suicide and active euthanasia is that the physician is not the direct cause of death in physician-assisted suicide; rather the patient is. The physician provides lethal drugs or some other means of death to a competent patient who then decides whether or not to use them.

A. Dr. Jack Kevorkian versus
Dr. Timothy Quill

Among the most controversial proponents of physician-assisted suicide is **Dr. Jack Kevorkian**. In June 1990, Dr. Kevorkian installed a homemade suicide device in the back of his automobile van and taught Janet Adkins, a middle-aged woman in the early stages of Alzheimer's disease, how to activate the machine to end her life. After saying her final goodbyes to her family, Adkins pushed a button that administered a sedative into her veins, which was followed by the drug potassium chloride to stop her heart.[36] Adkins was but the first of Dr. Kevorkian's many patients. In fact, before legal authorities decided to take action against him, he had already assisted 20 people to commit suicide.

In 1992, Michigan prosecutors decided to enforce a new law prohibiting anyone to intentionally assist someone else's suicide. Dr. Kevorkian was arrested, indicted, and tried for assisting the suicide of others. But jurors found him not guilty. They viewed him as a well-intentioned health care professional, intent on liberating suffering people from a hellish existence of unrelenting pain and suffering. The jurors' decision did not sit well with the majority of health care professionals and health care ethicists, however. In their estimation, Dr. Kevorkian was a medical renegade, willing to help virtually any adult commit suicide, whether or not they were both of sound mind and truly suffering from some awful, terminal disease. On the grounds that he was practicing bad medicine, the Michigan Medical Board revoked Dr. Kevorkian's medical license.

Undeterred by the Board's action, however, Dr. Kevorkian assisted at least 22 more people to commit suicide before he overstepped his limits. On the CBS television program *Sixty Minutes*, Dr. Kevorkian moved from physician-assisted suicide to voluntary active euthanasia. Over 15 million Americans watched Dr. Kevorkian as he administered a lethal injection to Thomas Youk, a 52-year-old man suffering from Amyotrophic Lateral Sclerosis (ALS), who could not kill himself because of the paralyzing nature of his disease. Dr. Kevorkian was promptly arrested and prosecuted for first-degree murder. The jury took pity on Dr. Kevorkian again, however. Pointing to what they viewed as his commitment to relieving people's pain and suffering, the jury found him guilty of only second-degree murder, and in 1999 a judge sentenced him to a prison term of 10–25 years.[37]

Significantly, not all physicians who openly admit practicing physician-assisted suicide are pursued by prosecutors or condemned by the health care community. For example, **Dr. Timothy Quill** publicly reported in the *Journal of the American Medical Association* that for many years he had treated a patient, for acute myclomonoscytic leukemia. When Quill could no longer help his patient control her pain, she requested barbiturates "for sleep." After several long consultations with his patient and her family, Quill prescribed the medication she needed to commit suicide.[38] Because of his long-term relationship with his patient and her family, and because he had really exhausted all available palliative treatments, most of the health care community did not condemn his actions.

B. Oregon's Death with Dignity Act

At present the only state where physicians may legally practice assisted suicide is Oregon. **Oregon's Death with Dignity Act (1998)** requires both the patient and the physician to meet several conditions for a legal physician-assisted suicide, including the following seven:

1. The patient must make two oral requests to his or her physician, separated by at least fifteen days.
2. The patient must provide a written request to his or her physician, signed in the presence of two witnesses.
3. The patient's diagnosis and prognosis must be confirmed by the prescribing physician and by a consulting physician.
4. The prescribing physician and a consulting physician must determine whether the patient is "capable."
5. The patient must be referred for a psychological examination if either physician believes that the patient's judgment is impaired by a psychiatric or psychological disorder.
6. The prescribing physician must inform the patient of feasible alternatives to assisted suicide including comfort care, hospice care, and pain control.
7. The prescribing physician must request, but may not require, the patient to notify his or her next-of-kin of the prescription request.[39]

Meeting all of the criteria listed above is no easy task, however. What's more, actually going through with the act of "medical" suicide, ordinarily demands an enormous effort of the will. No wonder, that of the thousand or so Oregonians officially qualified to commit suicide "medically," only 208 of them actually caused their own deaths between the years 1998 and 2004.[40]

Among the main reasons the 208 patients gave for their decision to commit physician-assisted suicide were fear of losing autonomy (84%), decreased ability to participate in enjoyable activities (84%), and losing control of bodily functions (49%).[41] Available empirical data provides the following interesting information about this group of people: 71% were men; 29% were women; 53% were married, 24% divorced, 18% widowed, and 5% single; 26% had college degrees or more, 64% had some college and 10% had high school diplomas only; 84% were suffering from cancer; and most were in their late sixties or early seventies. Information about the race and ethnicity of the assisted-suicide patients was lacking, although the demographics of Oregon suggest that most of them were probably White.[42]

C. The Elizabeth Bouvia Case

Supporters of physician-assisted suicide for competent persons with terminal, incurable, and painful diseases may not support it in cases like that of **Elizabeth Bouvia**, however.[43] Bouvia, who had suffered since birth from cerebral palsy, was a 25-year-old quadriplegic. She had had a difficult life and a failed marriage, but had a college degree and attempted to work. She was totally dependent on her parents for care; when her needs became too great for them to handle, they told her she had to find someone else to help her. Unable to find a way to live on her own (Bouvia was totally dependent on public assistance), Bouvia was forced to ask her father to drive her to Riverside General Hospital in California. Shortly after admission to the facility, she stated that all she wanted was pain relief and to be left alone.

Because they believed that Bouvia was not eating enough, and that she might be trying to starve herself to death, Riverside health care professionals decided to force feed her by means of a nasogastric feeding tube. Bouvia protested that she was eating enough and did not want to be force-fed. She contacted the American Civil Liberties Union (ACLU) to support her right to refuse treatment. A court battle ensued, and the judge ruled that the hospital could force-feed Bouvia, because there was some question whether she was competent to make decisions about her medical treatment.[44]

Bouvia responded to the court's ruling dramatically. She checked herself out of the hospital against medical advice and with an unpaid $56,000 bill. She got help to travel to a hospital in Tijuana, Mexico where health care professionals let her eat or not eat as she pleased. After several months, Bouvia got help to travel back to California. There she was admitted to Los Angeles County Medical Center from which she was subsequently transferred to High Desert Hospital, where force feeding was insisted on by the staff. Another court battle ensued. But this time Bouvia won her case. The court stated:

> The patient's mental and emotional feelings are entitled to respect. She has been subjected to the forced intrusion of an artificial mechanism into her body against her will. She has a right to refuse the increased dehumanizing aspect of her condition. The right to refuse treatment is basic and fundamental. It is recognized as part of the right of privacy protected by both state and federal constitution. It is not merely one vote subject to being overridden by medical opinion.[45]

Although the court solved Bouvia's problem, it did not solve the hospital's problem. They were confused whether they were obligated "to treat Bouvia selectively";[46] that is, to provide her with the painkillers and comfort assistance she wanted, but not the tube feedings they thought she needed in order to survive. Bouvia's health care professionals felt as if they were being forced to assist their patient's slow suicide, something they did not want to facilitate. As it so happened, Bouvia resolved her health care professionals' problem for them. She checked herself out of the hospital, found a way to secure adequate care for herself outside of a hospital setting, and, once again, proceeded to eat as much as she felt she needed to survive.[47]

IV. ADVANCE CARE DIRECTIVES

Because uncertainty about an incompetent person's treatment wishes often enters the end-of-life decision-making process, it is important that competent persons communicate their treatment preferences to trusted health care professionals, family members and friends in oral, or preferably, written form. As it stands, competent adults have the **right to refuse treatment** even if it is life-saving. Specifically, they have the right to refuse any or all of the following treatments: cardiopulmonary resuscitation, mechanical breathing or respirator, tube feedings, kidney dialysis, chemotherapy, intravenous therapy, surgery, diagnostic tests, antibiotics, transfusions, and even pain medication and palliative care. So enshrined is the right to refuse treatment in U.S. law that it may not be limited unless honoring it interferes with the common good. For example, the state may require an individual to be inoculated against certain life-threatening contagious diseases; it may require a pregnant woman (under certain limited circumstances) to submit to treatment to save the life of her fetus; or it may require an adult Jehovah Witness who is the single parent of several children to submit to a blood transfusion even though the procedure is forbidden by the religion he or she fervently embraces.

An increasingly popular way to make sure that one's right to refuse treatment will be honored when one is incompetent as well as when one is competent is the **advance care directive**. Currently, there are several types of advance care directives, the two most widely used ones being the **living will** and the **durable power of health care attorney**, sometimes called a medical power of attorney. Living wills are notarized documents produced by competent persons specifying what sorts of medical treatment they would want to refuse in the event they become unable to speak for themselves. As it stands, a living will becomes effective only when the incompetent patient is suffering from an incurable or irreversible disease and/or is permanently unconscious. The patient must also be terminal; that is, expected to die within a short period of time. All fifty states and the District of Columbia currently recognize living wills.

Because living wills do not give individuals the opportunity to be as specific about their medical treatment choices as they may want to be, and because they become effective only under a very limited set of circumstances, most states also provide competent adults with the opportunity to name someone their health care power of attorney or health care agent. Choosing the right health care agent, who need not be a family member, is important. Ideally, the health care agent's values should be similar to the patient's. In addition, the health care agent's knowledge of and commitment to the patient's treatment wishes should be great. Finally, the health care agent should have the courage to make the decisions the patient would make even if others disagree vehemently.

Of course, not every person has a living will, let alone a trusted person to name as his or her health care agent. If a person has neither a living will nor a durable power of health care attorney, most states specify who may make health care decisions for him or her. Usually the spouse is the legally recognized surrogate; however, if an incompetent patient has no spouse, or if her or his spouse is unable, unwilling, unworthy, or unavailable to make medical decisions for her or him, most states permit other family members (most often parents, children, and/or siblings) to call the shots. One state, Colorado, permits the consensus of "interested parties" to communicate the patient's wishes.[48] In the event that there are no surrogates for the patient at all, states typically authorize the attending physician, in consultation with another physician, to decide whether continued treatment is in the best interests of the incompetent patient.[49]

Despite the fact that an advance care directive constitutes a person's best chance to have his or her wishes honored in the event of incompetency, only about 20% of individuals across the United States have executed one.[50] Moreover, many persons with advance care directives have never explicitly discussed them with their families, physicians, and/or clergy members. For example, in a recent survey of 35,000 members of the North Carolina Chapter of the American Association of Retired Persons (AARP), the good news was that 50%, and not merely 20% (the national average) of this association's members had completed an advance care directive. But the bad news was that only half of them had ever talked to their families about their end-of-life treatment preferences. Even fewer had talked to their physicians (11%) and/or clergy persons (6%) about them.[51]

As a result of discussions *not had*, patients' wishes are not always honored; for, as they are currently phrased, advance care directives are merely "permissive" and "protective." In other words, advance care directives *permit* physicians to withhold and withdraw treatment without fear of state punishment. They do not, however, *require* physicians to withhold and withdraw treatment. Interestingly, there is some movement in the direction of subjecting physicians and/or health care facilities to professional penalties, civil suits, and even criminal sanctions if they fail to honor an advance care directive. Indeed, it has been argued that not honoring a patient's advance care directive is tantamount to committing battery on the patient, and that, at the bare minimum, patients subjected to such unwanted treatment should not incur financial liability for it.[52]

In recent years, there have been some second thoughts about advance care directives. There are some circumstances in which they may pose more harm than benefit to incompetent patients. Specifically, the present interests of an incompetent patient are not necessarily identical with the interests he or she had when competent. For example, at age 25, an athlete may think that life without a limb would be so awful that he or she would rather die "whole" than live without an arm or leg. But at the age of 80 that same person may decide that life in a wheelchair is better than no life at all. Two legs may not seem all that important to an octogenarian who stopped thinking about winning an Olympic medal long ago. In other words, just because someone has certain interests at age 25, it does not mean that he or she will have the same interests at age 80. Life experiences change our wishes and wants, and it is not clear that the wishes of a younger and healthier version of ourselves should necessarily trump the present wishes of an older and unhealthier version. Advance care directives should not be imposed on incompetent patients, who, in their *present* condition, would (if they could) express a wish to go on living. Past selves should not have unrestricted control over present selves.

Admittedly, as soon as the suggestion is made that past *competent* choice should not be automatically privileged over present *incompetent* choice, the value of advance care directives is put into question. Health care professionals and family members are forced back into the position from which they thought advance care directives had delivered them. Specifically, they are asked to decide what is best for the patient because the patient's current preferences are not known.

V. PALLIATIVE CARE AND HOSPICE

Opponents of assisted suicide and active euthanasia point out that if more was done to control people's pain and suffering, fewer people would feel a need to act on the basis of the kind of information provided in Derek Humphrey's do-it-yourself suicide manual, *Final Exit*.[53] In particular, they point out that patients who receive good **palliative care** are "more likely to accept a greater degree of nourishment, to be more active and less depressed and to be more open to other treatment possibilities."[54] That this should be the case is not surprising. For example, when I am in real pain all I can think about is the pain, and getting rid of it. Only after the pain is assuaged or eliminated, do I feel like living again.

In the past, health care professionals were reluctant to provide patients with adequate pain relief, particularly morphine and other barbiturates. They worried that legal authorities would view them as possible "drug dealers," selling narcotics illegally to drug addicts. They also worried that their colleagues would view them with suspicion. Most often, however, they worried that they would either addict their patients to pain remedies or inadvertently kill them in an effort to control their pain with strong narcotics. Because of these and other concerns, many health care professionals gave patients aspirins when they should have given them pain remedies far stronger than this over-the-counter panacea.

Fortunately, an increasing number of today's health care professionals realize that palliation is one of medicine's most important goals, and that they should be just as concerned about *underprescribing* as *overprescribing* pain remedies. Most medical schools now require their students to take palliative-care courses so that they can learn about which painkillers work best on which conditions. The narcotic that controls the pains of arthritis may have no effect on the pains that accompany ovarian cancer, for example. Palliative-care courses also teach physicians-to-be that titrating pain remedies is an art they can master. Patients rarely die as the result of a pain-medication overdose, a point that the AMA gladly emphasizes[55] as it encourages young physicians to consider making palliative care their specialty.

Important as it is to address patients' **pain**, it is equally important to address their **suffering**—that is, their depressions, fears, anxieties, bored feelings, and even suicidal thoughts. Hospice programs help do this. **Hospice** was imported from England to the United States in the 1970s. It is based on an ethics of service, dignity, and compassion. Originally designed for people in an advanced stage of cancer who wanted to die in a home-like environment, today many patients use hospice irrespective of their disease. Among the services hospice provides are assistance in daily living, respite care, spiritual counseling (if wanted), professional nursing care (if needed), palliative care, and family bereavement services following the patient's death. Hospice care is total care. The patient is served by an interdisciplinary team of nurses, social workers, therapists, pastoral counselors, dieticians, comfort keepers, and volunteers under the management of a physician with expertise in palliative care. In general, the hospice team involves the patient's family and friends in the patient's care, provided that they are willing and able to do so.

Given that hospice helps patients *live* through their dying process in as physically comfortable, psychologically stable, and spiritually nourished a condition as possible, it is surprising that only about 950,000 patients take advantage of its services in any year.[56] Among the reasons that more patients do not use hospice are that Medicare reimbursement policies require that patients not be referred for hospice care unless they have, in health care professionals' judgment, only 6 months or less to live. For fear of being accused of Medicare fraud, some health care professionals hesitate to refer patients who may live longer than 6 months to hospice. Clearly, the "6-month" rule undermines the overall purpose of hospice, which is to help patients come to terms with the ending of their existence. Because so many of the terminal patients that are sent to hospice are no longer capable of "thought-work," or even of saying goodbyes to their loved ones, hospice personnel strongly object to some of the Medicare policies that regulate them. Specifically, they argue:

> . . . Rather than penalizing hospices for helping patients live longer, more money could be saved by getting terminal patients into hospice program quicker. While fifteen percent of hospice patients live longer than six months . . . twenty-nine

percent of patients die within two weeks of entering hospice. These late enrollees miss the full effect of hospice, and they likely spend their last months in more-expensive hospitals.[57]

VI. CONCLUSION

Although people remain divided as to whether they would prefer a quick, sudden and unexpected death over a slow, steady, very expected death, there is much to be said in favor of a death process that provides the patient with the opportunity to reflect on the meaning of his/her life in the company of family, friends, and other compassionate caregivers. As our society ages, more people are living longer and experiencing the kind of disintegration and diminishment that usually accompanies the dying process. Most people do not die in the prime of their life, but at some point in the process of their withering. People need help saying their final goodbyes. They need physical help, psychological help, and spiritual help. Although most people fear dying in pain, they also fear dying totally dependent on others to feed, clean, and move them from place to place. They also fear losing their minds, their ability to communicate with others, indeed their very selfhood.

Most people do not want to get stuck in the dying process for years, dragging their families and friends in the tow that is pulling them towards the shores of nonexistence. But dying need not be utterly bleak if it is done in an appropriate setting such as hospice. But because even the best in the way of palliative care and hospice care will not be able to eliminate the suffering of some patients, carefully regulated physician-assisted suicide and active euthanasia should probably be legal options. These options should remain the courts of very last resort, however, used only because the combined human resources of one's self and one's caregivers are no longer sufficient to meet the challenges of the process of dying.

Discussion Questions

1. Explain how a physician's duties of beneficence and nonmaleficence can be reconciled with a patient's request for physician-assisted suicide. The patient argues that people have a right to control the time and manner of their death, for unless this right is recognized, human dignity and autonomy will be undermined.

2. Some ethicists have argued that there is no ethically significant difference between passive and active euthanasia, but only between acts intended to cause death on the one hand and acts not intended to cause death on the other hand. Given this view, if a physician's intention is to hasten death, is there any ethical

difference between his/her discontinuing a life-support machine and his/her providing terminal sedation?

3. Many requests for physician-assisted suicide are grounded on the patient's intractable pain and suffering. Would adequate pain management and palliative care eliminate the need for physician-assisted suicide? What is the difference between pain and suffering?

4. Strictly speaking, do patients have a *right* to die? If they do, do health care professionals have a strict obligation to help them die? What about family members and friends? Do they have a duty to help loved ones die when their lives become too miserable for them to tolerate?

Case Studies

1. Mr. Najiri, a Shiite Muslim and Arab-American, was put on life support following a massive cardiac arrest. He has only marginal brain activity and can only breathe with the assistance of a ventilator. He has no oral or written advance care directive. Within days, Mr. Najiri's family and friends arrive to lend emotional support. The physician assigned to the case speaks with the family about withdrawing life support when Mr. Najiri's brain dies. Mr. Najiri's family explains to the physician that for Shiite Muslims death means cessation of cardiac function rather than cessation of neurological function. A few weeks later, Mr. Najiri's condition worsens. He is now officially brain dead. At this point, the physician states to Mr. Najiri's family and friends that because Mr. Najiri is dead, the hospital will no longer continue to support his cardiac functions artificially. The family reminds the physician that for them brain death is not really death. The physician responds: "Fine, but here in the United States brain death is death. End of story."

a. May a physician invoke medical futility to justify discontinuation of artificial means of life support?

b. If medical futility is not a sufficient guide for end-of-life decision-making, what alternative concept or value should guide the decision-making process?

c. Is the physician in this case guilty of cultural imperialism? Why should brain death count as true death?

2. Rhonda is a 15-year-old who is diagnosed with acute lymphocytic leukemia. Her oncologist indicates that given the severity of her case, chemotherapy will probably extend her life at best for a year. To complicate matters, Rhonda already suffers from a congenital kidney ailment that will require a kidney transplant in the near future. A devout Christian, who is amazingly mature for her age, Rhonda refuses chemotherapeutic treatments, saying she has "reconciled herself to be with God." Her parents, however,

cannot bear the thought of her dying and tell the oncologist to proceed with the chemotherapy.

a. Whose wishes, Rhonda's or her parents', should be followed?
b. What is the most beneficent course of action for the physician to take?
c. Should minors be permitted to participate in their own end-of-life decisions? If so, to what extent and at what age?

3. As we noted in this chapter, the state of Oregon enacted the "Death with Dignity Act." It allows physicians to prescribe lethal drugs for terminally ill patients who express the desire to end their own lives. Some people think the law is too permissive; others think it is too restrictive. Use the following questions as an opportunity to solidify your own position on the "Death with Dignity Act."

a. Do you think the Oregon law is morally justified? Why or why not? Does physician-assisted suicide really constitute a dignified death? What, after all, makes a death "dignified"?
b. Do the provisions of the Oregon law safeguard against possible abuses of it?
c. Should physician-assisted suicide be legalized throughout the United States? Why or why not?

4. Mrs. M, who was in her mid-60s, had undergone a mastectomy for breast cancer. She received only three of the six originally recommended courses of adjuvant chemotherapy because of severe bone marrow suppression. Mrs. M was found to have bone and lung metastases, 14 months later. Her oncologist told her and her family that her illness was terminal and suggested that she enter hospice. He advised that further chemotherapy was not indicated because it would not improve her condition. Mrs. M had always been in control of her life and became angry and depressed that she was losing her battle against cancer and could do nothing. Morphine was prescribed for pain relief. Hospice workers saw Mrs. M weekly, but she did not respond well to the assistance they offered. They felt Mrs. M was denying the terminal nature of her illness when she refused to be a DNR (do-not-resuscitate) patient.

When Mrs. M returned for outpatient follow-up, she was in a wheelchair and extremely short of breath, and was described by her attending physician as being in a panic about her impending death. The next day she became more short of breath and called paramedics who brought her to the emergency department (ED). The staff tried to relieve her discomfort, but the ED physician told Mrs. M that there was not much medicine could do for her anymore. Mrs. M's denial of the inevitable was apparent. She reportedly told the ED physician "I want you to do everything possible to make me live. Give me the chemotherapy, now."

a. Should the attending physician put Mrs. M on a ventilator?

b. What is the likelihood of Mrs. M becoming a "medical futility" case down the line? How should the attending physician handle her case in the event that the situation gets worse than it already is? When, if ever, is enough *enough*?

c. Who should decide if Mrs. M. should get chemotherapy? Would it make a difference if she were willing to use her own money to pay for what physicians believe is medically futile treatment?

Endnotes

1. Gregory Pence, "Karen Quinlan," in: *Classic Cases in Medical Ethics*, 2nd ed. (New York: McGraw-Hill Publishing Company, 1995), p. 3.

2. In re Quinlan, 70 N.J. 10, 355, A.2d 647, 429 U.S. 922 (1976).

3. Marcia Angell, "The right to die in dignity," *Newsweek Magazine* (July 23, 1990): 9.

4. *Wendland v. Wendland*, S087265, Supreme Court of California, 2001 (Cal. LEXIS 6484, September 26, 2001).

5. Daniel Eisenberg, "Lessons of the Schiavo Battle," *Time Magazine* (April 14, 2005): 24.

6. Ibid., p. 25.

7. Ibid., p. 27.

8. Mark A. Hall, Ira Mark Ellman, Daniel S. Strouse, *Health Care Law and Ethics* (St. Paul, MN: West Group, 1999), p. 367.

9. In re Storar, 438 N.Y.S. 2d 266 (N.Y., 1981).

10. *Superintendent of Belchertown State School v. Saikcwicz*, 370 N.D. 2d 417 (MA, 1977).

11. Mark A. Hall, Ira Mark Ellman, Daniel S. Strouse, *Health Care Law and Ethics* (St. Paul, MN: West Group, 1999), p. 381.

12. Ibid, p. 391.

13. *Bowen v. American Hospital Association*, 476 U.S. 610 (1986).

14. *Child Abuse and Neglect Prevention and Treatment Program: Final Rule*, 50 Fed. Reg. 14877 (April 15, 1985).

15. Ronald E. Cranford, "Helga Wanglie's Ventilator," *Hastings Center Report*, 21, no. 4 (July–August 1991): 23.

16. Michael A. Rie, "The limits of a wish," *Hastings Center Report*, 21, no. 4 (July–August 1991): 24–25.

17. "Wanglie case decision," *Medical Ethics Advisor* 7, no. 8 (August 1991): 101–102.

18. Daniel Callahan, "Medical futility, medical necessity: the problem-without-a-name," *Hastings Center Report*, 21, no. 4 (July–August 1991): 34.

19. Council on Ethical and Judicial Affairs, American Medical Association, "Guidelines for the appropriate use of do-not-resuscitate orders," *Journal of the American Medical Association*, 265, no. 14 (April 10, 1991): 1868–1871.

20. Michael A. Rie, "The limits of a wish," *Hastings Center Report*, 21, no. 4 (July–August 1991): 26.

21. Pam Belluck, "Even as doctors say enough, families fight to prolong life," *New York Times* (March 27, 2005): 16.

22. Ibid.

23. Craig S. Smith, "France lets terminally ill refuse care, but still bans euthanasia," *New York Times* (April 14, 2005): A13.

24. Douglas Herbert, "Dutch law stokes death debate," CNN.com (April 11, 2001), *http://archives.cnn.com/2001/WORLD/Europe(04/11/euthanasizdebate* [accessed March 31, 2005].

25. Ronald Munson, *Intervention and Reflection: Basic Issues in Medical Ethics*, 6th ed. (Belmont, CA: Wadsworth, Inc., 2000), p. 208.

26. Andis Robeznicks, "A doctor chooses when to die," *American Medical News*, 46, no. 26 (July 14, 2003): 2.

27. *Parade Magazine* (February 9, 1992) (mail survey of 3,750 people aged 21 or older; 2203 respondents).

28. Ronald Munson, *Intervention and Reflection: Basic Issues in Medical Ethics*, 6th ed. (Belmont, CA: Wadsworth, Inc., 2000), p. 208.

29. Timothy E. Quill, *Midwife Through the Dying Process* (Baltimore, MD: Johns Hopkins University Press, 1996), p. 145.

30. James Rachels, "Active and passive euthanasia," *New England Journal of Medicine*, 292 (January 9, 1975): 78–80.

31. Willard Gaylin, Leon Kass, Edmund D. Pellegrino, and Mark Siegler, "Doctors must not kill," *Journal of the American Medical Association*, 259 (1988): 2139–2140.

32. John Hardwig, "Is there a duty to die?," *Hastings Center Report*, 27, no. 2 (1997): 35.

33. Henk A.M.J. ten Have and Jos V.M. Welie, "Euthanasia: normal medical practice," *Hastings Center Report*, 22, no. 2 (March–April, 1992): 34.

34. "It's over, Debbie," *Journal of the American Medical Association*, 259, no. 2 (January 8, 1988): 272.

35. Gregory Pence, "Karen Quinlan," in: *Classic Cases in Medical Ethics*, 2nd ed. (New York: McGraw-Hill Publishing Company, 1995), p. 64.

36. "Janet Adkins's suicide: reexamining the spectrum of issues it has raised," *Issues*, 5, no. 4 (July–August, 1990): 2.

37. "Kevorkian found guilty of second-degree murder," *CNN.com* (March 26, 1999), *http://www.cnn.com/US/9903/26/kevorkian.02/* [accessed March 31, 2005].

38. Russell L. McIntyre, "Physician-assisted dying: contemporary twists to an ancient dilemma," *Trends in Health Care, Law and Ethics*, 7, no. 2 (Winter 1992): 8–9.

39. The Oregon Death with Dignity Act (1998), Section 3.01 (1998).

40. Oregon Public Health Services, Center for Health Statistics and Vital Records, *Oregon's Death with Dignity Annual Report*, 2001, see *http://www.Ind.hr.stateor.us/chs/pas.*

41. Margot Roosevelt, "Choosing their time," *Time* (April 14, 2005): 32.

42. Andis Robenieks, "Assisted-suicide numbers continue to rise in Oregon," *American Medical News* (March 24/31, 2003): 15.

43. *Bouvia v. Superior Ct.*, 225 Cal. Rptr. 297 (App. 1986).

44. Mark A. Hall, Ira Mark Ellman, Daniel S. Strouse, *Health Care Law and Ethics* (St. Paul, MN: West Group, 1999), p. 343.

45. *Bouvia v. Superior Ct.*, 225 Cal. Rptr. 297 (App. 1986).

46. Mark A. Hall, Ira Mark Ellman, Daniel S. Strouse, *Health Care Law and Ethics* (St. Paul, MN: West Group, 1999), p. 343.

47. Gregory Pence, "Karen Quinlan," in: *Classic Cases in Medical Ethics*, 2nd ed. (New York: McGraw-Hill Publishing Company, 1995).

48. "Map of states with surrogate decision-making laws," *Choice in Dying, Inc.* (June, 1998).

49. Lance Stell, "The right to refuse treatment," in: Brunetti and Stell (eds.), *A Physician's Guide to Legal and Ethical Aspects of Patient Care* (Charlotte, NC: Carolinas Medical Center, 1994), p. S4.83.

50. Keith L. Stelter, Barbara A. Elliott, and Candace A. Bruno, "Living will completion in older adults," *Archives of Internal Medicine*, 152 (1992): 954–959.

51. Karen Garloch, "Survey asks for hopes, fears in end-of-life care," *Charlotte Observer* (July 15, 2003): 1A.

52. *First Healthcare Corp v. Rettinger*, North Carolina Court of Appeals, Health Law News, 1995; and Amicus Curiae Brief of Choice in Dying, *First Healthcare Corporation v. Rettinger*, North Carolina Supreme Court (1996).

53. Derek Humphreys, *Final Exit* (Eugene, OR: Hemlock Society, 1991).

54. Hastings Center, *Guidelines on the Termination of Life-Sustaining Treatment and the Care of the Dying* (Briarcliff Manor, NY: The Hastings Center, 1987).

55. Diane E. Hoffman and Anita J. Tarzian, "Achieving the right balance in oversight of physicians opioid prescribing for pain: the role of state medical boards," *The Journal of Law, Medicine, and Ethics*, 31, no. 1 (Spring 2003): 21–40.

56. "Almost one million dying received hospice care last year: new record," *Senior Journal* (November 3, 2004), *http://www.seniorjournal.com/NEWS/Eldercare/4-11-03HospiceMonth.htm* [accessed April 12, 2005].

57. Ibid.

chapter twelve

Organ Transplantation: Individual Allocation Decisions

I. INTRODUCTION

According to Renèe C. Fox and Judith P. Swazey, organ transplantation is "one of the most sociologically intricate and powerfully symbolic events in modern medicine."[1] The psyche of the U.S. public is captured by the "gift of life" drama that unfolds each time a person donates a part of himself or herself—blood, tissue, or an organ—to save the life of someone else. Being involved either as a donor or as a recipient of an organ transplantation, say Fox and Swazey, enmeshes one in a threefold act of obligation: "(1) to offer and give; (2) to receive and accept; and (3) to seek and find an appropriate way to pay."[2] Organ transplantation evokes images of people giving generous gifts that cause immense happiness and well-being to their recipients. Yet, as positive as the images may be, they still fail to motivate a sufficient number of people to organ donors.

In 2003, there were 86,355 U.S. adults, children, and infants on transplant waiting lists,[3] and, for lack of enough donors, 7,147 died.[4] Indeed, in 2003, 3915 kidney patients, 2071 liver patients, 582 heart patients, and 487 lung patients died while waiting for life-saving organ transplants.[5] As the shortage of available donor organs increases, people are taking desperate measures to secure them, including flying to developing nations where organs are available for sale.[6] Like the topic of health care reform policy, which we shall discuss in the next chapter, the topic of organ transplantation highlights issues related to the allocation of scarce medical resources. Who should get which life-saving or life-lengthening medical resource when there is not enough to go around? Are we obligated to share our organs with fellow citizens when we no longer need them? Why or why not?

II. Overview of Organ and Tissue Transplantation

A. History of Transplantation

Notable advancements in organ transplants did not begin until the 1950s. After several failed attempts, Dr. Joseph Murray performed the first successful kidney transplant in 1954 at the Peter Bent Brigham Hospital in Boston.[7] The donor of the kidney was the identical twin of the recipient. Earlier kidney transplants had failed because they were between relatives not closely enough related to prevent the recipient's immune system from rejecting the transplanted organ. Unable to solve the rejection problem, the only kidney transplants that surgeons performed in the United States between 1954 and 1957 were **isografts**—that is, transplantations between identical twins. **Allografts**—that is, transplantations between individuals who are not identical twins—became successful only after adequate antirejection drugs were developed; and not until the 1984 development of the powerful immunosuppressant drug, cyclosporine, did kidney transplantation become the remarkable success it is today.[8]

Of course, kidneys are not the only organs that can be transplanted successfully. In 1967, the first heart and the first liver transplantations were done successfully by Dr. Christian Barnard in Capetown, South Africa and Dr. Thomas Starzel in Denver, Colorado, respectively. Today about 1,800 heart transplants and about 3,900 successful liver transplants are performed annually.[9] Other organs that can be transplanted are the pancreas, the lungs, and the intestines. Pancreas, lung, and particularly intestine transplants are relatively few in number, however, and do not meet with the same success rates that heart and liver transplants do. Only 70 pancreas-alone transplants, 837 lung transplants, and 66 intestine transplants were performed in 1998.[10] Combination organ transplants were also performed, but, once again, they were few in number with mixed results. Only, 967 kidney–pancreas transplants and 46 heart–lung transplants were performed.[11]

In addition to organs, many tissues can be successfully transplanted, including the corneas, skin, bones, joints, heart valves, and bone marrow. Some tissue transplantations are **autografts**, as when burn victims have skin grafted from an unburned area of their body to a burned one; however, most tissue transplantations are **allografts**, with bone being the most common allograft transferred from one individual's body to another's.[12]

III. Ethical and Legal Issues Regarding Organ Donors

There are two types of organ donors: **cadaver donors** and **living donors**. Until very recently, most organ donors in the United States were cadaver donors; however, in 2001, the number of living donors slightly surpassed the number of cadaver donors for the first time.[13] This trend is continuing. In 2003, there were 6,821 living donors and 6,457 cadaver donors.[14] Not surprisingly, both cadaveric organ donation and living organ donation present complex ethical challenges.

A. Cadaver Donors

Although the difference between a cadaver donor and a living donor may seem obvious, determining whether someone is truly dead can be quite difficult. In the world of transplantation, it currently matters very much whether a donor is declared dead on cardiopulmonary criteria or on neurological criteria.

1. Heart-Beating Cadaver Donors (HBDs)

Before the 1970s, the only criterion that was used to determine death was the irreversible cessation of cardiopulmonary function. Individuals who suffered cardiopulmonary arrest lost the ability to breathe and, shortly thereafter, their brain function ceased. They died immediately or nearly immediately. The invention of mechanical ventilators destroyed this state of affairs, however. Persons with no brain function could go on breathing for quite some time. Suddenly, society was forced to reevaluate what it meant for a person to be dead. How was it supposed to treat individuals who lacked brain function, but whose hearts continued beating, thanks to the intervention of mechanical ventilators? Were they dead or were they alive? Would it be murder to detach them from their ventilators? Or would it be the only appropriate action to take, given that not persons but "corpses" were occupying hospital beds? Would it be permissible to use these "corpses" as organ donors or did they have to be buried intact instead?

In part, society answered these troubling questions by inventing a concept—in this instance, the concept of **brain death**. Death could now be determined by tests that showed irreversible cessation of circulatory and respiratory function *or* by tests that showed irreversible cessation of all functions of the entire brain. Surprisingly, within a very short period of time, the concept of brain death was accepted not only by all 50 states in the Union but also by the American people as a whole, even though a large percentage of them did not really understand the concept.

According to social historian, Martin Pernick, one of the main reasons for the public's quick acceptance of the concept of brain death was the way in which it was communicated to the public. As Pernick sees it, the notion of brain death was, to a great extent, motivated by the organ transplant community's interest in securing healthy organs for donation. Yet it was presented to the public as a way "to stop physicians from using futile machinery that prolonged and intruded upon a good death."[15] Before long most people came to view "brain death" as a friend of sorts, a final defense "against the invasive indignities of technological medicine."[16] Nevertheless, "pockets of resistance"[17] to brain death remained and exist to this day among conservative Catholics and Orthodox Jews. In fact, some critics of brain death are so vocal that many hospitals are reluctant to use brain-dead, heart-beating individuals as donors. Moreover, at least one state (New Jersey) that accepts brain death as true death nonetheless permits individuals to claim a religious exemption from this neurologically based criterion for death.[18]

Most experts maintain that a person is alive rather than dead ". . . if and only if he or she is a human body which is an integrated organic unity at the level of the 'organism as a whole.'"[19] Initially, the consensus was that *no* brain-dead individual was an integrated organic unity and, therefore, that *all* brain-dead individuals were truly dead. But over the years, several experts have challenged the view that *all* brain-dead individuals are necessarily unintegrated organic disunities. Michael Potts, for instance, believes that some brain-dead individuals, who survive for years on ventilators and feeding tubes, are integrated organic unities.[20] As he sees it, such individuals are not "fair game" for transplant purposes. Health care professionals must, absent their consent, keep them on "life support." To do otherwise would be to violate the **dead donor rule**, which "requires that patients not be killed in order to obtain their organs."[21]

Potts's critics reply to his line of reasoning in two basic ways. Some of them claim that the patients Potts labels "brain-dead" are not truly brain-dead but instead in a persistent vegetative state. People in a persistent vegetative state are classified as alive. They may not be killed for purposes of organ transplant. Other critics of Potts are bolder, however. They are weary of hair-splitting discussions about whether patients who have no higher-brain function are dead or alive. They think the time has come to abandon the whole-brain definition of death and to embrace in its stead a higher-brain definition of death. In their estimation, persons should be declared dead when the cerebrum (neocortex), which makes possible conscious thought, self-awareness, and interaction with the world outside of one's self, is no longer functional.[22] Were a higher-brain definition of death accepted, it would be permissible to use for transplant the organs of not only brain-dead individuals but also anencephalic infants and people in a persistent vegetative state. Anencephalic infants are born without a higher-brain structure. They have only a brain stem—that is, that portion of the brain that maintains the vegetative functions of the human body (respiration, heart rate, body temperance, blood pressure, and electrolyte balance). In contrast, people in a persistent vegetative state have a higher-brain structure. It is just that it is entirely dysfunctional.

Assuming that organs from anencephalic infants and people in a persistent vegetative state are healthy enough to be transplanted, adding them to the donor pool via definitional fiat might help alleviate our organ shortage problem. In addition, such a development might provide a measure of comfort both to parents who want their doomed infants' organs to go to good use[23] and to individuals who would rather give their organs to fully conscious people than keep them locked in their "vegetative," totally unconscious bodies for years on end. Yet, this very same development might also raise some red flags. Critics will likely point to the slippery slope that begins with using people with *nonfunctioning* higher brains as organ donors, and ends with using people with *poorly-functioning* higher brains as organ donors. Therefore, on balance, it may be best to leave anencephalic infants and people in a persistent vegetative state among the living.

2. Non–Heart-Beating Donors (NHBDs)

Failure to increase significantly the number of brain-dead, heart-beating organ donors has in recent years led health care professionals to reconsider their reluctance to go back to the "bad old days," when the only organs that were available for transplant came from the bodies of individuals who had been declared dead on cardiopulmonary criteria. Despite the fact that organs from such individuals, termed **non–heart-beating donors (NHBDs)**, are not always as good as organs from individuals declared dead by neurological criteria, they are usually quite good, if retrieved properly.

Transplant specialists divide NHBDs into four categories: (1) dead on arrival at the hospital (victims of an accident, cardiac arrest, or suicide, where resuscitation has either not been initiated or has been stopped en route to the hospital); (2) unsuccessful resuscitation (victim of an accident, cardiac arrest, or suicide, where resuscitation has been initiated either outside or inside the hospital only to fail); (3) awaiting cardiac arrest (patients from whom life-support machines are withdrawn); and (4) cardiac arrest in an HBD (patients who suffer an unexpected cardiac arrest sometime during or very shortly after being declared brain-dead).[24] Among these, NHBDs in categories one, two, and four are called **uncontrolled donors** because their hearts stop beating spontaneously and without warning. In contrast, NHBDs in category three are called **controlled donors**. Their hearts stop beating because life-support machines are withdrawn from them; their deaths are planned.

Before organs may be taken from an NHBD, there must be certitude that the donor's cardiopulmonary function has ceased irreversibly; that is, that autoresuscitation (self-resuscitation) is not possible. In the same way that experts have difficulty determining whether the whole brain has died, they have difficulty determining whether cardiac function is irretrievable. Compounding the experts' problems in pronouncing someone dead on cardiac criteria is the fact that it is notoriously difficult to define the term "irreversible." According to Stuart J. Younger and Robert M. Arnold, "irreversible" can mean the following:

1. There is no logical possibility of restoring a function now or in the future.
2. A function *cannot* be restored with present technology and clinical skills.
3. A morally defensible decision has been made not to restore the function even though that is technically possible.[25]

The first meaning of "irreversible" is uncontroversial; but both the second and third meanings of "irreversible" are controversial for at least three reasons. First, some minority communities fear that transplant teams, headed by largely White and/or otherwise privileged health care professionals, may prematurely declare disadvantaged patients dead in order to use their organs for advantaged patients. Second, certain religious groups fear that health care professionals may deliberately classify "vulnerable but biologically tenacious patients"[26] as dead for no other reason than to use their organs for fully conscious, mentally "with it" patients. Third, a particularly fearful segment of the U.S. population worries that unscrupulous health care professionals may snatch their organs from them during the course of routine, hospital-administered tests in order to sell them to the highest bidder on the organ black market.

Because they are well aware of the fears mentioned above, health care professionals are careful to rule out the possibility of autoresuscitation before they retrieve organs from an NHBD. Although most health care professionals believe autoresuscitation is not possible after a patient has been unresponsive, apnoeic and asystollic for 2 minutes, some think that autoresuscitation may be possible for as long as 10 minutes after this state of affairs occurs. The **Institute of Medicine (IOM)** recommends, as a compromise position, waiting 5 minutes before beginning organ retrieval procedures,[27] but a few daring experts suggest waiting zero minutes.

In defense of the boldness of their claim, this last group of experts invites us to consider two scenarios.

The first scenario is as follows:

> . . . Imagine two physiologically identical patients in adjacent beds [in a hospital that follows the wait-five minutes rule] who have simultaneous cardiac arrests after discontinuing respirator support. Patient A is DNR and is participating in a controlled NHBD protocol. Patient B wants to be resuscitated. According to the weakest construal of *irreversible* [a morally defensible decision has been made not to restore the function even though that is technically possible], the first patient is dead five minutes after the arrests but the second is alive.[28]

The second scenario is a variant on the first one:

> . . . imagine two physiologically identical patients who both request discontinuation of respirator support and refuse resuscitation. As above, patient A is part

of a controlled NHBD protocol. Patient C is simply DNR; he is not donating organs. Following an arrest, Patient A must be observed for five minutes with invasive monitors before death is declared. Consistent with practice in most deaths, however, Patient C is pronounced dead much earlier, at the moment when no heartbeat is heard or respiration observed.[29]

Reflecting on these two scenarios, it does seem puzzling that health care professionals should treat two biologically-identical cases so differently. If they are willing to declare non–organ-donating individuals dead as soon as their hearts stop, why are they so unwilling to make the same declaration about organ-donating individuals as soon as their hearts stop?

3. Reflections on the Use of HBDs and NHBDs

As we have just seen, the question "when does life officially end?" is not any easier to answer than the question "when does life officially begin?" Some experts are so reluctant to announce death's arrival that they refuse to declare a person dead either on neurological criteria or cardiopulmonary criteria until that person is nearly ready for transport to an undertaker and their organs are no longer fit for transplantation. Fearing that this state of affairs is unlikely to change unless we can determine the exact nanosecond of death's occurrence, Robert Truog recommends that we abandon the dead-donor rule and permit not-quite-dead persons to donate their organs if they so wish.[30]

The clear advantage of Truog's proposal is that, like the related proposal to declare anencephalic infants and individuals in a persistent vegetative state officially dead, it may increase the pool of organ donors. Truog's proposal has a serious disadvantage, however. It fails to address some people's fear that health care professionals may literally kill them in order to secure their organs for others to use. In view of this fear, most health care professionals think we should maintain the dead-donor rule for now.

B. Living Donors

Because the process for determining death seems to be getting more rather less complex, it is not surprising that the number of living donors has begun to outpace the number of cadaver donors. According to health care ethicist Lance Stell, one of the main explanations for this trend is that "[u]nlike deceased donation, which currently is presented as impersonal (nondirected) altruism, living donation is almost always 'directed,' i.e., the living donor not only knows personally and wishes to aid a particular recipient but most often is related to the recipient by marriage or blood."[31] Living donors may also have increased in number simply because the transplant community has become accustomed to using both living donors' whole, paired organs, such as the kidneys, and living donors' regenerative organs such as parts of livers, lungs, pancreases, and bowels. The only organs the transplant community rejects from living donors are nonpaired, nonregenerative organs. For example, the transplant community will not accept a living donor's heart, except in the rare instance when the living heart donor will receive a heart *and* lung from a third party at the time he or she gives their heart for a second party to use.

Although all types of living donors are increasing in number, living *kidney* donors remain the most numerous among living donors. Indeed, in 2003 over 40% of the kidneys transplanted in the United States came from living donors.[32] In contrast, only 5.9% of donated livers came from living individuals,[33] and only 1.3% of donated lungs came from living individuals.[34]

1. Related Living Donors

As might be expected, when one family member receives an organ from another family member, the organ recipient may feel he or she can never repay the gift he or she has been given. In fact, in some instances, organ recipients become so "tyrannized" by the gift they have received that they "have to sever relationships with the donor."[35] Another kind of human-relationship problem may occur if, instead of succeeding, the transplant fails. The organ donor may feel disappointed that their sacrifice was to no avail, while the organ recipient may feel regretful that they have weakened their family member's health for nothing. In one case with which I am personally familiar, a young woman received a kidney from first her father, then her brother, and finally a cousin. When another cousin offered his kidney to her, the young woman exclaimed, "No! I have caused enough trouble the way it is! I'd rather die than keep 'cannibalizing' the people whom I love."

Perhaps the most poignant problems associated with living related donors occur when parents want to donate organs to their children. Although health care professionals wish to honor parents' wishes about being kidney, liver, or lung donors for their children, and although society applauds parents who go beyond the call of duty for their children, parents are nonetheless not permitted to serve as sacrificial lambs for their children. Health care professionals will not violate the dead-donor rule to kill parents so that their children have a chance to live a long and healthy life. In fact, they will not even permit parents to seriously compromise their health in order to save their children from death or simply a very low-quality life. In this connection, consider the following case:

> In late December 1998, Renada Daniel-Patterson's father offered to donate a kidney to his daughter and ignited a controversy in the bioethics community. Renada had been born with only one kidney, which began to fail early in her childhood. At age six, Renada had to receive dialysis three times a week. She was

unable to attend school or venture very far from home. This pattern continued until Renada was 13, when Mr. Patterson called from prison to offer her his kidney. Renada was surprised to hear from her father, who was serving 12 years at California State Prison for burglary and drug convictions. Mr. Patterson was determined to be a compatible donor, and the family proceeded with the transplant operation. As a result of this surgery, Renada was able to live the life of a healthy girl for 2 years. Because the medication to prevent rejection of the transplanted organ made her feel ill and bloated and caused her to develop a hump on her back, Renada gradually began to skip doses. As a result, her donated kidney began to fail. It was under these circumstances that David Patterson offered to donate his second kidney to his daughter in 1998.[36]

Even if Mr. Patterson wants to make amends to his daughter for presumably having been a bad father, his life, as a life, is no less worth respect and consideration than his daughter's. Other compatible donors may yet be found for her. However much health care professionals may want to help Renada, they must not severely compromise her father's health in a possibly futile second attempt to help her escape the rigors of dialysis.

2. *Nonrelated Living Donors*

In the past, individuals who were not related to someone in need of an organ were not permitted to serve as donors. Health care professionals were suspicious of the ulterior motives of these volunteers, and/or they had concerns about whether they fully understood the risks of organ donation. But over the years, health care professionals came to the conclusion that just because someone volunteers to give an organ to a nonrelated recipient, it does not mean that he or she is looking for a financial reward or is ill-informed about the risks of organ donation. On the contrary, a living donor may fully understand the risks of organ donation and yet be entirely willing to accept them for purely humanitarian reasons and/or because he or she feels emotionally attached to the potential recipient. For example, someone may want to donate an organ to a close friend or to an admirable person who has contributed in exceptional ways to society.

Altruism of the type described above should not be dismissed as a sign of mental instability or outright "craziness." Yet, as Mark Anderson appropriately notes, "we might want to erect some barriers to ensure that the decision to donate is determined freely."[37] For instance, we might reject as organ donors individuals who have a history of seeking medical services excessively or whose motivation for donating seems out of sync with the rest of their lives. Or we might say "no thanks" to someone who wishes to give their organ to an individual who has power over them, be the power financial or psychological. To be sure, there will be exceptions to any rules we formulate. For example, in a case with which I am familiar, a transplant team initially refused a nanny's request to be used as a living donor for her employer. The man for whom she worked was in desperate need of a kidney and, as it turned out, her kidney was a better match for him than any one else he knew, including his family members. When the transplant team told her they were unwilling to use her kidney for her employer, she protested that she could not live with the thought that the children whom she loved as her own might lose their father for lack of a suitable donor.

The transplant team initially dismissed the nanny's protest speech. They told the nanny they thought she was the victim of extreme psychological and emotional pressure—of unnecessary "guilt feelings" and a hyper-inflated sense of duty. Outraged by the transplant team's well-intentioned, but nonetheless disrespectful words, the nanny icily commented, "You don't understand much about genuine love and affection. Do you?" Subsequent to their discussions with the nanny, the transplant team relented and told her they would use her kidney for her employer, after all. The administrators of the hospital at which the transplant was performed required both the nanny and her employer to sign documents attesting to the free and voluntary nature of the nanny's donation, however. In addition, the nanny and her employer were required to sign papers assuring all concerned that the nanny would not be financially rewarded or punished on the basis of her decision to donate/not donate her kidney to her employer.

IV. ETHICS OF TRANSPLANT TEAMS AND END-OF-LIFE TEAMS

Important as it is to be sure that the organ donor–organ recipient relationship is appropriate, it is just as important for the health care community to develop policies that separate clinicians' duties to organ donors (particularly organ donors who are in the process of dying) on the one hand from transplant teams' duties to organ recipients on the other. The primary ends and aims of each of these two groups of health care professionals differ, and they must be balanced against each other in order to achieve a satisfactory organ transplant—that is, one about which everyone "feels good" or at least, "at peace with themselves." No one should be a party to a situation in which, for example, family members feel that their loved one's dying process is being expedited in order to secure his or her organs for transplant purposes.[38]

After death has been established by means of neurological criteria, the leader of the end-of-life team should explain to family members that their loved one is indeed dead, and that the time has come to remove any and all machines from their loved one's body, unless he or she wanted to be an HBD. In the event that the deceased patient did indeed want to be an organ donor, the end-of-life team should immediately contact the local **Organ Procurement**

Organization (OPO) and, if there is one, the hospital transplant team. Then they and/or representatives of the OPO need to explain to the family why, for purposes of organ retrieval, certain machines must be kept on even though the patient is dead. If the family wishes no more information about the organ-retrieval process than this, health care professionals should respect their wishes; however, if the family wishes more detail about the organ-retrieval process, that information should be provided to them in a thorough and sensitive matter.

Depending on where the machines will be removed—in the deceased patient's hospital room or in the operating room where the organ retrieval will occur—it may or may not be advisable to have the family present. Some families want to be at their loved one's side when the life-support machines are turned off. For them, this action serves as the true period to the last sentence of their loved one's life. Sensitive to such human sentiments, some health care professionals have developed policies that permit interested families' members to be present at the machine removal process, whether the removal occurs in the decreased patient's hospital room or in the operating room. Suffice it to say that every effort is made to handle such scenarios respectfully as well as efficiently.

Although it is challenging to develop good organ-retrieval policies for HBDs, who remain the cadaver donors of choice, it is even more difficult to develop such policies for NHBDs. As we noted above, NHBDs are identified in either uncontrolled or controlled contexts. A person who suffers a cardiac arrest at the scene of an accident, at home, in an ambulance on the way to the hospital, in an emergency room or in another uncontrolled context, and who cannot or should not be resuscitated is declared dead by cardiac criteria. If health care professionals think that the deceased person's organs are healthy, they may send his or her body to an operating room for ventilation and artificial cardiac support. They may also initiate cold perfusion via femoral cannulas to keep the deceased person's organs viable for transplant. Meanwhile, they will try to contact the family for instructions about how or how not to proceed, even if the deceased person was a registered organ donor. If family members are found and object to the deceased person's organs being used, health care professionals will discontinue their efforts to preserve the person's organs and give orders to transport the body to the morgue.

To the degree that health care professionals have concerns about using NHBDs who have died in uncontrolled contexts as organ donors, they have even more concerns about using NHBDs who have died in controlled contexts as organ donors. Typically, the latter NHBDs are patients from whom life-support machines have been deliberately withdrawn. Not wanting to give the impression that they have hastened such patients' death for reasons other than the patients' wishes, health care professionals have, for the most part, not used their organs for transplant purposes in the past. Many health care professionals have had a recent change of heart, however, in some measure due to family members' incredulous reactions to their reluctance. A case in point is the following one:

> Christine Frank knew one thing for certain on that horrible day when she was told neither of her teenage sons would survive a car accident. "I said, 'Listen to me now. They are to be organ donors. That was their wish'," said Frank, who lost James, 18, and Christopher, 15, in 1998. "When you're hit with tragedy, if you're any kind of survivor, you're going to find something to hold on to, to find it made sense."
>
> Christine Frank, of Cincinnati, had talked about organ donation with her sons not six months before they died and knew that is what they wanted. Retrieving organs from James was relatively straightforward. A ventilator kept his heart pumping and lungs moving while doctors conducted tests that showed he had no brain function, meaning he was brain dead. To preserve James's organs, the ventilator stayed on until surgeons could begin harvesting.
>
> A ventilator also was keeping Christopher's heart pumping. But he had minimal brain function. When a CT scan showed his brain stem was critically injured, indicating no chance for survival, his parents told doctors to end life support. Doctors turned off the machine, waited for his heart to stop beating, then waited five more minutes to be sure it would not start again. At that point, Christopher was officially dead, and doctors could begin harvesting his kidneys.
>
> Thinking of the two women who received kidneys from Christopher, Christine Frank is baffled that cardiac donation is so rare. "I don't understand why it's not being done everywhere," she said.[39]

Part of the answer to Christine Frank's bafflement is that, like many other people, many health care professionals are uncertain about when death actually occurs. The most important response to Christine Frank's question is, however, that health care professionals do not want to pressure either family members or patients to stop life-sustaining treatments in order to precipitate cardiac arrest and death. In addition, they do not want uninformed individuals to get the wrong idea if they happen to witness the medical procedures that occur when machines are about to be withdrawn from a patient who is a designated organ donor. While still alive, the patient may be prepped for surgery. Moreover, in some instances, anticoagulants and vasodilators may be administered to the patient, not to benefit the patient but to preserve the quality of his or her organs. Similarly, while the patient is still alive, perfusion and cooling cannulas may be inserted into him or her, once again for the purposes of organ donation. Unless these procedures are carefully explained to interested parties, it is possible to convey the impression that the patient's death is being hastened.

In an effort to avoid misunderstandings about using NHBDs in controlled contexts as organ donors, many hospitals require that the patient or the patient's surrogate initiate the conversation about the possibility of organ donation. Specifically, the IOM recommends that the "decision to withdraw life-sustaining treatment or to stop cardiopulmonary resuscitation should be made before the option of organ and tissue donation is discussed."[40] In addition, the IOM advises health care professionals not to use medications simply to sustain organ quality or to insert lines into the patient before life-support machine withdrawal unless it is truly necessary to do so and the family is in full agreement.

V. INCREASING THE SUPPLY OF ORGANS

Clearly, health care professionals would not find it necessary to use organs to which serious ethical question marks are attached if the pool of organ donors, particularly cadaver donors, was far larger than it is today. According to several polls, more than 70% of American adults say they want to donate their organs after their death,[41] yet relatively few actually sign donor cards.[42] The main reasons people do not sign donor cards include not liking the idea of being cut up, lingering fears that health care professionals may hasten their death in order to secure their organs, and a general reluctance to confront matters related to death. Other reasons include lack of information about how to become an organ donor. Were we as aggressive about getting people to be organ donors as we are about getting people to give blood, perhaps we could go a long way to resolving the organ shortage problem. Only recently have advertisements about the benefits of organ donation appeared in the print and electronic media. In addition, a variety of more formal, usually legal, remedies have been suggested to increase the number of organs available for transplant. They include required request laws, routine notification laws, mandated choice laws, presumed consent initiatives, financial incentive laws, and even consideration of a full-scale organ market.

A. Required Request

Because many people do not have organ donor cards and/or an advance care directive identifying themselves as organ donors, health care professionals are faced with the task of asking grieving family members about their loved one's desire to be an organ donor. Not surprisingly, many health care professionals find this task so difficult that they fail to perform it. In an effort to remedy this state of affairs, federal and state laws were passed requiring health care professionals and/or other designated persons to approach all families of donor-eligible patients about their loved one's organ donation wishes. Although hospitals have complied with these laws, "it has been demonstrated that consent to organ donation is obtained in no more than half of cases."[43] Among the reasons for this 50% failure rate are that some health care professionals make the organ donation request in an abrupt, awkward, or alienating manner; some families are not sure about their loved one's wishes; and some families simply refuse to honor their loved one's organ-donation wishes. They either cannot bear the thought of their loved one's body being "cut up" or they want to make funeral arrangements as quickly as possible.

B. Routine Notification

Realizing that because most health care professionals are not specially trained to make organ-donation requests, they may be unable to properly execute required request laws, US health care authorities now require hospitals to report all deaths to a local OPO. In some instances, hospitals have asked OPO personnel to make the initial organ-donation request as well as to explain in detail the organ-donation process to families. A notable percentage of families view this way of handling their situation as somewhat cold and impersonal, however. Numerous studies show that organ-donation requests are most likely to succeed when the deceased patient's attending physicians and/or nurses make the initial request and OPO personnel simply add further explanation. Apparently, many patients' families want the "person who knows the patient's condition best"[44] or who has spent the most time with them to make the initial request.

C. Mandated Choice

Because families do not always honor their loved one's organ-donation wishes, and because health care professionals and OPO personnel are very reluctant to proceed without the family's consent, organ donors' wishes to give the gift of life are sometimes defied in death. In an effort to take the family out of the organ-donation consent process as much as possible, some experts have proposed that everyone, or at least the majority of the adult population, be required to identify themselves as either organ donors or organ nondonors when they apply for a driver's license or are admitted to a hospital or other health care facility. After identifying themselves as organ donors/organ nondonors, individuals would be assured that their organ-donation wishes would be honored irrespective of their family preferences.

Although the AMA favors mandated choice laws, experiments to implement them have had "counterproductive" results so far.[45] For example, Texas decided to repeal its mandated choice law when it discovered that subsequent to the passage of the law, there was a drop in the number of individuals identifying themselves as organ donors. Rather than increasing the pool of organ donors, as had been hoped, the law decreased the pool to only 20% of eligible Texans. Apparently, the mandated choice law heightened Texans' fear that if someone identified themselves as an organ donor, physicians would not "do as much [as they should] to save their lives."[46] Moreover, despite the fact that many people do not want their family members to trump their organ-donation decisions, others (indeed as many as 56.8% in one study) prefer their family members to make the final judgment call.[47]

D. Presumed Consent

Very popular in European nations, presumed consent policies rely on the assumption that unless individuals have taken "proactive, explicit, and legally sanctioned measures to register their refusal,"[48] it is safe to assume they would want to be organ donors. The reasoning behind this assumption is inspired by the altruistic thought that the bulk of the population is willing to give the "gift of life" to someone when they no longer need them for their own use, and that only a few persons would want to take every piece of their body to the grave.

Interestingly, despite all the reports that Europeans are far more communitarian than individualistic Americans are, European presumed consent laws have not actually worked any better than U.S. required request/mandated choice laws. Like U.S. health care professionals, European health care professionals are reluctant to proceed with the organ retrieval process if family members protest. In fact, if family members provide oral testimony that their loved one had no interest in serving as an organ donor, European health care professionals halt the organ-retrieval process. As they see it, family protest nullifies the *presumption* of patient consent to organ donation.

Even if European presumed consent laws worked perfectly in European nations, the U.S. citizenry would probably resist the passage of similar laws in the United States. When U.S. citizens are polled about presumed consent laws, less than one-fourth show support for them.[49] Given the fact that many U.S. citizens do not fully trust health care professionals' motives when it comes to securing organs for transplant purposes, a presumed consent law may cause large numbers of them to document an unwillingness to serve as organ donors. Critics of presumed consent laws also note the unsettling fact that although educated, privileged people would have the advantage of opting out of the organ donor pool, less educated people, many of whom belong to economically and/or racially disadvantaged populations, may not be aware of "opt-out" procedures. As a result of the disparity just described, the organs of a disproportional number of individuals from an economically and/or racially disadvantaged population might find themselves in the bodies of advantaged individuals willing to use others' organs but not to share their own.

E. Financial Incentives

Because required request, routine notification, mandated choice, and presumed consent regulations and laws have not been able to meet the demand for organs, some experts recommend rethinking the assumption that altruism and voluntarism must be the exclusive or primary motivations behind organ donation. As they see it, the 1984 **National Organ Transplant Act (NOTA),** which forbids ". . . any person knowingly to acquire, receive, or otherwise transfer any human organ for valuable consideration for use in a human transplantation if the transfer affects interstate commerce,"[50] should either be repealed or amended to permit certain sorts of financial incentives for organ donation, particularly cadaver organ donation. Proposed financial incentive policies for cadaver organ donation include providing a small funeral expense benefit to organ donors' family; sending a modest contribution to organ donors' favorite charity or designated beneficiary; reducing declared organ donors' health care costs in return for "future rights" to their organs upon death; and giving preferential treatment to declared organ donors who find themselves in need of an organ while still alive.[51] Each one of these proposals is beset by one or another ethical concern, most of which have to do with enticing people of limited means to "share" their own or family members' organs in return for some monetary benefit, however small, and/or disrupting the present system of organ allocation which tries to make its decisions on medical criteria alone.

F. Commercialization of Organs

Even more controversial than the financial incentives for organs we just discussed are proposals to offer patients on the verge of death a lump sum for access to their organs upon death and/or offering families a lump sum for their deceased loved one's organs. Depending on the amount of this lump sum, inappropriate acts of heroism and/or inappropriate acts of profiting from the death of one's relatives might occur. A woman with just a short time to live may willingly refuse costly, beneficial treatment if she knows that, upon her death, her struggling family will inherit money they desperately need. Or a family, who knows their loved one did not want to be an organ donor, may nonetheless hide this fact from health care professionals in order to sell his or her organs for the going rate.[52]

Concerned as critics are about paying lump sums to *cadaver donors* and/or their families, they are even more concerned about paying lump sums to *living donors* for their organs. The main argument against permitting living donors to sell their organs is that such sales would lead to the further commodification of the human body; however, many people believe that their body is their property and that they should be able to sell parts of it if they so choose. They point out that we already permit people to sell their hair, blood, sperm, and eggs. Why, then, should we prohibit them from selling their organs, whole or in part, if they understand the attendant risks? After all, people do all sorts of risky things for money.[53]

To the argument that people have a right to sell parts of their body if they so choose, responses include the point that even if this right exists, it is not unlimited. The law forbids people to sell themselves into slavery not only because it is morally wrong for one person to own another a person, as if persons were just things to add to one's pile of possessions, but also because the ability to transfer ownership of one's own body or parts of it to another person "may result in unacceptable exploitation of the poor."[54] In a 2004 *New York Times* article on the global organ market, reporter Larry Rohter detailed how a U.S. woman received a kidney in South Africa from a poor Brazilian man as part of a global network of **organ traffickers**. Although the 48-year-old woman knew that it is illegal to buy a kidney in the United States and in many other nations, she had been on kidney dialyses for 15 years and on two kidney transplant lists for 7 years. Her health was getting very bad and her physicians allegedly told her to get a kidney any way she could. The woman's husband heard about an organ trafficking ring in Israel. Desperate for help, he contacted the leader of the ring, Ilan Peri, who, because of the woman and man's relatively modest means, asked them for $60,000 (half the ordinary fee of $130,000 for a kidney). Peri then contacted Shushan Meir, an Israeli-born South African, to find a kidney donor for the woman. In turn, Meir contacted his agents in Brazil who recruited a willing donor. A poor man from the slums of Recife, Brazil was flown to South Africa for the procedure. He received $6,000 for his kidney (the other $54,000 went to the organ traffickers).

Although all the middle-men in the scheme were eventually prosecuted under one or another nation's laws, the South African hospital and its transplant team escaped sanctions. Adding to the ethical complexity of the case just described is the fact that the donor's payment was stolen from him on his way home and he is now far less healthy than he used to be. Nevertheless, the man maintains that he would do it again not only for the money but also for the woman whose life he saved.[55]

The woman is doing well and is extremely grateful to her donor. Her only regret is that he did not get his money. She and her husband plan to send him money whenever they have extra funds. None of the woman's U.S. physicians have asked her about how she got her kidney, even as they willingly provide her with needed follow-up care. Although some ethics experts regard this state of affairs as a win–win situation for both donors and recipients, others regard it and situations like it as fraught with moral peril. They note with concern that before all the middlemen in the organ-trafficking ring were caught in the nets of one legal system or another, poor men in Recife were "volunteering" to sell their organs for $3,000.[56]

VI. ALLOCATION OF ORGANS

So far we have focused on organ donors. As expected, the ethical and legal issues that surround organ recipients are no less complex. Because organs are such a scarce resource, there have always been questions about the fairest way to distribute them. Before kidney transplants became as successful as they are today, the only other option individuals in end-stage renal disease had was kidney dialysis. In the 1960s, however, there were far more patients in end-stage renal disease than kidney-dialysis units could accommodate. As we mentioned in Chapter 2, in the early 1960s, a Seattle hospital that could accommodate only a handful of the city's end-stage renal disease patients established an advisory committee (composed of laypersons and health care professionals) that would decide on criteria for selecting kidney dialysis patients. The committee interviewed prospective kidney dialysis patients and made decisions that were in large measure based upon the "social worth" of each candidate. For example, in making his selections, one committee member later confessed that he remembered "voting against a young woman who was a known prostitute. I found I couldn't vote for her, rather than another candidate, a young wife and mother. I also voted against a young man who, until he learned he had renal failure, had been a ne'er-do-well, a real playboy."[57] When the larger public discovered that the selection committee was "playing God" with people's lives and using allocation criteria that reflected "middle-class suburban value system(s)," health care ethicists and policymakers realized that something had to be done to distribute scarce, life-saving resources more fairly.

Eventually, policymakers resolved the kidney dialysis controversy in a dramatic way. In 1972, after intense lobbying pressure, the U.S. Congress decided to fund all patients needing renal dialysis or renal transplantation. It passed the **End-Stage Renal Disease Act (ESRDA)**.[58] At the time the act was passed, its advocates claimed that its high initial costs would decline, as technology developed. This optimistic prediction proved false.[59] By 1991, the program cost more than 6 billion dollars per year.[60] Today it costs more than 22 billion dollars a year and there is no reason to think it will cost less in the future.[61]

Clearly, the ESRDA experience underscores the fact that saving lives can be a very expensive endeavor. As we shall discuss in Chapter 13, total health care costs are so high in the United States that public officials are no longer inclined to promise everyone in the United States expensive medical treatments on demand. Moreover, even if United States public officials had the will to fund all organ transplants and not just kidney transplants, they would not be able to provide enough organs for transplantation, short of requiring individuals to "donate" their organs at death and/or permitting individuals, while alive, to sell their organs for considerable sums of money.

Reluctant to force citizens to be either cadaveric organ donors or living organ donors, US federal and state authorities have tried to devise fair ways to allocate the organs that are available for transplant. In 1984, the U.S. Congress passed the **National Organ Transplant Act.**[62] This act created the **Organ Procurement and Transportation Network (OPTN)**[63] which is managed by the **United Network for Organ Sharing (UNOS)**, a private non-profit organization.[64] The organization UNOS determines the criteria for organ allocation in the United States and coordinates the efforts of the 69 **OPOs.**[65] When an organ becomes available for transplant, UNOS initially offers it to rank-ordered, qualified medical matches in the geographic area from which the organ came. If no one in that geographic area is a medical match for the available organ, it is then offered within the larger region (eleven nationwide) from which the organ came. Finally, if no one in that region is a medical match for the available organ, it is offered nationwide.

On paper, UNOS's allocation system seems ideal. Unfortunately, like all the systems human beings devise, UNOS's allocation system is flawed. For example, some people may live in geographic areas where the number of organ donors is high, but the number of patients waiting for organs is low. In contrast, other people may live in geographic areas where the number of organ donors is low, but the number of patients waiting for organs is high. Thus, people who need organs in organ-scarce geographic areas may seek wait-list status in several geographic areas in order to maximize their chance of getting an organ. In addition, UNOS may alter its system to become more national in focus. As soon as an organ becomes available, it would be offered nationwide irrespective of its place of origin.[66]

A. Criteria for Placement on an Organ Waiting List

As we just noted above, some patients get wait-listed at more than one transplant center. Getting on one waiting list—let alone several waiting lists—is no easy task, however.[67] Individual transplant centers are permitted to set their own waiting list criteria. Most centers use criteria such as "the prospects for successful surgery, the duration of the expected benefit, and the post-transplantation quality of life."[68] They do not want to give an organ to someone who is in such poor physical condition, for instance, that they cannot benefit from a transplantation. In addition, some transplant centers exclude from their waiting lists people over a certain age, people who have committed serious crimes, or people who are already wait-listed at another transplant center.[69] In contrast, other transplant centers do not object to waitlisting elderly persons, felons, or multilisted individuals provided they can benefit from a transplant. Instead, they refuse to wait-list patients without supportive familial networks, or patients whom they perceive as unable and unwilling to follow medical orders. For example, Hall, Ellman, and Strouse describe a very troubling case in which a prestigious heart and lung transplant center refused to wait-list a 34-year-old woman with Downs Syndrome "because physicians thought she was not sufficiently intelligent to comply with the complicated post-transplant drug regimen."[70] Still other transplant centers refuse to wait-list patients whom they perceive as somehow personally responsible for the failure of their organs. Specifically, some liver transplant centers exclude all alcoholics and smokers from their wait lists, unless these individuals enter and stay in treatment programs for their addiction. Other transplant centers think that it is "ill-advised" to base wait-list standards on the concept of individual responsibility because of "inadequate consensus about virtue, undue selectivity about what behaviors will deserve eligibility, and invasions of privacy."[71] They point out that if transplant centers reject individuals addicted to alcohol and smoking, they should also reject individuals addicted to food, particularly high-cholesterol food.

Sad to say, ability to pay is probably the single factor which prevents otherwise qualified patients from being wait-listed at a transplant center. Over a decade ago, health care ethicist Arthur Caplan noted that the costs for transplants were very steep: $35,000 for a liver transplant; $60,000–$100,000 for a heart transplant; and $150,000–$250,000 for a liver transplant.[72] These costs have all gone up, and as Caplan points out, they do not typically include travel costs (which can be considerable if the transplant is to take place out of town), family visitation costs, time out of work, and child care.[73] Although Medicare currently covers heart, liver, and bone marrow transplants in addition to kidney transplants, it does not cover transplants it considers experimental. Medicaid pays for several kinds of transplants in some states, but only for bone marrow transplants in other states. Moreover, private health care insurance plans may or may not cover some or all of the costs for certain transplants. Patients are often not aware that their private health care insurance plans do not cover, for example, a pancreas transplant procedure until they are in desperate need of one. The only recourse such patients have is to pay out of pocket and/or rely on the charity of others.

Although most transplant centers try to include a certain number of "charity cases" on their transplant lists as a matter of public duty and/or institutional conscience, they cannot provide a "free" organ transplant to anyone who needs one. Whether it is permissible to use patients' financial status as a criterion for exclusion on a transplant waiting list is, of course, highly debatable. Some health care ethicists think that public monies and charity monies should not be spent on very expensive transplants for small numbers of poor people, when large numbers of poor people lack basic health care. In response to this point, other health care ethicists note that society cannot expect relatively poor people to donate their organs at death if they routinely land in the bodies of relatively rich people, unsympathetic to the plight of those who cannot pay their own medical bills.

B. Criteria for Receiving an Organ

As we noted above, as soon as a patient gets on a transplant list, their position on it will be determined not only by the length of time they have spent on the list, but also by medical criteria such as their need for the transplant and/or the likelihood of their actually benefiting from it. Patients awaiting transplant are put into one of six categories. Category One includes the least sick individuals, people who are still able to work or attend school, whereas Category Six includes the sickest patients, people who are often on life-support of one type or another. In general, the sickest patients have first priority for an organ transplant, which fits well with Americans' adherence to the **rule of rescue**. Our emotions are such that we want to rescue a person from death if we are able to do so, even though our reason tells us that it probably does not make good sense to give precious organs to very sick individuals who are not likely to have nearly as good outcomes as less sick individuals. For example, in 1991 the 1-year success rate for liver transplant was only 47.0% in Class Six recipients, whereas it was 79.1% in Class One recipients.[74] Because of outcome studies such as this one, many health care ethicists think that very sick patients should have transplant priority only if they are likely to do as well postoperatively as less sick patients would. For this reason, Mickey Mantle, sick as he was, should probably not have received a liver transplant on June 8, 1995. The baseball legend, who had both pickled his liver with alcohol and blackened his lungs with smoke, died of complications associated with lung cancer on August 13, 1995. Mantle's physicians must have known about their patient's total health profile when they placed him at the top of their institution's liver transplant list. Thus, their ultimate goal in transplanting Mantle may have been "limelight" rather than "rendering appropriate care to their patient while upholding the standard of medical care."[75]

Not only do emotions govern transplant lists in cases like that of Mickey Mantle, they also play a strong role in **retransplantation** cases. Although patients who need a retransplant because their bodies rejected the first or even second organ that was given to them are usually very sick, and unlikely to respond well to a third organ, many transplant teams nonetheless accord such patients' preferential treatment. In theory, retransplant patients should go to the bottom of Class Six, the overall class of patients to which they will probably be assigned; however, in practice, they often find themselves at the top of Class Six because the health care professionals who originally tried to help them may be unwilling to give up on them, or may feel some special duty to them. For example, when a transplant team at Duke University gave, by mistake, an incompatible lung to a young patient named Jesica Santillan who promptly rejected it, they felt a special obligation to retransplant her even though they suspected that the retransplant was probably futile in her case. Due to the hospital's "lack of redundancy," which amounted to not comparing Jesica's blood type to the organ donor's, Jesica's transplant was not compatible, and her immune system began to attack the organs within 40 minutes of the procedure. A second set of organs became available for Jesica 13 days later. Surgeons performed another transplant, but it was too late. Jesica had suffered from brain damage following the first transplant, and she died 2 days later from internal bleeding.[76]

VII. Conclusion

Americans' need for organs is likely to increase in the future because of the aging of the U.S. population. Regrettably, the cost of organ transplants is not likely to decrease; and, short of coercive laws or, preferably, an epidemic of altruism in the United States, there will never be a large enough supply of human organ donors, cadaver or living, to meet the demand for them. Putting aside the cost issue for a moment, the organ-supply problem might be resolved by developing better artificial organs than the ones developed in the past, a major breakthrough in xenograft research, or growing organs from stem cells programmed to accomplish this feat. So far, there is considerable reason to think that it will take an extended period of time before large numbers of individuals are walking around with totally implantable artificial hearts, pig livers, or stem cell derived lungs in their bodies. But there is a real possibility that researchers may be able to develop treatments and/or drugs for failing organs in the same way that they have developed treatments and/or drugs for other life-threatening conditions such as cancer, diabetes, and HIV-AIDS. Such treatments and drugs are likely to be expensive, however. Even if we solve the organ-supply problem, we cannot solve the organ-demand problem without spending a conceivably disproportional portion of our total health care budget on organ-transplant operations and follow-up care. In the future, one of the best ways to solve the organ-demand problem might be by *not* meeting it in all cases, but only in some. Rationing may prove to be the court of last resort in the world of transplantation.

Discussion Questions and Case Studies

1. Jacob Wilson, in his mid-fifties and father of four children, received a kidney transplant in 2001. In early 2003, his body rejected the kidney. In late 2003, he received a second kidney that lasted until early 2004. Mr. Wilson received a third kidney in late 2004 after a local television station recounted his story. From this case four moral perspectives emerge.
   a. Mr. Wilson should not have received the third kidney because he had already received two other kidneys, both of which failed. He should have been placed at the very bottom of the waiting list.

  b.   Because Mr. Wilson's medical team had invested so much time and effort into saving him, he should have received the third kidney, even if he was moved ahead of patients who had not received even one kidney.

  c.   Organ transplantations should be based on a blind lottery. Therefore, Mr. Wilson's opportunity should not be based on history, but on random selection. To do otherwise constitutes discrimination.

  d.   Mr. Wilson's selection was influenced by the media and gave him an unfair advantage in obtaining a transplant. While no one advocates his returning the kidney, neither can the receipt of it be deemed moral.

   1.   Assess the relative strengths and weaknesses of the four moral perspectives described above.

   2.   What value assumptions are relevant when prioritizing organ recipients?

   3.   What role, if any, should the "rule of rescue" have in moral deliberations concerning organ transplantations?

2. Some parents of anencephalic infants request discontinuation of life-sustaining measures in order to donate of their infant's organs to infants whose lives can be saved. In this way, families find their infants' death more tolerable.

  a.   Is it wrong to hasten the death of anencephalic infants so that their organs can be used for infants who have a chance to lead a "more meaningful" life?

  b.   Are you for or against defining not only anencephalic infants but also individuals in a persistent vegetative state as officially dead, so that their organs can be retrieved for transplant purposes? Why or why not?

3. In 1991, Governor Robert Casey of Pennsylvania suffered a heart attack. He also suffered from amyloidosis, a hereditary heart disease that causes the liver to produce a protein that weakens other organs. By 1993, Governor Casey was placed on a waiting list for a heart–liver transplant. He received both in less than a day even though the average waiting time was 67 days for a liver and 198 days for a heart. Governor Casey's selection for transplant bypassed eight other candidates ahead of him who required either a heart or a liver.

  a.   Should someone needing two transplants take priority over someone needing only one?

  b.   Should priority be given to public officials ? What about celebrities?

  c.   Does the likelihood of a favorable medical outcome affect the moral rightness or wrongness of such a selection practice?

4. A woman was advised that she needed a bone marrow transplant and radiation therapy to halt the progression of breast cancer. Her health plan refused to pay for the procedure on the grounds that bone marrow transplants for breast cancer are experimental procedures and not proven accepted treatment's. The woman's appeal to the insurance company was rejected. However, the Medical Center at which she was being treated agreed to absorb the cost, enabling the woman to have the transplant. Unfortunately, she died 18 months later.

  a.   Did the health care insurance company act in a morally responsible or irresponsible way? Must health care insurance companies cover all life-saving treatments, no matter how expensive?

  b.   Does the fact that the woman lived only 18 *months* after the transplant affect your answer to (a) in one way or another? What if she had lived only 18 more *days*? What if she had lived 18 more *years*?

5. What role, if any, should "social worth" and "lifestyle choices" have in the allocation of organs? Do you think alcoholics, heavy smokers, and/or extremely obese individuals should be put on organ waiting lists, and if so, under what conditions, if any? Do you think prisoners on death row should be transplanted? Why or why not?

6. Do you favor rationing organ transplants on the grounds that they are very expensive? Why or why not?

Endnotes

1. Renée C. Fox and Judith P. Swazey, "Organ and tissue transplants," in: Warren T. Reich (ed.), *Encyclopedia of Bioethics* (New York: Simon and Schuster, 1995), p. 1982.

2. Ibid.

3. Friedrich K. Port, Dawn M. Dykstra, Robert M. Merion, and Robert Wolfe, "Trends and results for organ donation and transplantation in the United States, 2004," *2004 OPTN/SRTR Annual Report (Organ Procurement and Transplantation Network and the Scientific Registry of Transplant Recipients), Table 1.3* (2004), *http://www.ustransplant.org/annual_reports/2004/chapter_i_AR_cd. htm* [accessed April 19, 2005].

4. Ibid., *Table 1.6*.

5. Ibid.

6. Lois LaCivita Nixon, "Dirty pretty things: a narrative frame for black market organ sale," *Lahey Clinic Medical Ethics*, 11, no. 2 (Spring 2004): 9.

7. National Kidney Foundation, "Milestones in organ transplantation," *National Kidney Foundation, Inc.* (December 27, 2002), *http://www.kidneysocal.org/ milestones.html* [accessed April 19, 2005].

8. Friedrich K. Port, Dawn M. Dykstra, Robert M. Merion, and Robert Wolfe, "Trends and results for organ donation and transplantation in the United States, 2004," *2004 OPTN/SRTR Annual Report (Organ Procurement and Transplantation Network and the Scientific Registry of Transplant Recipients), Table 1.1* (2004), *http://www.ustransplant.org/annual_reports/2004/chapter_i_AR_cd.htm* [accessed April 19, 2005].

9. Ibid., *Table 1.11a*.

10. Ibid.

11. Ibid.

12. Steven L. Solomon, "CDC response to infections related to human tissue transplantation," *Centers for Disease Control* (May 14, 2003), *http://www.cdc. gov/ washington/testimony/ps051403.htm* [accessed April 19, 2005].

13. Lance K. Stell, "Organ transplantation: how far have we come, how far should we go?" *The Ethical View: A Publication of the Medical Humanities Program of Davidson College* (March 2005): 5.

14. Ibid., p. 6.

15. Martin Pernick, "Brain death in a cultural context: the reconstruction of death 1967–1981," in: Stuart J. Youngner, Robert M. Arnold, Renie Schapiro (eds.), *The Definition of Death: Contemporary Controversies* (Baltimore, MD: Johns Hopkins University Press, 1999), pp. 3–33.

16. Ibid.

17. Stuart J. Youngner and Robert M. Arnold, "Philosophical debates about the definition of death: who cares?" *Journal of Medicine and Philosophy*, 26, no. 5 (October 2001): 528.

18. Ibid.

19. Michael Potts, "A requiem for whole brain death: a response to D. Alan Shewmon's 'The brain and somatic integration,'" *Journal of Medicine and Philosophy*, 26, no. 5 (October 2001): 481.

20. Ibid., p. 485.

21. John A. Robertson, "The dead donor rule," *Hastings Center Report*, 29, no. 6 (1999): 6.

22. Robert M. Veatch, "The dead donor rule: true by definition," *The American Journal of Bioethics*, 3, no. 1 (Winter 2003): 10.

23. Eileen P. Flynn, *Issues in Health Care Ethics* (Upper Saddle River, NJ: Prentice Hall, 2000), p. 172.

24. G. Kootstra, J. H. C Daemen, and A. P. A Oomen, "Categories of non-heart beating donors," *Transplant Procurement*, 27 (1995): 2893–2894.

25. Stuart J. Youngner and Robert M. Arnold, "Philosophical debates about the definition of death: who cares?" *Journal of Medicine and Philosophy*, 26, no. 5 (2001): 531.

26. Stuart J. Youngner, Robert M. Arnold, and Michael A. DeVita, "When is 'dead'"? *The Hastings Center Report: Organ Transplantation*, 29, no. 6 (November– December 1999): 19.

27. John A. Robertson, "The dead donor rule," *Hastings Center Report*, 29, no. 6 (1999): 11.

28. Stuart J. Youngner, Robert M. Arnold, and Michael A. DeVita, "When is 'dead'"? *The Hastings Center Report: Organ Transplantation*, 29, no. 6 (November– December 1999): 17.

29. Ibid.

30. Robert D. Troug, "Is it time to abandon brain death?" *Hastings Center Report*, 27, no. 1 (1997): 29–37.

31. Lance K. Stell, "Organ transplantation: how far have we come, how far should we go?" *The Ethical View*, 4, no. 1 (2005): 6.

32. Marsha Rule, "Living organ donors improve the lives of others," *UW Medicine* (Winter/Spring 2005), *http://depts.washington.edu/mnw/organdonor.html* [accessed May 22, 2005].

33. Friedrich K. Port, Dawn M. Dykstra, Robert M. Merion, and Robert Wolfe, "Trends and results for organ donation and transplantation in the United States, 2004," *OPTN/SRTR Annual Report* (March 30, 2005), *http://www.optn.org/AR2004/chapter_i_AR_cd.htm* [accessed May 22, 2005].

34. Ibid.

35. Renèe C. Fox and Judith P. Swazey, *Spare Parts: Organ Replacement in American Society* (Oxford: Oxford University Press, 1992), p. 40.

36. Ryan Sauder and Lisa S. Parker, "Autonomy's limits: living donation and health-related harm," *Hastings Center Report*, 10, no. 4 (2001): 399.

37. Mark F. Anderson, "The future of organ transplantation: from where will new donors come, to whom will their organs go?" *Journal of Law Medicine*, 5, no. 2 (Summer 1995): 31.

38. Eileen P. Flynn, *Issues in Health Care Ethics* (Upper Saddle River, NJ: Prentice-Hall, 2000), pp. 171–172.

39. "Non-beating hearts an obstacle for organ donation," *Organ Transplant Association* (August 28, 2002), *http://organtx.org/ethics/nonheart.htm* [accessed May 18, 2005].

40. Institute of Medicine, *Non-Heart Beating Organ Transplantation: Practice and Protocols* (2000), p. 42.

41. Advisory Committee on Organ Transplantation (ACOT) Members, "U.S. Department of Health and Human Services Advisory Committee on Organ Transplantation," *Donate Life* (May 23, 2003), *http://www.organdonor.gov/acot5-03.html* [accessed May 17, 2005].

42. Ibid.

43. Laura A. Siminoff and Mary Beth Mercer, "Public policy, public opinion, and consent for organ donation," *Cambridge Quarterly of Healthcare Ethics*, 10, no. 4 (Fall 2001): 378.

44. Ibid., p. 379.

45. Ibid., p. 380.

46. Ibid.

47. Ibid.

48. Ibid, p. 381.

49. Ibid.

50. National Organ Transplant Act. Pub. Lit. No. 98-507, 3 Usc 3ol.2, 1984.

51. Laura A. Siminoff and Mary Beth Mercer, "Public policy, public opinion, and consent for organ donation," *Cambridge Quarterly of Healthcare Ethics*, 10, no. 4 (Fall 2001): 381–383.

52. A.H. Barnett and David L. Kaserman, "The shortage of organs for transplantation: exploring the alternatives," *Issues in Law and Medicine*, 9, no. 2 (1993): 117.

53. Lori B. Andrews, "My body, my property," *Hastings Center Report*, 16, no. 5 (1986): 28.

54. Lori Andrews et al., "Sacred or for sale?" *Harper's Magazine* (October, 1990): 47, 50.

55. Larry Rohter, "Tracking the sale of a kidney on a path of poverty and hope," *New York Times* (May 23, 2004): 1, 8.

56. Ibid.

57. Mark A. Hall, Ira Mark Ellman, and Daniel S. Strouse, "Defining death and transplanting organs," in: Hall, Ellman, and Strouse (eds.), *Health Care Law and Ethics* (St. Paul, MN: West Group, 1999), pp. 298–299.

58. "Timeline: pertinent events regarding medical resource allocation and kidney dialysis," *"Seattle's God Committee": Allocation of Limited Medical Services* (April 24, 2005), *http://medicine.creighton.edu/idc135/2004/Group6b/Timeline.htm* [accessed May 18, 2005].

59. Robert S. Lockridge, "The direction of end-stage renal disease reimbursement in the United States," *Seminars in Dialysis* (March 2004), 17, no. 2: 125–130, *http://www.blackwell-synergy.com/links/doi/10.1111/j.0894-0959.2004.17209.x/abs/* [accessed May 18, 2005].

60. Azza M. Jayaprakash, "Can medicare keep its contract?" *American Medical Association,* 6, no. 4 (April 2004), *http://www.ama-assn.org/ama/pub/category/12186.html* [accessed May 22, 2005].

61. Ibid.

62. Mark A. Hall, Ira Mark Ellman, and Daniel S. Strouse, "Defining death and transplanting organs," in: Hall, Ellman, and Strouse (eds.), *Health Care Law and Ethics* (St. Paul, MN: West Group, 1999), pp. 295.

63. Ibid.

64. Ibid.

65. Ibid.

66. Mark A. Hall, Ira Mark Ellman, and Daniel S. Strouse, "Defining death and transplanting organs," in: Hall, Ellman, and Strouse (eds.), *Health Care Law and Ethics* (St. Paul, MN: West Group, 1999), pp. 298.

67. Arthur Caplan, "Organ and tissue transplants: ethical and legal issues," in: Warren T. Reich (ed.), *Encyclopedia of Bioethics* (New York: Simon and Schuster, 1995), p. 1892.

68. Mark A. Hall, Ira Mark Ellman, and Daniel S. Strouse, "Defining death and transplanting organs," in: Hall, Ellman, and Strouse (eds.), *Health Care Law and Ethics* (St. Paul, MN: West Group, 1999), pp. 296.

69. Ibid., pp. 296–297.

70. Ibid., p. 297.

71. Ibid., p. 296.

72. Arthur Caplan, "Organ and tissue transplants: ethical and legal issues," in: Warren T. Reich (ed.), *Encyclopedia of Bioethics* (New York: Simon and Schuster, 1995), p. 1892.

73. Ibid.

74. UNOS Policies, *1993 Annual Report* supra note 130, app. at E-12.

75. Eileen P. Flynn, *Issues in Health Care Ethics* (Upper Saddle River, NJ: Prentice-Hall, 2000), p. 177.

76. David Resnick, "The Jesica Santillan tragedy: lessons learned," *Hastings Center Report,* 33, no. 4 (July–August 2003): 16–17.

chapter thirteen

Health Care Reform: Social Distribution Decisions

I. INTRODUCTION

In 1960, U.S. health care expenditures amounted to $120 billion; in 1970, they were up to $251 billion; in 1980, they increased to $431 billion; in 1990, they escalated to $805 billion; in 2000, they skyrocketed to $1,214 billion; and, then, in 2002, to $1.4 trillion.[1] Americans now spend more than 15% of their dollars, or $5,035 per capita on health care each year.[2] As a percentage of the gross national product (GNP), the cost of U.S. health care is about 14%, nearly twice as high as the percentage in most other developed nations.[3]

How did the costs of health care get so high in the United States? Why do people in the United Kingdom, Germany, and Canada pay only about half of what we pay for health care? And why is it that the United States is the only developed nation in the world that does not provide universal health care coverage to its citizens? Although 241,000,000 U.S. citizens are covered by either public health care insurance (Medicare or Medicaid) or private health care insurance (mostly employer provided, but in some instances privately purchased), 44,000,000 U.S. citizens have no health care insurance at all?[4] As we will see in this chapter, answers to these questions are not uniform. But unless we confront their dizzying complexities and politics, we cannot hope to understand the array of health care reform proposals that have emerged in recent years.

II. HEALTH CARE COSTS IN THE UNITED STATES

As we might expect, experts disagree with each other about the factors that contribute to the high cost of health care in the United States. Still, most of them lay a measure of the blame at the doorstep of one or more of the following culprits.

First, the U.S. population is aging. When the baby boom of 74 million people born in the United States between 1946 and 1964 reaches old age in 2030, people aged 65 and older will constitute at least 20% of the U.S. population. Those aged 85 and older will number 9 million, a threefold increase from the late 1970s. Because older people need more frequent health care than younger people do, the total cost of health care in the United States will rise each year as the combined number of the elderly increases.[5]

Second, today's elderly individuals tend to die not swiftly from an acute episode of cardiac arrest or pneumonia, for example, but slowly from a chronic condition like diabetes or Alzheimer's disease. We have learned how to prolong peoples' lives by keeping their illnesses under control for years, even decades. The home–health care, skilled nursing, and assisted living industries thrive, as more and more members of the U.S. population require their costly services. Given that 24% of people aged 85 and older, for example, are currently in skilled nursing homes at a per capita cost of $46,000[6] a year, the total elder care bill is likely to be extremely high by 2030 when the percentage of people in skilled nursing homes will have doubled.

Third, U.S. patients and/or their families demand aggressive treatment, and health care professionals provide the same, at both the end of life and the beginning of life. In this respect, health care ethicist Daniel Callahan notes, "[p]atients in general say they do not want excessive treatment, or to have their dying prolonged. But when the time for dying comes, they are perfectly capable of matching their physicians in their desire to see if just a *little* bit more might be done to gain a little more life."[7] No wonder, then, that at present almost 30% of patients' total costs are incurred within the last year of their lives, as progressively more aggressive and costly therapies are used.[8] Reluctance to give up on life is no less manifest at the beginning of life than it is at the end of life, however. Specifically, in 1995, the cost to save one extremely premature baby was approximately $158,000, and the total bill for neonatal intensive care was $2.6 billion[9] (admittedly, a relatively small amount compared to the $106.5 billion bill for long-term care in 1995,[10] but still one that shows how much Americans are prepared to spend to save a few lives).

Fourth, because "[t]echnology that would only be available in regional medical centers in some countries is available not only in community hospitals but in clinics and even physicians' offices in the U.S.,"[11] U.S. health care professionals often use it even when it is unlikely to medically benefit their patients. For example, in 1999 U.S. physicians performed 388.1 coronary angioplasties per 100,000 population. In contrast, German physicians performed only 165.7 of these procedures per 100,000 population, while U.K. physicians performed only 51 for the same number of people.[12] Statistics such as these help explain why per capita health care *technology* costs in the United States have increased by an astronomical 791%, compared with the more modest increase of 269% for health care spending in general.[13]

Fifth, the cost of prescription drugs in the United States is outrageously high,[14] largely because U.S. pharmaceutical companies claim they need to make their largest profits in the United States, where the costs of researching and designing to bring a single drug to market average more than 16 years and 800 million dollars.[15] Pharmaceutical companies engage in patent fights to get the exclusive rights to sell popular drugs like Claritin, which enriched Schering–Plough's coffers by $2.5 billion,[16] for wallet-breaking sums. In addition, these companies lobby lawmakers to prevent U.S. citizens from getting less expensive supplies of their name-brand products from other nations, particularly Canada,[17] and/or generic versions of their products, developed in poor nations that cannot afford to pay top-dollar for U.S. name-brand drugs. Finally, pharmaceutical companies visit physicians' offices with free supplies of their products and "sweeteners" such as free meals and "educational trips" to the Caribbean and other resort destinations. They also spend untold millions on TV advertisements directed to the public at large. These high price ads promise people not only health but, very often, productive, happy, and even "sexy" lives.

Sixth, because the U.S. health care insurance system is fragmented, some of it public (Medicare and Medicaid discussed below), but most of it private, it is administered not only by federal and state bureaucrats but also by private health care insurance agents, each of whom carries a different form to fill out in triplicate or more. Unable to fill out myriad forms, let alone haggle with health care insurance companies about their ever-changing policies, health care professionals and institutions have been forced to hire billing personnel. So costly are these office helpers that by the 1990s, one-eighth of every U.S. dollar spent on health care went to cover administrative costs. This state of affairs has only gotten worse since then. Indeed, according to health care economist Milton Fist, the amount of money now being spent on health care administrative costs is so large, it is enough to buy every uninsured individual in the United States, $3,000 worth of health care insurance per annum.[18]

Seventh, unlike health care professionals in most other developed nations, where physicians, for example, are not "fair game" for lawyers, U.S. health care professionals and institutions often practice medicine "defensively." For fear of civil suits, they order an excessive number of tests, refer their patients to specialists even when they know they do not need them, and keep detailed records of patient visits (for example, immediately after seeing me, my physician tape-records the results of my tests and his instructions to me on audiotape). In this connection, Dr. James Gordon recounts the story of a physician treating a patient in a military hospital. Explaining his treatment orders to a group of medical students, the physician noted that because he was in a military hospital that protected him from most civil malpractice suits, he had to order only the tests that were "really necessary"[19] for his patient. Were he in a civilian hospital, he would feel compelled to order unnecessary tests for fear of litigation.

So great is health care professionals' fear of being dragged into court that by the early 1990s they were paying a total of $5.6 billion per annum for malpractice insurance.[20] These costs have further soared in the 2000s, so much so that many physicians, for example, have either limited their scope of practice or dropped out of practice altogether. Very recently, some physicians have even gone on strike to demonstrate to patients the potentially disastrous consequences of excessive malpractice suits. They claim that soon it will be too expensive and emotionally harrowing for them to practice medicine. Indeed, in 2002, malpractice premiums for neurosurgeons averaged $71,200 per annum across the country, peaking in Philadelphia at $267,000. Premiums for obstetrician-gynecologists were also exceptionally high. They averaged $56,546 per annum across the country, peaking at $210,576 in Miami. Emergency physicians were also hit particularly hard. Their average malpractice insurance cost was $53,500 across the country, peaking, once again, in Miami at $150,000.[21]

Eighth, adding further avoidable costs to the health care bottom line is the fact that Americans assume little responsibility for their own health status, and health care professionals continue to practice a style of medicine that opts for a pound of cure over an ounce of prevention. Comment Joseph L. Bast, Richard C. Rue, and Stuart A. Wesbury: "Americans lead lifestyles that expose them to much higher rates of disease and health complications than faced by the people of most other nations. Sometimes we deliberately kill ourselves—suicide is the third leading cause of death among teenagers and young adults—but more often we eat, smoke, drink, or couch-potato ourselves to death."[22] Americans indulge their physical and psychological urges, fully expecting a miracle cure when it is time to pay the piper for their health "sins." So dependent are some Americans on the god "medicine" that they expect it to make them as beautiful as models, as sexy as movie stars, as fit as Olympic athletes, as smart as mathematical wizards, and as wealthy as Wall Street tycoons.

Ninth, there are far more specialists than primary care physicians in the United States, and specialists' fees are very high compared to those of primary care physicians. Whereas a primary care physician typically makes under $140,000 a year,[23] cardiologists, radiologists, and anesthesiologists are accustomed to making twice or even three times that much per annum.[24]

Understanding some of the factors that shoot health care costs to astronomical levels is helpful, but it does not explain why the U.S. citizenry and government, for that matter, continue to pay them with only half-hearted efforts to control them. Part of the reason for our willingness, however grudging, to spend what seems like a disproportional amount of our GNP on health care costs may be our cultural belief that the cost of health care goods and services operates like the cost of any kind of goods and services. Supposedly, "you get what you pay for," and, with respect to U.S. health care, you get the highest quality health care in the world. But this belief is just that, a belief, founded more on faith than fact. As it so happens, the **World Health Organization (WHO)** ranks the U.S. health care system number 37 on a list of 191 health care systems.[25]

Among the factors that WHO takes into account when it ranks health care systems are the quality of medical training, the development and use of medical technology, people's overall health status, and people's overall access to health care in a nation. Although the United States gets high marks for its medical schools and technological feats, it gets mediocre marks for its citizens' overall health status and overall access to health care. Significantly, a nation's overall health status seems to be closely connected to whether its citizens have universal health care coverage or not. Thus, it is not surprising that the IOM Committee on the Consequences of Uninsurance, has concluded that the United States' failure to provide its citizens with universal health care coverage is a failure it must address. Comments the Committee:

> The costs to society of having a large uninsured population do not come primarily from the costs of providing health services free of charge to them [$99 billion in 2001]. Rather, the major economic costs are the loss health and longevity by the uninsured due to their inadequate health care. In order to estimate the value of these poorer health outcomes, the Committee adapted an analytic strategy used by regulatory agencies such as the Environmental Protection Agency and the Food and Drug Administration to value the health benefits of environmental or safety interventions. The years that someone expects to enjoy over the course of a lifetime in particular states of health can be thought of as that person's stock of "health capital." Using its estimate of the mortality difference between insured and uninsured populations and estimates of health status differences between these groups as reflected in the nationally representative Health Interview Survey, the Committee calculated the value of health capital lost due to the lack of coverage. Assigning a value of $160,000 to a year of life in perfect health (a midrange estimate of values used by federal regulatory agencies and studies of individuals' willingness to pay for reductions in the risk of dying), the Committee estimated the value of forgone health among the uninsured as between $1,645 and $3,280 for each additional year without insurance. For 40 million uninsured Americans, the aggregate, annualized cost is between $65 and $130 billion.[26]

If we add this last cost of $65 to $130 billion to the $99 billion we pay out each year to cover the cost of care for people with health care insurance, the true annual cost of health care in the United States is somewhere between $174 billion and $229 billion. This last sum is more than enough to support a universal health care system in the United States; but because of largely political reasons, U.S. public officials cling to a health care insurance system that seems out of sync with "widely accepted democratic cultural and political norms of equal consideration and equal opportunity."[27] We have a class-stratified society in which those with adequate health care insurance have more opportunities to live their lives in good health than those who lack it.

A recent *New York Times* article entitled "Life at the top in America isn't just better, it's longer: three heart attacks, and what came next" dramatically documents the state of affairs noted above.[28] Each of three New Yorkers had a heart attack. The first New Yorker, a very well-off architect, was rushed to one of the best hospitals in New York City, had an angioplasty, got excellent follow-up care including help from a health-conscious wife, and significantly altered his health habits, so much so that his overall health status was better than it had been before he had his heart attack. The second heart attack victim, a middle-class, African-American with a job as a transportation coordinator, was initially taken to a hospital that did not do angioplasties, but was eventually transferred to one that did, when he made it clear that he was not in the mood for second-class treatment. He left the hospital with several prescriptions, including one for the same statins that his cardiologist had prescribed following his first and second heart attacks. Although his attempts to exercise and eat a healthy diet were somewhat sabotaged by his love of fried foods, he got his cholesterol levels down by faithfully taking his statins and reminding himself that his fourth heart attack might very well kill him before his 50th birthday. The third heart attack victim, a working-class domestic maid, originally from Poland, initially resisted going to a hospital. She protested that she did not have the time or money to be sick. Eventually, she relented and wound up in a large public hospital. She left it with one prescription for a statin. She stopped taking the drug when she realized her health care insurance plan did not cover the hefty price. Because she went back to work too soon after her heart attack, and because she was intent on satisfying the many demands of her newly acquired husband, the woman's health condition rapidly deteriorated. Her heart condition worsened and she developed diabetes.

III. HEALTH CARE INSURANCE ACCESSIBILITY IN THE UNITED STATES

A. Employer-Based Health Care Coverage

Although we might not realize it, our present system of health care coverage, in which most insured Americans obtain health care insurance through their employers rather than the government (Medicare and Medicaid being the exception), is not the result of a political debate during which it was decided that (1) employers should provide health care insurance to their employees and dependents and (2) the government should provide coverage only to individuals who cannot or should not work. Rather employer-based coverage was the result of employers volunteering to provide health care insurance to employees as a way "to improve incentives in the face of national wage freezes in the 1940s."[29] Health care coverage is a voluntary benefit. Employers do not have to offer it, a fact that should send chills down the spines of the 159,600,000 U.S. employees who rely on it for coverage.[30]

In the past, employers were able to comfortably provide health care insurance for both their employees and employees' dependants. But with the escalation of health care costs, many employers have found it increasingly difficult to offer adequate health coverage to their employees, let alone their dependents. In fact, by the 1990s, employers' health-care insurance bills were so high that in order to maintain profit margins on their products, some employers shrunk their workforce size, shifted their workers from full-time status with benefits to part-time status with no benefits, and/or charged consumers more money for their products (in 1990, for instance, over $675 of the cost of a Ford vehicle went to pay for Ford employees' health care coverage).[31]

Not wanting to engage in the cost-saving tactics described above, other employers saw in emerging **managed care organizations (MCOs)** their best opportunity to reduce their employees' health coverage costs. These organizations supposedly compete among themselves to offer employers the least expensive package of quality health care services and goods possible for their employees. They try to control the costs of their plans in three ways: (1) by restricting patients' access to expensive or medically unnecessary tests and treatments; (2) by limiting health care professionals' ability to provide their patients with the best/most care possible; and (3) by limiting patients' choice of health care professionals and health care institutions to those that are willing to charge less than their competitors.

Although MCOs were able, for a time, to reduce employers' health care insurance bills, their cost-controlling powers diminished over time. As a result of patients' and health care professionals' complaints about health care coverage restrictions and low-quality health care, MCOs started to include more goods and services in their packages, to make it easier for patients to access the health care professionals of their choice, and to reimburse health care professionals more amply for patient care. Predictably, the MCOs passed their additional costs on to employers, so much so that at the beginning of the 2000s employers' health care costs had increased an average of 11%. The worst hit employers faced bills that were 20% higher or more. For example, in 2003, MCOs presented the California Public Employees' Retirement System (next to the federal government, the second highest purchaser of health care goods and services in the United States) with a bill 25% higher than the one it had submitted to the system in 2002.[32]

Not wanting to do what they had done in the past to cover their health care costs, many employers decided neither to raise the price of their products nor to downscale their businesses but instead to ask their employees to pay a greater share of their health care insurance bills. According to Gregg Lehman, president of the National Business Coalition, when an employer's health care costs went up 15%, they typically "pass[ed]" along fifty to eighty percent of the increase to employees."[33] Faced with having to pay more for their health care insurance, a noticeable number of employees began to disenroll from their companies' health care coverage plans.

Truth be told, an employee's decision to disenroll from his or her company's health care insurance plan can be quite reasonable. In 2003, for example, employees paid an average of 27%, or $2,412, for a family plan cost at a total of $9,068. Were the total cost of this family plan to increase by 15%, to around $11,448, and if employers asked their employees to pay 50%–80% of the $1370 increase, then employees' contribution would increase anywhere from $685 to $1,196 in that year. Paying up to $3,608 of their own money a year for health care insurance is often more of a burden than the lower-paid employees of a business can shoulder.[34] There comes the financial straw that finally breaks the back of an individual's budget, be that individual an employee or an employer.

Finding themselves, like many of their poorer employees, unable to pay their share of increased health care insurance bills, many owners of small-sized, struggling businesses felt forced to drop their health care benefits. They reasoned that their employees needed jobs more than health care coverage. Increasingly, it is only big and successful businesses that are able to provide their employees with adequate health care insurance plans. Whereas 99% of businesses with 1000 employees or more offer health care insurance to their employees, only 83% of businesses with 25–99 employees do.[35] Worse, just 67% of businesses with 10–24 employees, and only 29% of businesses with 10 employees or less offer health care benefits to their workers.[36]

B. Individually Purchased Health Care Coverage

Between 1987 and 2002, the percentage of Americans with employee coverage dropped from 70.1% to 64.2%.[37] Contrary to common perceptions, however, persons without employer-based health care insurance are not necessarily out of work. On the contrary, 83% of the uninsured are members of families in which one or more of the adults in them work one or more part-time or full-time jobs.[38] Only 1% of uninsured workers who are eligible for employer-provided health care insurance turn it down so that they can spend the saved money on luxuries.[39] Most working individuals who lack health care insurance lack it either because they work for employers who do not offer it to them, or because they work for employers who require employees to pay dearly for their health care insurance. Important as health care insurance is to most individuals, it is not usually as important to them as shelter and food.

Individuals who want to purchase health care insurance will not be able to find an affordable policy in the **individual market** easily, however. On the average, policies purchased in the individual market are 20%–30% higher than ones purchased in the workplace because employers do not have to pay taxes on the health care premiums they purchase for their employees. Therefore, a family policy that costs $9,068 in the workplace, might cost anywhere from $10,871 to $11,468 in the individual market. For the average low-income family in the United States, family policies in this price range constitute at least one-third, and, in some instances, nearly one-half of their yearly income.[40] As a result of this state of affairs, some low-income working families elect to cover only the primary worker in the family. His or her dependents, including children, go without coverage, a situation that upsets many parents who do not know what else to do. Other low-income families are even worse off than this, however. They cannot even afford to cover their main breadwinner. They avoid physicians until they are so sick that they must seek services at a hospital emergency department, where their bill will be far higher than the one they would have received had they been able to see a regular primary care physician instead.

C. Government-Subsidized Health Care Coverage: Medicare

If an individual survives to age 65, he or she will probably qualify for **Medicare**. Established in 1965, Medicare, which is funded by the federal government, is predicated on the assumption that when people retire from work, someone other than their families or former employers may have to help them pay for their medical bills. Currently, Medicare covers 35 million elderly Americans, 6 million disabled Americans, and, as we noted in Chapter 11, any U.S. citizen who needs kidney dialysis or a kidney transplant.[41]

Medicare health insurance coverage is quite good, though there are some serious gaps in it. It is also a costly program, for which the federal government pays with mandatory payroll taxes. Specifically, in 2005, the federal government's Medicare costs were $278 billion (about 13% of the total U.S. health care bill).[42]

Medicare is a tripartite plan. **Part A** covers inpatient hospital costs and, as we noted in Chapter 10, 100 days of rehabilitative care in a skilled nursing facility (SNF), a limited amount of home–health care subsequent to a hospital or SNF stay, and, very recently, hospice care. **Part B** covers outpatient hospital costs, physicians' fees, and some medical supplies, surgical services, and diagnostic tests. **Part C**, sometimes called **Medicare + Choice**, is a relatively new part of Medicare. It permits individuals to remain in Medicare's traditional fee-for-service program or select from a variety of managed care plans. Individuals who select Medicare + Choice have more control over which health care professionals treat them, and, in some instances, get more and better medical goods and services. Fewer and fewer managed care plans are willing to provide Medicare + Choice plans, however, because the federal government is as "penny-pinching" with them as it is with health care institutions and health care professionals in general.

Medicare reimbursements to health care institutions are limited by a number of rationing strategies, including one called **diagnosis-related groups (DRGs)**. Medicare takes all medical diagnoses and groups them according to their relative medical-resource consumption. It then assigns each medical diagnosis to one of 480 DRGs. Each DRG is "weighted" for its average patient cost. Mark A. Hall, Ira Mark Ellman, and Daniel S. Strouse provide the example of the DRG for *major* chest surgeries, which are weighted at 3.0, signaling an expensive hospitalization. *Minor* chest surgeries are placed in one of two other groups, depending on whether they are accompanied by complicating conditions. These two groups of minor chest surgeries are weighted at 2.5 and 1.5, respectively. With an average cost per case of about $7,000, the first DRG pays the hospital $21,000 ($7,000 × 3); the second pays $17,500 ($7,000 × 2.5); and the third pays $10,500 ($7,000 × 1.5). In each case, this amount of money is what the hospital gets, whether the patient's actual hospital bill is higher or lower than the allotted DRG amount.[43]

Similarly, with respect to the reimbursement of health care professionals, Medicare officials have developed a system known as the **resource-based relative-value scale (RB-RVS)**. The scale regulates the amount that health care professionals can charge Medicare for their services. It measures the relative costs of each service provided according to the time, mental effort, and technical skill it requires, as well as differences in the health care professionals' insurance and specialty training. In general, the amount that health care professionals are reimbursed for their Medicare patients on the RB-RVS scale is lower than the amount they receive for their privately insured patients, a situation that causes some health care professionals to set limits on the number of Medicare patients they serve.[44]

Reimbursement rates are not the only sore spots in Medicare coverage, however. As we repeatedly stressed in Chapter 10, Medicare does not cover much in the way of long-term care, precisely the kind of care an aging population needs most. In addition, Medicare has not covered prescription drugs until recently when powerful lobbies such as the **AARP** began to protest that elderly Americans were no longer able to pay their pharmacy bills. They stressed that many low-income seniors were skipping meals in order to pay for their medications, taking bus trips to Canada where prescription drugs can be purchased for a fraction of what they cost in the United States, splitting their medications in half to make them last longer, or simply doing without.

Well aware that elderly Americans are both large in number and active voters in elections, the U.S. Congress passed a $400 billion prescription drug benefit in 2004. High as the price tag for this legislation was, the drug benefit it provides to individual Medicare beneficiaries is generally viewed as "not generous by most standards," however.[45] The **Prescription Drug Plan**, which costs Medicare beneficiaries an additional $420 a year of their own money, also has a deductible, a 25% co-pay from $250 to $2,250, and *no coverage* from $2,250 to $5,100. Only when a Medicare beneficiary's prescription drug bill soars over $5,100 to catastrophic heights does the government provide adequate relief. Indeed, at this point, the government foots 95% of the bill.[46]

D. Government-Subsidized Health Care Coverage: Medicaid

Previously, we noted that many individuals simply cannot afford health care insurance. Some, but by no means all of them, may qualify for **Medicaid**, a government-subsidized entitlement program that pays for medical care for certain low-income individuals and families. Contrary to common misconceptions, Medicaid does not cover medical care for all poor people but only for so-called "deserving" poor people—that is, people whom society regards as poor through no fault of their own.[47] Its recipients are divided into two types: the categorically needy and the medically needy. According to Saul Wurtzman, categorically needy individuals include:

-Individuals who meet the requirements of the Aid to Families with Dependent Children (AFDC) program that were in effect in their state on July 16, 1996,

-Children under age 6 whose family income is at or below 133% of the federal poverty level (FPL),

-Pregnant women whose family income is at or below 133% of the FPL (services to these women are limited to their pregnancy and aftercare),

-Supplemental security income (SSI) recipients in most states,

-People who get adoption or foster care assistance from Social Security,

-Children under age 19, in families with incomes at or below the FPL.[48]

To the degree that women and children constitute most of the individuals in the *categorically needy* group, most of the individuals in the *medically needy* group are among this nation's elderly poor. As we noted in Chapter 10, these elderly individuals have either always been poor or they have become poor by using their life savings to pay their long-term health care bills.

Medicaid is financed by both the federal government and state governments. States do not have to provide *any* of their poor citizens with Medicaid assistance; if a state does decide to establish a Medicaid program, however, it is entitled to federal matching funds to which many strings may be attached. Medicaid is a very expensive program. In 2004, it covered 50 million people for a total of $305 billion, accounting for 17% of all U.S. health care expenditures.[49]

Notably, in that same year as in years past, Medicaid did not cover any *childless* adults, no matter how poor. Among these uncovered individuals were millions of single women and men who work very hard and yet remain very poor because their wages are so low.

Many health care professionals refuse to see Medicaid patients or see them reluctantly because government reimbursement rates for Medicaid patients are even lower than government reimbursement rates for Medicare patients. They protest that a "Medicaid practice" is an extraordinarily poor practice and, truth be told, this statement is accurate.[50] Moreover, many states are finding it difficult to support their Medicaid programs, which typically account for about 16% of a state's general-fund spending.[51] Given the fact that the ranks of Medicaid will swell as one baby boomer after another exhausts their life-savings on medical care, states may be spending as much as 20% of their general funds on Medicaid by 2020. Such a financial burden may tempt legislators to disband their state's Medicaid program, instructing their Medicaid recipients to seek charity care or free care instead. Unfortunately, it is doubtful that the supply of uncompensated care would be able to meet the demand for it under such circumstances.

IV. HEALTH CARE SYSTEM REFORM PROPOSALS

The high cost of U.S. health care, in combination with a labyrinth health care financing system that fails to cover 44 million U.S. citizens with health care insurance, is enough to convince most people that the U.S. health care system needs not simply to be tweaked here and there but to be substantially overhauled. Yet finding a reform proposal that pleases most of the people most of the time, let alone all of the people all of the time, has proved frustrating. Each of the three major approaches—the private-market approach, the employer-based approach, and the government approach—has both strong defenders and fierce opponents. Therefore, we need to assess them as objectively as possible to determine which one of these "medicines" is the least bitter for the American people to swallow.

A. Private-Market Approach

One proposed remedy for the U.S. health care system, known as the **private-market** or **tax credit/voucher** remedy, encourages individuals to use government tax credits, tax deductions, and/or vouchers to purchase health care insurance at their workplace or in the private market. This approach to health care reform aims to extend coverage to more U.S. citizens and to control costs by limiting government subsidies to an amount large enough to purchase *basic* health care goods and services but not *luxury* health care goods and services. Motivating the private-market approach is the vision of free, responsible, and rational individuals, shopping in the health care insurance market for the best health care "buy for their bucks," where even the worst buy is still an acceptable buy. It is also motivated by two other visions: (1) that of efficient health care insurers competing among themselves to supply low-cost, high-quality health care insurance policies to individuals and institutions and (2) that of health care professionals striving to provide low-cost, high-quality health care to patients.

In an ideal world, this scenario would play out perfectly. Unfortunately, we do not live in an ideal world; and there may be reasons to fear that, in our real world, the story the private-market approach tells would not end with everyone living happily ever after. In the first place, the more the government gives by way of tax credits, tax deductions, and vouchers, the less funds it has to fund Medicare and Medicaid. In other words, the government may find itself "robbing Peter to pay Paul." Second, no matter the incentives offered, some individuals may fail to buy health care insurance unless they are *required* to do so by government mandate. But enforcing such a mandate would require much government effort and imagination. It is easy enough to require all drivers to purchase motor vehicle insurance in order to be able to operate a motor vehicle legally, but how would the government operationalize the equivalent of this requirement in the health care arena? Third, some individuals may not be savvy health care insurance shoppers. They may not realize just how bad one policy is compared to another. Fourth, some health care insurance companies may engage in fraud and false advertising, requiring much greater government monitoring of the health care insurance industry. Fifth, and probably most significantly, health care insurance companies may not be able to provide *basic* plans inexpensive enough for government tax credits, tax deductions, and/or vouchers to cover.[52]

That this last possibility is a real one is manifest in the way in which the private-market's solution to controlling the spiraling costs of health care—namely, managed care organizations—fared. As we noted above, managed care organizations were created as cost-control mechanisms. Initially, many people were enthusiastic about MCOs because the health care insurance plans they offered were considerably less expensive than traditional health care insurance plans. But, when patients realized that MCOs prevented them from getting all the care they wanted from their preferred health care providers, they began to rebel.[53] "What do you mean I have to pay everything or extra to go see good old Doc Jones? What do you mean that you don't cover the expensive/cutting-edge treatment I need? How dare you compromise my health!!!" Rather than fighting patients armed with lengthy bills of rights, the MCOs decided to increase the cost of their plans, which, as a result, became almost expensive as the plans they were meant to replace.[54]

B. Employer-Based Approach

A second proposed remedy for the U.S. health care crisis builds upon the current largely **employer-based health care insurance system**, as we discussed above. Instead of providing citizens with tax credits, tax deductions, and/or vouchers, the government uses its monies to make it easier for more, even all, employers to provide health care insurance to their employees and dependants. Strategies to accomplish this difficult task include (1) pooling small companies into groups large enough to have leverage in the health care insurance purchasing market; (2) making employees pay more for health care insurance through higher co-payments and deductibles; (3) offering employees personal health care savings accounts designed to sensitize them to the true costs of medical services so that they will use these services sparingly; and (4) offering employees disease management programs that provide them with better-coordinated as well as more cost-effective health care for expensive chronic diseases such as diabetes or asthma.[55]

The major advantage of the employer-based approach to health care reform is that it builds on the present system which, despite its flaws, seems to work well enough for most Americans. Indeed, two-thirds of Americans under age 65 still get their health care insurance at work, or as the dependent spouse or child of a worker.[56] In 2000, the annual total cost for an average health care insurance policy at work was $2,246 for individuals and $6,351 for families.[57] Although high, these costs are, as we noted above, about 20%–30% lower than the costs for health care insurance purchased outside the workplace.[58] Were all employers, large and small, able to offer affordable and adequate health care insurance to all their employees, part-time as well as full-time, then the health care insurance crisis in the United States could be ameliorated, though certainly not resolved.

Interestingly, former President William Clinton and his wife, Hillary Rodham Clinton tried to resolve the U.S. health care insurance crisis by means of an employer-based approach to health care insurance. Under the 1993 **Clinton Plan**, also known as the "play-or-pay" plan, every American would have received health care insurance from either their employer or the government. Employers would have had to "play" by providing insurance to all their employees, or "pay" by providing tax dollars to help defray the costs for a government plan for employees without employer-based health care insurance coverage. In order to make it possible for all employers, including small ones, to "play" the health care insurance game, the Clinton

Plan included provisions to pool small employers together into groups that could collectively buy affordable health care insurance for their employees. Among the more controversial aspects of the Clinton Plan were a recommendation to set across-the-board budgets at the national level as well as several proposals to severely limit insurance companies, sales of reform and restrict insurance companies' sales of private health care insurance policies.[59]

Viewing the Clinton Plan as a definite threat to their profits, the health care insurance industry launched a clever television-advertisement campaign called "Harry and Louise." The ads portrayed the Clinton Plan as a choice-squashing version of "socialized medicine." Enough Americans were persuaded by the advertisements' message to express disapproval of the plan to their congressional representatives and senators who obligingly voted it down.[60]

C. Government-Based Approach

The third remedy for the woes of the U.S. health care system is sometimes referred to as a **government-based** or **single-payer approach**, although it is often called **national health insurance**. Under this approach, the government becomes the sole payer for a basic package of health care services and goods provided to all U.S. citizens. Employers no longer have to provide employees with health care insurance because everyone receives tax-subsidized health care insurance. Some versions of the government-based approach replace Medicare, Medicaid, and all private insurance plans with a national health trust fund paid for through taxes. Other versions expand Medicare to include all age groups, eliminating the need for other government systems of health care coverage.[61]

Over and beyond the fact that it erases the problem of the uninsured, the advantages of the single-payer approach to health care insurance are at least threefold, according to health care ethicist Gregory Pence. He notes that:

> . . . a single-payer system eliminates the wasteful duplication and conflicting rules that seem inevitable with multiple insurers. Second, such a system can control costs: It has enormous power in negotiating with physicians and hospitals; it can essentially say, "Take it or leave it." Third, a single-payer system eliminates cost-shifting to other payers.[62]

But, like the private-market approach and the employer-based approach, the single-payer approach also has disadvantages. First, it increases taxes, perhaps substantially. Second, it puts the federal government in charge of the whole health care insurance industry, a situation which could lead to major cost constraints affecting choice, quality, and availability of health care. Third, it either eliminates the private health care insurance industry or limits it to providing elite or boutique care to individuals who can afford to pay for all the miracles and marvels of modern medicine out of pocket. Fourth, and finally, because it is public, government-based health care insurance gives "political and ideological biases more power to influence scientific decisions, curtail experimentation and limit coverage."[63]

V. CONCLUSION

Whether the health care crisis will be addressed through the private-market, the employer-based, or the single-payer approach remains a question. But one thing is certain: the health care crisis cannot be resolved unless Americans accept some form of health care rationing and learn how to limit their increasingly insatiable appetite for health care. Among the most instructive lessons in health care rationing is the so-called **Oregon Plan**. In the late 1980s, the state of Oregon experienced a budgetary shortfall in the funding of health care services for Medicaid recipients. The Oregon Legislature needed to get cost efficient and fast. It chose to eliminate funding for very costly organ transplants, including bone marrow transplants, in order to use the money saved for services such as prenatal care for over a thousand pregnant women who could not otherwise afford it. One of the admittedly sad consequences of this decision was that a 7-year-old boy named Coby Howard was denied the $100,000 he needed for a bone marrow transplant. He died, and rapidly became the "poster child" for those opposed to rationing health care goods and services in ways that sacrifice a small number of high-cost patients to benefit a large number of low-cost patients.[64]

Realizing that it may have been a mistake to remove one type of treatment from Medicaid funding without consulting the public at large, the Oregon Legislature passed the **Oregon Basic Health Services Act (OBHSA)** in 1989.[65] The purpose of this Act was not only to limit the number of Medicaid health care services and goods rationally, but also to extend Medicaid coverage in Oregon from 58% to 100% of the federal poverty level and to require all employers to provide health care insurance to their employees. The legislature assured the public that decisions to exclude items from Medicaid coverage would be both democratic and medically sound. Treatments would be ranked not simply on the basis of their clinical effectiveness but also in terms of their value to Oregonians. To this end, the governor appointed an 11-person Health Services Commission composed of five physicians (three family physicians, an obstetrician, and a pediatrician), a public health nurse, a social worker, and four lay persons, one of whom was the chairperson.

The Commission decided to use cost-effectiveness methods to rank Medicaid goods and services from the most important to the least important.

But because cost-effectiveness methods determine the importance of a health care item primarily on the basis of its dollar cost and the number of people it can benefit, the Commission made some initial mistakes. For example, it ranked scheduled tooth-cappings higher on its list of priorities than emergency appendectomies. Embarrassed by counterintuitive determinations such as this one, the Commission eventually rejected its overly "objective" cost-effectiveness approach in favor of a more "subjective" approach. It arranged for over 60 public hearings. They were attended by members of vulnerable populations such as elderly persons, disabled persons, mentally ill persons and low-income persons as well as by health care professionals and public authorities. It oversaw 47 state-wide meetings organized and conducted by Oregon Health Decisions, a nonprofit, citizen-led grassroots organization, and it monitored a University of Oregon telephone survey, the purpose of which was to assess Oregonians' attitudes about falling victim to certain diseases and disabilities.[66]

Using all of the information it gathered, the Commission then proceeded to rate, from most to least essential, 16 categories of health care services (half of which related to acute and chronic diseases, and half of which consisted in special categories such as preventive health care, maternity care, and comfort care). Throughout the rating process, the Commission appealed to three criteria; (1) the *value* of the category to the individual; (2) the *value* of the category to society; and (3) the medical necessity of the category. The result of the Commission's effort was a priority list much more in tune with Oregonians' views on the importance of various health care services to them.[67]

At the top of the 16-category, 709-item list of Medicaid health care services were "essential services," such as those that treat acute fatal conditions, preventing death and promising full recovery (for example, an appendectomy for appendicitis), and those that provide care most people regard as basic (for example, an annual physical exam). Toward the middle of the list were found "very important services," such as those that treat acute nonfatal conditions, returning the patient to previous health (for example, fillings for dental cavities), and those that address chronic nonfatal conditions where one-time treatment improves the patient's quality of life (for example, a hip replacement for someone who would otherwise be wheel-chair dependent or even bedridden). At the bottom of the list were services "valuable to certain individuals," such as treatment for acute nonfatal conditions (for example, costly IVF treatments for infertility).[68]

After studying this list and checking its coffers, the Oregon Legislature funded the first 567 items on the 709-item list. Three treatment categories were altogether excluded from funding: (1) treatments for largely self-improving conditions (for example, the common cold); (2) treatments of questionable effectiveness (for example, liver transplants for nonrecovering alcoholics, aggressive treatment for late-stage cancer or AIDS patients, and aggressive treatment for extremely premature infants) [less than 500 grams and less than 23 weeks gestation]; and (3) cosmetic surgery (for example, benign skin lesions or, more controversially, breast reconstruction after mastectomy). Although the Commission was grateful that the state legislature funded all the services it regarded as "essential" and "very important," it was predictably disappointed that it did not fund all of the 709 of the items on its list.[69]

When Oregon submitted its health plan to the federal government for Medicaid matching funds, it was faulted on several accounts. Among the most serious objections to the Oregon Health Plan were that its findings were applicable only to poor people on Medicaid. Many political activists saw the plan as a scheme created to serve the majority's well-being at the expense of vulnerable minorities' rights. After much back-and-forth haggling, however, the state of Oregon finally secured federal approval and matching funds for its Medicaid plan. Still in effect, the Oregon Health Plan has added 130,000 low-income persons to Medicaid's roster, a remarkable feat in cost-constrained times. Just as significantly, reports indicate that the quality of care for Medicaid patients in Oregon has improved subsequent to the plan's implementation.[70]

Discussing the Oregon Health Plan is perhaps the best note on which to end this book. Our challenge as a nation is to devise a U.S. Health Plan modeled on the best features of the Oregon Plan. We need to decide which health care services and goods we view as essential, which we think are very important, and which we are willing to do without. Each one of us has to ration himself or herself so that our health care system does not implode on itself. So long as we continue to demand *all* that medicine has to offer and then some, the U.S. health care system will continue to falter. Health care costs will not go down and coverage will not increase until we learn how to say no to ourselves. In this connection, health care ethicist Dan Callahan wisely observes that "the only effective way to cope" with our often unrealistic health care demands is to

> . . . keep before the public eye the needs of other sectors and aspects of [our] society. A society with ever-improving health but inadequate parks and schools will not be a well-functioning society. Healthy but unemployed people will not find their lives satisfactory nor will the economy be in good shape if unemployment is too high. We lack as a society a good sense of the proper balance among the various needs of society, some kind of integrated and coherent picture with which to work in public policy. It is not too soon to begin attempting to develop one, particularly in order that the demand for better health, usually insistent, is not allowed to increase its already undue power.[71]

Callahan's message makes sense to me. His worldview is one that I share. But whether his message and mine will fall on closed or open ears remains an open question. Will we kill ourselves as a society in the pursuit of our individual health and separate well-being? An affirmative answer to this question would constitute a tragedy of tsunamic proportions, made worse by the fact that we had it in our power to avoid it.

Discussion Questions

1. Should more funds be spent on providing life-extending treatments for adults over the age of 80 or on providing preventive medicine for children under the age of 18? Which use of funds is best? How would you feel if your 80-year-old grandmother was denied a liver transplant so that a thousand children could get a standard battery of vaccines?
2. Some health care reformers favor a two-tiered health care system. In the lower tier, a basic package of health care goods and services would be provided for everyone. In the higher tier, those who wanted supplemental or expedited care would be permitted to buy it. Is this system unfair to those who cannot afford the higher tier, even if access to the lower tier ensures them a minimum level of well-being?
3. Reports indicate that 50% of the people on Medicaid smoke. Yet Medicaid does not pay for counseling or services that assist people in stopping their smoking habit. Given that smoking is linked to many chronic diseases, evaluate suggestions that Medicaid should pay for smoking-related counseling services.
4. Is health care a right or an entitlement? Support your position.

Case Studies

1. Cape Fear Endocrinology and Metabolic Associates are the only endocrine specialists in their county. For cost-control measures, they do not accept either Medicare or Medicaid patients. As a result of Cape Fear's policy, people in the county do not have access to specialists for treatment of their chronic diseases (for example, diabetes, hyperthyroidism, and gout).

    a. Is Cape Fear's policy ethical? Evaluate it by drawing upon the various ethical theories discussed earlier in the text.
    b. If an employee of Cape Fear opposes this policy, yet needs to keep their job, how should the employee deal with their predicament? Keep quiet, protest, or try to reason with the physicians?

2. Mrs. Archer has been diagnosed with Alzheimer's disease and has recently taken up residence in a nursing home. Medicare will cover treatment for her Alzheimer's disease, but not for the routine care she receives at the nursing home. She is required to spend her private savings for the later care. Only after she exhausts all her personal assets will Mrs. Archer be

eligible for Medicaid, which offers services that are sometimes less high-quality than those Medicare offers. Mrs. Archer's children hate the idea of their mother being on Medicaid, but they are unwilling to use their own money to subsidize better care for their mother. Instead they start lobbying Congress to spend more money on Medicaid so that their mother can have high-quality "free" health care.

    a. Should family members be required by law to help pay the health care costs of other family members?

    b. Would it be ethical to withhold care from Mrs. Archer, since her condition will gradually worsen and normal functioning will not be restored? After all, were care withdrawn from her, everyone would save.

3. Another alternative for providing health care to as many people as possible is the idea of a health-voucher program. Such a program would grant a fixed amount of money to each person below a certain level of income. This would permit someone to shop around for the most affordable health care.

    a. What are the advantages of such a program? What are the disadvantages?

    b. Would such a system create more injustices (owing to people being unable to have costly procedures) than actual equal access?

4. Jane Miller, a retired, 70-year-old widow, belongs to Provident HMO. She lives alone on a fixed income and cannot afford any other supplemental plans. Recently, she broke a hip. Her medications left her in a confused state of consciousness. A visiting nurse was assigned to assist her. As a result of the nurse's help, Mrs. Miller's physical condition improved and her mind totally cleared. Nevertheless, her physician ordered a few more visits from the nurse in order to insure there were no problems. Because her HMO did not consider those extra visits "medically necessary," however, it refused to pay for them.

    a. Is Provident HMO acting ethically in denying the nurse's extra visits?

    b. Should insurance companies be able to restrict health care ordered by a physician? If so, what are the limits to the restrictions they may impose?

    c. What is "medically necessary" care for someone like Mrs. Miller who has trouble taking care of herself (for example, shopping, cleaning, cooking, bathing, walking, and getting in and out of bed)?

Endnotes

    1. Robin Toner and Sheryl Gay Stolberg, "Decade after health care crisis, soaring costs bring new strains," *New York Times* (August 11, 2002): 19.

2. "Health care spending soars," *Charlotte Observer* (January 8, 2003): 10A.

3. Timothy Stoltzfus Jost, "Why can't we do what they do? National health reform abroad," *Journal of Law, Medicine, & Ethics*, 32, no. 3 (Fall 2004): 435.

4. Catherine Hoffman, Diane Rowland, and Alicia L. Carbaugh, "Holes in the health insurance system—who lacks coverage and why," *Journal of Law, Medicine, and Ethics*, 32, no. 3 (Fall 2004): 390–396.

5. Robert H. Binstock, "The financing and organization of long-term care," in: Leslie C. Walker, Elizabeth H. Bradley, and Terrie Wetle (eds.), *Public and Private Responsibilities in Long-Term Care: Finding the Balance* (Baltimore: Johns Hopkins University Press, 1998), p. 4.

6. Ibid., pp. 4–5.

7. Daniel Callahan, *False Hopes: Why America's Quest for Public Health is a Recipe for Failure* (New York: Simon and Schuster, 1998), pp. 257–258.

8. Jack Meyer, Sharon Silow-Carroll, and Sean Sullivan, *Critical Choices Confronting the Cost of American Health Care* (Washington, D.C.: National Committee for Quality Health Care, 1990), p. 52.

9. Ernle W. D. Young and David K. Stevenson, "Limiting treatment for extremely premature low-birthweight infants (500 to 750g)," *American Journal of Diseases of Children*, 144 (May 1990): 549–552.

10. Robert H. Binstock, "The financing and organization of long-term care," in: Leslie C. Walker, Elizabeth H. Bradley, and Terrie Wetle (eds.), *Public and Private Responsibilities in Long-Term Care: Finding the Balance* (Baltimore: Johns Hopkins University Press, 1998), p. 5.

11. Timothy Stoltzfus Jost, "Why can't we do what they do? National health reform abroad," *Journal of Law, Medicine, & Ethics*, 32, no. 3 (Fall 2004): 436.

12. Ibid., p. 436.

13. Daniel Callahan, *False Hopes: Why America's Quest for Public Health is a Recipe for Failure* (New York: Simon and Schuster, 1998), p. 91.

14. Jeff Gerth and Sheryl Gay Stolberg, "Drug makers reap profits on tax-backed," *New York Times* (April 23, 2000): A1.

15. Carmelo Giaccotto, Rexford Santerre, and John Vernon, "Explaining pharmaceutical R & D growth rates at the industry level: new perspectives and insights," *AEI-Brookings Joint Center for Regulatory Studies, http://www.aei.brookings.org/admin/authorpdfs/page.php?id=312* [accessed May 28, 2005].

16. Robert Pear, "Rise in health care costs rests largely on drug prices," *New York Times* (November 14, 2000): A18.

17. Robin Toner and Sheryl Gay Stolberg, "Decade after health care crisis, soaring costs bring new strains," *New York Times* (August 11, 2002): 19.

18. Milton Fisk, *Toward a Healthy Society: The Morality and Politics of American Health Care Reform* (Lawrence, KA: University Press of Kansas, 2000), p. 77.

19. James S. Gordon, *Manifesto for a New Medicine* (New York: Addison-Wesley Publishing Co., Inc., 1996), p. 266.

20. Ibid., pp. 266–267.

21. Daniel Eisenberg and Maggie Sieger, "The doctor won't see you now," *Time Magazine* (June 9, 2003): 55.

22. Joseph L. Bast, Richard C. Rue, and Stuart A. Wesbury, Jr., *Why We Spend Too Much on Health Care* (Chicago: The Heartland Institute, 1992), p. 37.

23. "Economic boom a bust for physician income: average physician income dropped between 1995 and 1999, as other professionals' earnings rose," *Center for Studying Health Care System Change* (March 26, 2003), *http://www.hschange.com/CONTENT/548/?topic=topic03* [accessed June 10, 2005].

24. Ibid.

25. Richard D. Lamm, "Good health care is more than medicine," *The Chronicle of Higher Education* (September 22, 2000): B17.

26. Dianne Miller Wolman and Wilhelmine Miller, "The consequences of uninsurance for individuals, families, communities, and the nation," *Journal of Law, Medicine, and Ethics*, 32, no. 3 (Fall 2004): 402.

27. Ibid., p. 403.

28. Janny Scott, "Life at the top in America isn't just better, it's longer: three heart attacks and what came next," *New York Times* (May 16, 2005): A1, A18–A19.

29. Catherine Hoffman, Diane Rowland, and Alicia L. Carbaugh, "Holes in the health insurance system—who lacks coverage and why," *Journal of Law, Medicine, and Ethics*, 32, no. 3 (Fall 2004): 391.

30. Ibid., p. 390.

31. Jack K. Shelton and Julia Mann Janois, "Unhealthy health care costs," *Journal of Medicine and Philosophy*, 17, no. 1 (February 1992): 8.

32. "The unraveling of health insurance," *Consumer Reports* (July 2002): 49.

33. Ibid.

34. Catherine Hoffman, Diane Rowland, and Alicia L. Carbaugh, "Holes in the health insurance system—who lacks coverage and why," *Journal of Law, Medicine, and Ethics*, 32, no. 3 (Fall 2004): 391.

35. Sherry A. Glied and Phyllis C. Borzi, "The current state of employment-based health coverage," *Journal of Law, Medicine, and Ethics*, 32, no. 3 (Fall 2004): 405.

36. Ibid.

37. Catherine Hoffman, Diane Rowland, and Alicia L. Carbaugh, "Holes in the health insurance system—who lacks coverage and why," *Journal of Law, Medicine, and Ethics*, 32, no. 3 (Fall 2004): 392.

38. Sherry A. Glied and Phyllis C. Borzi, "The current state of employment-based health coverage," *Journal of Law, Medicine, and Ethics*, 32, no. 3 (Fall 2004): 405.

39. Ibid., p. 406.

40. Catherine Hoffman, Diane Rowland, and Alicia L. Carbaugh, "Holes in the health insurance system—who lacks coverage and why," *Journal of Law, Medicine, and Ethics*, 32, no. 3 (Fall 2004): 392.

41. Cindy Mann and Tim Westmoreland, "Attending to Medicaid," *Journal of Law, Medicine, and Ethics*, 32, no. 3 (Fall 2004): 417.

42. Ibid.

43. Mark A. Hall, Ira Mark Ellman, and Daniel S. Strouse, *Health Care Law and Ethics*, 2nd ed. (St. Paul, MN: West Group, 1999), p. 66.

44. Ibid., p. 68.

45. Jeanne M. Lambrew, "Numbers matter: a guide to cost and coverage estimates in health reform debates," *Journal of Law, Medicine, and Ethics*, 32, no. 3 (Fall 2004): 451.

46. Ibid.

47. Cindy Mann and Tim Westmoreland, "Attending to Medicaid," *Journal of Law, Medicine, and Ethics*, 32, no. 3 (Fall 2004): 417.

48. Richard Saul Wurman, *Understanding Healthcare* (Newport, RI: TOP, 2004), p. 302.

49. Cindy Mann and Tim Westmoreland, "Attending to Medicaid," *Journal of Law, Medicine, and Ethics*, 32, no. 3 (Fall 2004): 417.

50. Ibid., p. 419.

51. Ibid.

52. Rashi Fein, "Health-care reform: is it time for our medicine?" *Modern Maturity* (August/September, 1992): 26.

53. Christine Gorman, "Playing the HMO game," *Time Magazine* (July 13, 1998): 24.

54. Jill Wechsler, "Rising healthcare premiums challenge MCOs to cut costs," *Managed Healthcare Executive*, 14, no. 10 (October, 2004): 14.

55. "The unraveling of health insurance," *Consumer Reports* (July, 2002): 50–52.

56. Institute of Medicine, *Coverage Matters: Insurance and Health Care* (Washington, D.C.: National Academy Press, 2002), p. 39.

57. Ibid.

58. Ibid., p. 41.

59. Merrill Matthews Jr. and Molly Hering, "The Clinton plan," *National Review* 45, no. 24 (December 13, 1993): 4–11.

60. Mollyann Brodie, "Impact of issue advertisements and the legacy of Harry and Louise," *Journal of Health Politics, Policy and Law*, 26, no. 6 (December, 2001): 1353–1361.

61. Rashi Fein, "Health-care reform: is it time for our medicine?" *Modern Maturity* (August/September, 1992): 29.

62. Gregory E. Pence, *Classic Cases in Medical Ethics* (New York: McGraw-Hill Companies, Inc., 2000), p. 458.

63. Rashi Fein, "Health-care reform: is it time for our medicine?" *Modern Maturity* (August/September, 1992): 29.

64. Laurie Zoloth, *Health Care and the Ethics of Encounter: A Jewish Discussion of Social Justice* (Chapel Hill, NC: The University of North Carolina Press, 1999), pp. 30–31.

65. John D. Golenski and Stephen M. Thompson, "A history of Oregon's basic health services act: an insider's account," *Quality Review Bulletin*, 17, no. 5 (May 1991): 144–149.

66. Ibid.

67. Laurie Zoloth, *Health Care and the Ethics of Encounter: A Jewish Discussion of Social Justice* (Chapel Hill, NC: The University of North Carolina Press, 1999), pp. 32–47.

68. Oregon Basic Health Services Program, HSC Categories and Rankings, 22 February 1991, *Hastings Center Report* (May/June 1991), p. 10.

69. David C. Hadorn, "The Oregon priority-setting exercise: quality of life and public policy, *Hastings Center Report* (May/June 1991), pp. 10–16.

70. Institute of Medicine, *A Shared Destiny: Community Effects of Uninsurance* (Washington, D.C.: National Academy Press, 2003), p. 66.

71. Daniel Callahan, *What Kind of Life?* (New York: Simon and Schuster, 1990).

Index